OPD-CA-2

OPD-CA-2

Operationalized Psychodynamic Diagnosis in Childhood and Adolescence

Theoretical Basis and User Manual

Edited by
OPD-CA-2 Task Force, Franz Resch, Georg Romer,
Klaus Schmeck, and Inge Seiffge-Krenke

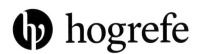 hogrefe

Library of Congress Cataloging in Publication information for the print version of this book is available via the Library of Congress Marc Database under the Library of Congress Control Number 2016954775

Library and Archives Canada Cataloguing in Publication Data

OPD-KJ-2 operationalisierte psychodynamische Diagnostik im Kindes- und Jugendalter. English

    OPD-CA-2 operationalized psychodynamic diagnosis in childhood and adolescence: theoretical basis and user manual / edited by OPD-CA-2 Task Force, Franz Resch, Georg Romer, Klaus Schmeck, and Inge Seiffge-Krenke.

Translation of: OPD-KJ-2 operationalisierte psychodynamische Diagnostik im Kindes- und Jugendalter. Includes bibliographical references.
Issued in print and electronic formats.
ISBN 978-0-88937-489-8 (hardback).--ISBN 978-1-61676-489-0 (pdf).--
ISBN 978-1-61334-489-7 (epub)

    1. Psychodiagnostics--Handbooks, manuals, etc. 2. Psychological tests for children--Handbooks, manuals, etc. 3. Teenagers--Psychological testing--Handbooks, manuals, etc. I. Resch, Franz, 1953-, editor II. Romer, Georg, 1963-, editor III. Schmeck, Klaus, 1956-, editor IV. Seiffge-Krenke, Inge, editor V. Title. VI. Title: Operationalized psychodynamic diagnosis in childhood and adolescence. VII. Title: OPD-KJ-2 operationalisierte psychodynamische Diagnostik im Kindes- und Jugendalter. English.

| RC469.O6213 2016 | 616.89'075 | C2016-906452-2 |
| | | C2016-906453-0 |

This present volume is an adaptation and translation of *OPD-KJ-2 – Operationalisierte Psychodynamische Diagnostik im Kindes- und Jugendalter* by Arbeitskreis OPD-KJ-2 (2016, ISBN 978-3-456-85652-0), published under license from Hogrefe AG, Bern, Switzerland. © 2016 by Hogrefe AG, Switzerland. Translated and revised by Theodore Talbot and the OPD-CA-2 Task Force, 2016.

The authors and publisher have made every effort to ensure that the information contained in this text is in accord with the current state of scientific knowledge, recommendations, and practice at the time of publication. In spite of this diligence, errors cannot be completely excluded. Also, due to changing regulations and continuing research, information may become outdated at any point. The authors and publisher disclaim any responsibility for any consequences which may follow from the use of information presented in this book.

© 2017 by Hogrefe Publishing
http://www.hogrefe.com

PUBLISHING OFFICES

USA:	Hogrefe Publishing Corporation, 7 Bulfinch Place, Suite 202, Boston, MA 02114
	Phone (866) 823–4726, Fax (617) 354–6875; E-mail customerservice@hogrefe.com
EUROPE:	Hogrefe Publishing GmbH, Merkelstr. 3, 37085 Göttingen, Germany
	Phone +49 551 99950–0, Fax +49 551 99950–111; E-mail publishing@hogrefe.com

SALES & DISTRIBUTION

USA:	Hogrefe Publishing, Customer Services Department,
	30 Amberwood Parkway, Ashland, OH 44805
	Phone (800) 228–3749, Fax (419) 281–6883; E-mail customerservice@hogrefe.com
UK:	Hogrefe Publishing, c/o Marston Book Services Ltd., 160 Eastern Ave., Milton Park,
	Abingdon, OX14 4SB, UK
	Phone +44 1235 465577, Fax +44 1235 465556; E-mail direct.orders@marston.co.uk
EUROPE:	Hogrefe Publishing, Merkelstr. 3, 37085 Göttingen, Germany
	Phone +49 551 99950–0, Fax +49 551 99950–111; E-mail publishing@hogrefe.com

OTHER OFFICES

| CANADA: | Hogrefe Publishing, 660 Eglinton Ave. East, Suite 119–514, Toronto, Ontario, M4G 2K2 |
| SWITZERLAND: | Hogrefe Publishing, Länggass-Strasse 76, CH-3000 Bern 9 |

Hogrefe Publishing
Incorporated and registered in the Commonwealth of Massachusetts, USA, and in Göttingen, Lower Saxony, Germany

Printed and bound in Germany

ISBN 978-0-88937-489-8 (print) • ISBN 978-1-61676-489-0 (PDF) • ISBN 978-1-61334-489-7 (EPUB)
http://doi.org/10.1027/00489-000

Contents

The OPD-CA-2 Task Force

Steering Committee of the OPD-CA-2 Task Force

Franz Resch, Georg Romer, Klaus Schmeck, Inge Seiffge-Krenke

Coauthors of the Manual

Petra Adler-Corman, Cord Benecke, Oliver Bilke-Hentsch, Carola Cropp, Veronika Diederichs-Paeschke, Heiko Dietrich, Rainer Fliedl, Christine Forkel, Tanja Göttken, Ulrike Held, Cordula Jaletzke, Florian Juen, Eginhard Koch, Franz Resch, Christine Röpke, Georg Romer, Susanne Schlüter-Müller, Klaus Schmeck, Inge Seiffge-Krenke, Bruno Stafski, Annette Streeck-Fischer, Helene Timmermann, Matthias Weber, Ruth Weissensteiner, Katharina Weitkamp, Kerstin Westhoff, Klaus Winkelmann, Sibylle Winter

Editorial Committee

Oliver Bilke-Hentsch, Eginhard Koch, Franz Resch, Georg Romer, Susanne Schlüter-Müller, Klaus Schmeck, Inge Seiffge-Krenke, Annette Streeck-Fischer, Matthias Weber, Katharina Weitkamp, Sibylle Winter

Working Groups for the Individual Axes

Interpersonal Relations Axis
Spokesperson: Rainer Fliedl
Rainer Fliedl, Tanja Göttken, Brigitte Seifert, Matthias Weber, Ruth Weissensteiner

Structure Axis
Spokesperson: Eginhard Koch
Cord Benecke, Carola Cropp, Florian Juen, Eginhard Koch, Franz Resch, Susanne Schlüter-Müller, Klaus Schmeck, Annette Streeck-Fischer, Klaus Winkelmann

Conflict Axis

Spokesperson: Inge Seiffge-Krenke

Petra Adler-Corman, Heiko Dietrich, Christine Röpke, Inge Seiffge-Krenke, Helene Timmermann, Sibylle Winter

Prerequisites for Treatment Axis

Spokesperson: Oliver Bilke-Hentsch

Oliver Bilke-Hentsch, Georg Romer, Katharina Weitkamp, Kerstin Westhoff

Scientific Editor: Katharina Weitkamp

Members of the original OPD-CA Task Force (1996–2007) who are also coauthors of the first Manual (2003) and its revised 2nd edition (2007): Birgit Atzwanger, Walter Bauers, Alfred Behnisch, Oliver Bilke, Gertrude Bogyi, Karl Heinz Brisch, Dieter Bürgin, Manfred Cierpka, Barbara Diepold, Heiko Dietrich, Reinmar du Bois, Michael Karle, Kai von Klitzing, Ulrich Knölker, Eginhard Koch, Franz Resch, Rainer Richter, Georg Romer, Gerd Rudolf, Susanne Schlüter-Müller, Klaus Schmeck, Michael Schulte-Markwort, Gerhard Schüßler, Inge Seiffge-Krenke, Rainer Georg Siefen, Georg Spiel, Anette Streeck-Fischer, Margot Völger, Matthias Weber, Klaus Winkelmann, Gisela Zeller-Steinbrich, Renate Zimmermann

Foreword

The entire OPD Task Force is pleased to congratulate the group members of the Child and Adolescent OPD Task Force on the second edition of *Operationalized Psychodynamic Diagnosis in Childhood and Adolescence* (OPD-CA). The work has been a great success and we congratulate the group members on this enormous achievement!

The second edition of OPD-CA has not only been revised but has been redesigned in many areas. The experiences gathered in training seminars over the past several years have contributed significantly to OPD-CA-2 being more user-friendly and more theoretically sound than its predecessor.

The revised version presents a diagnostic system for children and adolescents which, among other things, allows the determination of therapeutic goals. It is possible to use the tool to formulate points of focus in therapy and to develop therapy plans.

For a child who seeks and requires therapeutic help psychodynamic formulations can be developed which not only determine the symptoms but explain them as well. Such formulations are the core of a case report that must be able to record and describe the currently active psychological dimensions. OPD does exactly that by evaluating these dimensions on 4 axes. In addition, OPD can help to explain why a patient developed a specific problem at a given time and why he or she maintains it. This is clinically relevant because the psychological factors involved in the development of the problem or the onset of symptoms are often the same factors on which therapy should focus.

OPD can also capture the attachment and relationship representations a child has acquired in the family or in other developmental contexts, his or her internal conflicts and mental structure. OPD describes these aspects as psychodynamic case formulations in relation not only to the present but also to past and future circumstances. Based on the biography of the patient, key psychodynamic concepts that shape current relationships can be understood; wishes and desires for the future can be explained. Formulations developed with the help of this manual prove their clinical validity by allowing practitioners to make predictions about the individual's mental functioning in future situations. This makes it possible to develop hypotheses as to how a child or adolescent will react in certain situations and which therapeutic approaches will be effective.

This new manual is now used for OPD-CA training seminars and will be used in a number of research projects. We hope that many researchers and practitioners in the field of child and adolescent psychiatry and psychotherapy will make use of this manual. We look forward to the results! On behalf of the entire OPD group, I hope that OPD-CA-2 will play an integral role in psychotherapeutic practice, continuing education, and research.

Manfred Cierpka, OPD Spokesperson

Foreword

The diagnostic categories of the DSM and the ICD systems provide important information geared to formulate therapeutic intervention for psychopathological syndromes. However, only an enriched psycho-dynamic diagnostic formulation permits to institute a highly person-alized, individually tailored therapeutic program for these conditions. The problem is the often imprecise, impressionistic quality of psycho-dynamic formulations. This problem becomes greater in the diagnostic evaluation of children and adolescents, where a developmental per-spective and an assessment of environmental constraints and resources are crucial contributors to the formulation of a comprehensive and practical therapeutic approach.

The OPD-CA-2 diagnostic approach responds effectively to these chal-lenges. The present, English version of that approach presents a clear and comprehensive diagnostic approach that includes both the categorical, descriptive phenomenology of standard psychiatric classification and a clear, updated system of psychodynamic inquiry that enriches psychi-atric diagnosis with the formulation of four psychodynamic axes. These axes integrate a developmental perceptive with specific assessment of interpersonal relations, dominant conflicts, intrapsychic structure, and prerequisites for treatment. It is a comprehensive, empirically based and clinically tested approach to the diagnosis and treatment indications for the entire field of child and adolescent psychopathology. I warmly rec-ommend it to all child and adolescent psychiatrists, psychologists, and social workers as an essential contribution to clinical practice.

Otto F. Kernberg, Professor Emeritus of Psychiatry

Preface

Diagnostics for children and adolescents have multiple functions. Disentangling between normative development and psychopathology, and clarifying the indication for psychotherapy are essential elements of the diagnostic process, after which practitioners also have to decide about which specific therapeutic technique is most appropriate for a child or adolescent patient. Given the recent development towards evidence-based medicine, the appropriate assignment to specific therapeutic techniques has become more and more important and is one of the corner stones of therapeutic success.

However, current diagnostic systems are too limited to answer all these clinically and empirically relevant questions. Nosological classification via DSM-5 or ICD-10 is important, but not sufficient for therapeutic work. Furthermore, we need specific indices to measure therapeutic progress. With this book, we present the first empirically based assessment tool for psychodynamically relevant dimensions in child and adolescent psychotherapy.

The OPD-CA-2 provides helpful tools for the indication of treatment, the planning of treatment and its evaluation. Important dimensions such as the quality of relationships to significant others (including the therapist), structural functioning of the patient (such as his or her capacity for emotion regulation), prevailing intrapsychic conflict issues which hinder functional development as well as treatment requirements (such as treatment motivation) can be assessed. The instruments presented cover a wide range of assessment which can be applied to the child and his or her parents. They relate diagnostic questions to the main developmental areas in childhood or adolescence, such as school, family, peers, and health. Starting from the diagnostic interview, these tools allow all relevant diagnostic categories to be coded. Correspondingly they can also be used for the evaluation of treatment.

This book presents the results of 30 years of collaborative work of practitioners and researchers from different fields such as child and adolescent psychiatry, child and adolescent psychotherapy, and developmental psychology. The OPD-CA Task Force has, over the decades, refined the conceptual work in all diagnostically relevant dimensions, improved the reliability and validity of the instruments, documented its empirical significance in a number of studies with various clinical samples, and provided helpful clinical tools and case studies for practical application. After several revisions of the instrument and extensive usage in Germany, we now want to make the instrument available to colleagues in research and practice in other countries. On behalf of the Task Force OPD-CA-2, we wish you every success with the implementation of the instrument and we are eager to learn about your experiences and results with the instrument. Feel free to contact us whenever questions or suggestions arise from your work with the instrument, be it in clinical practice or research. This will help us to make the future OPD-CA even more applicable in different cultural contexts.

Franz Resch
Georg Romer
Klaus Schmeck
Inge Seiffge-Krenke

Part 1: The OPD-CA-2

1. Introduction

Beginning in 1992, the *Operationalisierte Psychodynamische Diagnostik* (in English *Operationalized Psychodynamic Diagnostics,* OPD) for adults was developed for German-speaking countries (Arbeitskreis OPD, 1996) and then later revised (Arbeitskreis OPD, 2006). The English versions of the Manual were published a bit later (OPD Task Force, 2001, 2008). The OPD is a system with psychodynamically based diagnostic axes for supplementing and expanding nosological classification schemes (such as DSM-5 in the USA, American Psychiatric Association, 2015; ICD-10 in Europe, World Health Organisation, 1992).

The result is an instrument that both takes into account psychodynamic theory and attempts to improve interrater reliability in the psychodynamic assessment of mental states. This instrument is intended to remedy the fuzziness of psychoanalytic concepts – often criticised by other therapy approaches – through definitional principles. Of course, the reduction of fuzziness and ambiguity necessarily entails a curtailment of some theoretical models, which is appropriate given the practical diagnostic and therapeutic considerations.

From the outset, the OPD and the *Operationalized Psychodynamic Diagnosis in Childhood and Adolescence* (OPD-CA; in German *Operationalisierte Psychodynamische Diagnostik im Kindes- und Jugendalter* [OPD-KJ]; Arbeitskreis OPD-KJ, 2007) aimed at complementing the categorical approach (in terms of diagnoses) with a dimensional view of mental disorders in terms of ratings of severity along different axes (or dimensions). This approach to the classification of mental disorders has proven to be forward-thinking and ground-breaking, as the current developments in the new DSM-5 show, in which dimensional perspectives and assessments of severity have now been integrated into the categorical system of psychiatric diagnoses (APA, 2015).

In the case of children and adolescents, the continued development of the ICD-8 and ICD-9 very early on led to a multiaxial nosological framework (Remschmidt & Mattejat, 1994; Remschmidt, Schmidt & Poustka, 2008; Rutter, Shaffer, & Sturge, 1975). This allowed diagnostics on several levels: Along the first axis the clinical-psychiatric syndrome is described, while the second axis allows coding of developmental disorders, the third records intelligence, and the fourth diagnostically classifies physical illnesses as well as disabilities. The fifth axis captures associated abnormal psychosocial circumstances, and a sixth axis ascertains the level of psychosocial functioning. A task force was established in 1996 with the aim of developing a German instrument for the Operationalisierte Psychodynamische Diagnostik im Kindes- und Jugendalter (OPD-KJ; Arbeitskreis OPD-KJ, 2003, 2007; Operationalized Psychodynamic Diagnostics in Childhood and Adolescence [OPD-CA] in English). The aim was to capture, similar to the adult version, psychodynamic aspects of childhood and adolescence, extending beyond the multiaxial classification system, as an aid to appropriate treatment planning.

Based on the OPD instrument for adults, profound modifications were necessary for childhood and adolescence. The central issue was the influence of developmental processes on the psychodynamics. The second edition of the German classification system OPD-KJ-2 combines psychodynamic, developmental, and clinical psychiatric perspectives (Resch & Koch, 2012; Resch, Schulte-Markwort, & Bürgin, 1998; Windaus, 2012). Multidimensional models of the origins of mental disorders are included (Herpertz-Dahlmann, Resch, Schulte-Markwort, & Warnke, 2008) and integrated in an overall biopsychosocial model open to dynamic perspectives (see Chapter 2 *Developmental Concepts and Ages*). The OPD-CA-2 should accordingly take into account the following special therapeutic considerations: It should allow a good differential indication for therapy and treatment planning given psychodynamic considerations, as well as provide information for a relationship-based foundation for parental work, and, for practical purposes, maintain a sufficiently high level of differentiation and comprehensibility despite the high level of complexity. The psychodynamic approach to the child indeed requires correspondingly complex, multidimensional, and development-oriented diagnostics, and may not remain at the level of nosological assessment.

The identification of specific psychiatric disorders through questionnaires and interviews has a long clinical tradition, with increasing attention in recent years to developmental aspects and resources in childhood and adolescence. The diagnostic approach in the OPD-CA goes beyond an integration of developmental diagnostics on the one hand and psychiatric classification on the other hand. The OPD-CA aims at a complex identification of psychodynamic processes that takes into account the child's or adolescent's subjectivity and attempts to render the symptoms also hermeneutically accessible and understandable in a developmental context. The developmental perspective is central to all aspects of the diagnostic process, from the type of assessment and selection of relevant diagnostic categories to the process of assessment along various substantive dimensions – where, at the end of the process, a recommendation for treatment can be made integrating psychiatric symptomatology, level of development, and psychodynamic aspects.

In the OPD-CA too we specify, as an orientation aid, certain age groups in which developmental adjustment or maladjustment as well as structural resources become visible. Although compared with adults, children still seem incompletely structured, since at certain ages they cannot fully perceive the causal relationships in the world, some insights and background information remain hidden to them, and their affect regulation depends on significant attachment figures, each child at any given age will possess an optimal structure. At each age, a person has available to him or her a repertoire of experiential and behavioral capacities that also takes into account internal conflicts and allows the active formation of relationships. The view of children as generally not optimally adjusted to their environment or as immature according to some adult ideal is inappropriate. Dysfunctional types of behavior and fantasies always need to be compared against age-appropriate requirements. A child is not an incomplete adult. In order to identify psychodynamic disorders in children of different ages, mentally impaired children have to be compared with healthy children of the same age (Resch & Koch, 2012).

The developmental aspect is relevant at all levels of the diagnostic process. The collection itself of diagnostically relevant information, i.e., the settings the persons are interviewed in as well as the different levels at which information is obtained (play, observation, dialog, scenic understanding) was adapted to the different developmental stages. The collection of relevant psychodynamic information along the axes of *in-*

terpersonal relations, conflict, structure, and prerequisites for treatment is differentiated according to the levels of development. As development is always considered contextually, developmentally relevant areas such as family, play, school, peer group, etc., need to be included as well.

The numerous experiences from trainings and information from empirical studies of the German instrument informed the development of the OPD-KJ into the OPD-KJ-2. An English version of the first edition of the Manual was not published so we shall henceforth refer to the second edition as the OPD-CA-2 but use the abbreviation OPD-CA to refer to the the original German version or to the instrument generally. Items and definitions that had proven to be insufficiently clear and selective were revised or even removed. The thorough revision of the axes and their dimensions also incorporated factor-analytic findings, so that significantly improved reliability and construct validity can be expected compared with the original OPD-KJ Manual. The partially new nomenclature of the conflicts is intended to increase comprehensibility of the key conflict themes. The structure axis now shows similarities with the alternative model for personality disorders in Section III of the DSM-5 (American Psychiatric Association, 2015), which incorporates a scale for the level of personality functioning on four dimensions: *identity, self-direction, empathy,* and *intimacy.* This has significant similarities with the four dimensions of the *structure* axis of the OPD-CA-2: *identity, control, interpersonality,* and *attachment.*

The basic concern of the OPD to reduce the fuzziness and ambiguity of some psychoanalytic concepts and constructs through operationalization is also a central concern for the child and adolescent version. It is vital that the operationalization of theoretical constructs is based on practical experience. The reduction of fuzziness and ambiguity within the OPD-CA was therefore necessary to meet the needs of diagnostic practice and psychotherapeutic activities. The revised OPD-CA-2 also does not attempt any reformulation of psychodynamic constructs, but refers, for the most part, to concepts largely accepted as clinical theory within psychodynamic discourse. Users identifying with a particular psychoanalytic approach may then have the impression of a lack of theoretical clarity due to the emphasis on pragmatics. However, the aim of the OPD-CA is to serve psychoanalytic discourse independently of any approach and to be applicable across approaches in order to have an empirically verifiable operationalization of psycho-dynamic constructs.

Even if a more operationalized diagnosis cannot capture the overall form of a mental disorder in a specific instance and in the context of a individual's life with all the varied aspects of that disorder, we assume that the operationalization of psychodynamic diagnostics will allow an improvement in communication between different therapists as well as, in particular, an optimization of contact between psychodynamic perspectives and other therapy approaches. On top of this, the clarity and transparency of diagnostic and psychotherapeutic processes should be increased and therefore be beneficial when applied to clinical work and research. The OPD-CA-2 could only disappoint those therapists who believe that psychodynamic processes as dyadic communication phenomena are fundamentally not amenable to empirical approaches or methods of verification and not subject to agreement between different therapists. On the other hand, therapists concerned with the empirical testing of their own thoughts and actions and who advocate operationalization and manualization in the interest of greater transparency towards the patient will welcome the further development in the OPD-CA-2.

The psychiatric and psychological study of children and adolescents generally includes their most important attachment figures. Besides the specific diagnosis, the diagnostic assessment of the relationship dynamics between parents and children is also clinically relevant. The younger the patient, the more interlaced are the intrapsychic and interpersonal levels. For this reason, the OPD-CA-2 also includes an *interpersonal relations axis* for assessing the child's or adolescent's relationships to the examiner and to the relevant familial attachment figures, as well as for assessing the family dynamics.

The *mental structure* construct embodies two ideas in particular: on the one hand, capturing lived functions in experiential schemata and, on the other hand, making available this experience through actualization, which allows the transfer of the experience to new and meaningful functions. Accordingly, *mental structure* is an individually typical disposition to experience and behavior that is available to the individual when faced with making a decision about different interactional options. The OPD-CA-2 describes four dimensions within this structure: reflective (self) functions form the *identity* axis, communicative qualities form the *interpersonality* axis, internalized attachment experiences form the *attachment* axis, and finally there is the *control* axis (Goth et al., 2012; Resch & Koch, 2012).

In selecting the construct *conflict* our idea was that, besides interactional aspects and individual experience, essential aspects of the unconscious also play a role in coping with the environment. In particular, in work with children and adolescents, the combination of internal and external mental conditional factors (that is, of conflict and interaction) becomes especially important (Seiffge-Krenke, 2012a).

Finally, the *prerequisites for treatment* axis represents the areas that, in addition to psychodynamic constructs, are of great importance for treatment planning. They include subjective dimensions of the children and adolescents as well as their resources. The incorporation of these items was a particular concern as the diagnostic view all too quickly focusses on the pathological in the sense of deficiency.

The OPD-CA-2 makes no claim to completeness regarding the dynamic constructs. The reliability of individual items was examined on the basis of practice as well as empirical studies. The corresponding modifications to definitions and anchor-point descriptions result from the experiences of recent years. The psychometric quality of the OPD-CA instrument proved altogether empirically satisfactory; single weaknesses were remedied through specific changes in the OPD-CA-2. The OPD-CA has thus become established in the research world, despite the focus on clinical applications.

In fact, the OPD-CA has established itself over the years as a very successful concept, as evidenced by the great interest both in the Manual and in trainings. We hope that the revised OPD-CA-2 will stir great interest and offer an exciting expansion of diagnostic potential to people already familiar with the first version of the OPD-CA. We would be greatly pleased if this new instrument also proved useful in your everyday diagnostic and therapeutic work.

2. Developmental Concepts and Ages

Which developmental concept forms the basis for the attempt by the OPD-CA-2 to bring together psychodynamic concepts with ontological developmental phenomena?

Only a working definition can come into question that clarifies the scope while at the same time allowing for sufficient openness to the varieties of experience and behavior of the child. According to Montada (1987), the temporal aspect of development is especially important. All changes that can be meaningfully related to the temporal dimension of the different age groups thus become the subject of development. Whereas development was primarily viewed as a process of maturation in the early 20th century, with, for example, Karl Bühler (1918) stating that the concept of development includes both predisposition as well as a plan or objective of growth, nowadays the following characteristics are thought to govern the developmental process: The emphasis lies on aspects of differentiation, namely subtle formation and refinement, and the emergence of more and more degrees of freedom in decision-making. Integration that over time compiles increasingly more details into a new whole also forms a crucial facet of development. Environmental stimuli are perceived with increasing selectivity, and the interaction between rapid, holistic responses and search responses down to the last detail becomes increasingly complex. In the course of development, function and structure enter into close interplay, with structural consolidation of experiential content being an essential feature of development.

2.1 Theoretical Foundations of the Developmental Concept in the OPD-CA-2

The developmental concept underlying the OPD-CA-2 is based on an interactionist model of development (Oerter, 1995). The concept is further based on the stages of cognitive development according to Piaget (1952), and integrates the concept of developmental lines from psychoanalytic theory (A. Freud, 1965) and the developmental tasks from empirical developmental psychology (Havighurst, 1972), while incorporating more recent advances. As the OPD-CA-2 is intended for clinical use, a developmental-psychopathological approach is also urgently needed. The following sections present in detail these theoretical elements underlying our view of development.

The Interactionist Model of Development

Early conceptions of development were governed by stage models nowadays largely considered as outdated. The psychodynamic developmental idea of the OPD-CA-2 is based on an interactionist model of development (Oerter, 1995). This model ties an active, self-motivated subject advancing his or her own development to an equally demanding and influential object world. Cultural techniques, standards, attachment figures' expectations, and physical environmental conditions serve as developmental incentives or challenges that must be dealt with by the individual in a process of adaptation. The interactionist theory thus concedes to the individual an active role in the shaping of his or her environment – the individual looks for and shapes the environmental conditions– in the same way as he himself or she herself is shaped by these environmental conditions (Resch, 1999a).

The Concept of Developmental Lines and its Further Development

Anna Freud worked on the interaction between the ego and the id at different levels of development (A. Freud, 1936). A prototypical developmental line can run from the infant's full emotional dependency through partial object relations to mature object relations. Another further developmental line runs from the baby's body as shared with the mother to bodily self-determination in adolescence. Other developmental lines, such as that running from the young child's egocentric world view to empathy, reciprocity, and camaraderie, have been replaced in the OPD-CA-2 by modern contemporary concepts of mentalization (Fonagy, Gergely, Jurist, & Target, 2006) such that from the outset the child exists in a state of dialectical tension between egocentricity and reciprocity (see overview in Dornes, 2006). The developmental line running from erotic play with the child's own body or the mother's body through transitional objects to toys, hobbies, and finally to work have been superseded by contemporary activity-theoretical considerations indicating an increasing integration of the inclination towards pleasure and the assumption of responsibility in human actions (Resch, 2012). Fundamental for the concept of psychodynamic developmental lines is the integration of cognitive, social, and emotional learning processes leading to differentiation in the sense of appropriate sequencing.

The Concept of Developmental Tasks

The concept of developmental tasks from Havighurst (1972) shares with Anna Freud's concept the ideas of normative development, continuity, and sequencing. Noteworthy, however, is the emphasis on active achievement on the individual's part during development. Solutions to age-specific developmental tasks can advance the individual's own development. The focus thus lies on individual activity. The mastery of adaptational demands becomes clear in various forms of progression, namely, in successfully continued development on the one hand and in developmental standstill or regression on the other. Solving age-specific developmental tasks necessarily involves the integration of requirements from three areas (physical condition, social norms, and personal skills). Havighurst bases his approach on a division of the course of human life into six segments:

- *Infancy and early childhood*, from birth to 5–6 years
- *Middle childhood*, from 5–6 to 12–13 years
- *Adolescence*, from 12–13 to 18 years
- *Early adulthood*, from 18 to 35 years
- *Middle adulthood*, from 35 to 60 years
- *Later maturity*, 60 years and older

For each of these six stages of development Havighurst defines age-specific developmental tasks connected with one another across the entire lifespan. The eight developmental tasks of adolescence (such as reconceptualization of the self, development of a mature bodily concept, separation from parents and development of mature relationships with close friends and the beginning of romantic relationships) rest on the accomplished developmental tasks of late childhood (such as learning physical skills, developing a positive attitude towards oneself as a growing organism, learning an appropriate masculine or feminine role, and attaining personal independence). Accomplishment of the developmental tasks is, in turn, the precondition for approaching the stage-specific developmental tasks of the next age group.

Much more clearly than in Anna Freud's work, Havighurst's concept stresses the normative demand of society on development. Many developmental tasks involve normative expectations such as entering school, the transition to a secondary school, graduation, etc. Explicitly operationalized is also the sequencing of the developmental tasks. Compared with developmental lines, developmental tasks have been especially well studied for childhood and adolescence (Seiffge-Krenke, 1998). On the other hand, Anna Freud's consideration of the course of development is more complex and more difficult to operationalize, but then more suitable for the complexity of psychodynamic relationships.

The Developmental-Psychopathological Perspective

Another conceptual element of the OPD-CA-2 is the developmental-psychopathological perspective that attempts to reformulate the aetiopathogenesis of mental symptoms on the basis of developmental aspects. The developmental idea is intended not only to change the view on aetiology, epidemiology, type, and severity of mental disorders, but also to reconceptualize diagnostics, therapy, rehabilitation, and prevention in a flexible and dynamic way. The basic idea is to focus on the influences of normal development on the aetiopathogenesis of psychopathological symptoms in different periods of life, as well as the influence of psychopathological adaptive mechanisms on the normal course of development in the life cycle. Given their somatic, cognitive, and emotional make-up, children in different stages of life possess different resources for responding to different forms of mental irritation. This variety can be reflected in different age-related anxieties, such as separation anxiety and fear of the dark at early ages and social anxieties and existential anxieties in later childhood. If, on the other hand, mental problems have effects modulating development, the job is to determine to what extent psychopathological symptoms in children and adolescents present a risk factor for normal development (Resch, 2012). Five points are especially important in this regard:

1. Psychopathological phenomena exhibit subclinical forms and dilution levels 10 to 20 times more often compared with complete clinical pictures, and psychopathological symptoms do not always represent preliminary stages of serious illnesses. There exist transient, reactive, and subclinical response phenomena to normal life stress.
2. Psychopathological response patterns must be considered in terms of functionality. Psychopathological symptoms do not conclusively express pathological disorders, but rather indicate forced adjustment processes. Most intrapsychic symptoms are meaningful in ways accessible through hermeneutic interpretation.
3. The transition from normality to pathology is fluent.
4. Pathology is not defined by the symptom alone, but by a reciprocal relationship between the necessity of adaptation (the problematic situation) and possible resources to cope with it. All forms and varieties of psychopathology can therefore be meaningfully explained only in relation to the conditions of life.
5. The path from normality to pathology is not simply reversible. All forms of improvements and healing eventually lead to new integration as part of the developmental path.

Risk factors are events and experiences most likely leading to later mental disorders. There exist both external (familial and socio-cultural) and internal (psychological and dispositional) risk factors (see Herpertz-Dahlmann et al., 2008). Protective factors can protect the child from a negative development under conditions of risk. Such factors can not only prevent illnesses, but also delay or ameliorate illnesses or accelerate autoregulatory processes and healing tendencies. Such protective factors can be effective in either an internal-constitutional way, a familial-social way, or an extra-familial, social way (Fegert & Resch, 2012). The interplay of risk factors and protective factors influences the child's developmental process.

"Vulnerability" is defined as the disposition to follow a negative course of development under risk conditions. In contrast, we speak of resilience when coping with life succeeds even under adverse conditions of development (Resch, Mattejat, & Remschmidt, 2006).

The development of mental structures is, in turn, inconceivable without the development of memory. All experiences recorded in the subject's representational store and therefore contributing to the further development of mental structure are closely tied to a functioning memory. Squire (1982) distinguishes between two forms of memory: declarative and nondeclarative memory. While declarative memory stores experiences that are explicitly recorded through the working memory, learned and eventually consciously reproducible, nondeclarative memory contains experiences controlling our behavior implicitly (that is, below the threshold of consciousness). Nondeclarative memory is available to people from birth on, and is characterized by different priming effects, conditioning processes, habituation, and sensitization responses as well as by different routines of action, thought, and perception. Such implicit experiences (also known as nondeclarative experiences) have a lasting influence on human experience and behavior, although they are not directly accessible to self-knowledge and awareness. The structural disposition to act in interpersonal relationships is based on both implicit and explicit memory mechanisms and is therefore characterized by unconscious procedural action potentials as well as by conscious declarative representations (reviewed by Resch, 2009). Declarative memory may be divided into episodic and semantic memory. In episodic memory (also known as experience memory), personal events and experiences are stored in a spatial-temporal reference system with affective, cognitive, and self aspects. In contrast, semantic memory contains old and newly acquired factual knowledge as well as general knowledge in the sense of verbalized knowledge of the world that is accessible to and well communicated verbally in narratives. Declarative memory is in principle accessible to self-reflection, developing only during the first few years of life and attaining a new level of complexity as language develops.

Conceptions of the unconscious as consisting of procedural memory structures (unconscious experiences are not explicitly accessible to reflective processes, but do influence the child's experience and behavior) also explain why early childhood experiences are left to explicit access by memory functions only from age 3 on, while early life experiences are procedurally anchored and are not directly accessible to consciousness, and yet can control experiential and behavioral dispositions (see Dornes, 2006). While in the early stages of memory development explicit storage and the conscious retrieval of memory content are still not possible in a sustainable way, tendencies in action and styles of perception are procedurally stored. These implicit experiences can be narratively modified repeatedly and subsequently associated with early years in explicit images and stories.

The empirically supported assumption that mental injuries (traumas) lead to a decoupling of procedural and explicit memory storage may explain why under such extreme psychological conditions unconscious behavioral tendencies and premonitions develop into responses to certain triggering events without associated images. Nor is the emergence of unconscious conflicts conceivable without a correlation with memory processes. Psychodynamic researchers in particular could benefit from an intensive dialog with cognitive neuroscientists regarding these issues.

The *concept of mentalization* is currently the most explored model as to how people mentally process and represent their interpersonal experiences. Peter Fonagy and his research group developed this concept by combining and integrating elements of psychoanalytic theory with considerations of attachment theory and the empirical results of mind-theoretical research (Fonagy et al., 2006). The concept of mentalization is closely tied to reflective self-functions and characterizes the ability to regard other people and one's own person as individuals with mental and emotional states, emerging during the course of ontological development. Mentalization makes intersubjectivity possible, allows adopting others' perspectives, and culminates in self-reflective cognition (reviewed by Resch, 2009).

In the reflexive space created through mentalization, conflicts can emerge between different value commitments, needs, tendencies in action, and preferences. Disruptions of mentalization processes lead to structural difficulties and to the unavailability of the mental space, so that persons with structural disorders will tend to contain their conflicts less within themselves than to act them out in their immediate interpersonal field.

Another element of the developmental concept of the OPD-CA-2 is *attachment theory*, which, since the extraordinary work of Bowlby

(1988) and Ainsworth and colleagues (1978), has made important contributions to the diagnostics of relationships and enabled a wealth of insights into the parent-child relationship. Attachment is characterized by the fundamental confidence in an attachment figure. All three aspects play a special role: the search for and preservation of closeness, the creation of a human refuge that can provide comfort, support, and security, and, finally, the formation of a secure basis for the child's exploratory behavior. Attachment is thus not only a quality of the adult or child him-/herself, but characterizes primarily an interpersonal relationship. From the experiences of attachment the child ultimately develops internal representations of important emotionally charged relationships; these representations are also known as "inner working models." Such internal relationship models form a part of the mental structure.

The development of the child manifests itself as a process of bidirectional interactions between the child's own experiential potentials on the one hand and challenges of the (social) environment on the other. The development of the self and emotional regulation in the intersubjective context is extensively discussed in Resch and Koch (2012).

Following Stern (1985), we can describe the development of the self as a path proceeding from the emergence of self-perception through the core sense of self to the autobiographical self after attainment of the ability to symbolize. A review of the literature is provided in Dornes (2006). We assume that children from the age of 3 years develop, together with verbal self-perception, an increasingly clearer mental representation of themselves and of others. Ultimately, the child will also be able to give a name to this internal representation of him-/herself. The result is an initial narrative self-concept that renders experiences of self. As of this stage, the mental structure has a self-reflexive quality that can enter into interaction and communication.

2.2 The Age Groups

All the aforementioned developmental concepts form the basis of a division into the age groups of the OPD-CA-2. The foundation is provided by Piaget's stages of cognitive development (Piaget, 1952). We have adopted Piaget's key assumptions of phase-specific development, the adherence to basic age-specific anchors (such as enrolment in school, puberty), and the universality of phase processes, despite our awareness of the abbreviated and simplified character of this view of developmental processes given the actual and tremendous variances within the individual stages of development. Nevertheless, Piaget's approach seems useful as a conceptual framework that, however, must be modified with regard to mentalization and self-development, as the child's assessment stages commence only in the third year of life. From this point on the child – even if only to a limited degree – is able to provide information about him-/herself and his/her emotional states in his/her interaction with others. Different to previous editions of the OPD-CA, Age Group 1 therefore ranges no longer from 1.5 to 5 but from 3 to 5 years. Age Group 2 ranges from 6 to 12 years and Age Group 3 comprises the period of adolescence from 13 to 18 years of age. These stages have a moderate level of differentiation and can also be related to important normative milestones such as preschool age, school, and the onset of adolescent changes. They also covary with major changes in socio-emotional development, such as the development of empathy, perspective taking, and attachment development in families. Similarly, these developmental steps apply to the perception of illness and stress management. A focus on the sequence of cognitive stages which, as indicated below, also includes a focus on affective and social developmental processes, therefore appears useful in the OPD-CA-2 as well.

Age Group 0 (0 to 2 years)

The period from 0 to 2 years of age should not form the basis of an overall assessment according to the axes in the OPD-CA-2. In this age group, besides the individual factors of the child, especially aspects of the relationships with parental figures and other reliable people play a fundamental role. This phase of life is characterized by rapid changes in the self and in relationships: (pre-)stages of object relations, emergence of the experience of self, differentiation of affective experience and the handling of relationships, development of the symbolization function, and the incipient development of autonomy with increasing mobility. We assume that an increasingly differentiated subjective inner world of the child with early forms of representation and fantasies will emerge in this phase of development. However, immediate access to this inner world through language, play, and drawing is only partially available, so that the child's subjective experiencing can be disclosed only indirectly. In clinical contexts, too, ages 0 to 3 are often especially salient, so that separate psychopathological terminology has been devised. While in this age group relationship analyses are useful, structural assessments with the present Manual do not seem appropriate. In the age group from 1 to 3 years we find preforms of conflict, and the prerequisites for treatment can be evaluated in discussions with the families. The development of a separate instrument of psychodynamic assessment for this age group has been planned in a separate task force.

Age Group 1 (3 to 5 years)

This period basically corresponds to the late pre-operational period of development of the kindergarten and preschool child at the transition to concrete operations. Self–object differentiation has occurred, intentionality and language may be presupposed, and role changes and role playing are possible. Even if the child can name and recognize many different emotions, the ability to regulate emotions is still basically tied to the interaction with significant attachment figures. Relationships with others, especially friends, are viewed on the level of the greatest possible similarity and personal advantage. In the cognitive area, both empirical thinking skills, such as causality and logic, as well as magical thinking with finalism, animism, and cognitive egocentrism are observed. Especially under increased affective pressure empirical-logical thought processes will be replaced by magical thinking. This may lead, in the attribution of causes of illness, among other causes, to a personal perception of the illness as punishment.

Age group 2 (6 to 12 years)

This period of time roughly corresponding to the concrete operational stage is characterized by the adoption of a social perspective. The child is able to consider experiences and relationships from different points of view. Private and generally imposed worlds of experience become differentiated from one another. Feelings are understood as something that can be triggered by external and/or internal events and as something increasingly controllable by the child; this ability for emotional regulation and, therefore, also for hiding emotions from about the age of 10 years may be regarded as a sign of maturity. At the level of relationships with friends, the exchange of material goods is important, and the child stabilizes his/her identity and self-worth both within the family and among peers by comparing differences in qualities and achievements. On the cognitive level, classificatory skills, size relations and mastery of numerical space develop. External as well as internal causes may be assumed as the causes of illness.

Age Group 3 (13 to 18 years)

The child or adolescent has acquired higher-order self-reflective skills and metacognitive processes that can lead to a particular preoccupation with him-/herself. From the perspective of others, these periods of self-preoccupation are sometimes misinterpreted as withdrawal. The insight into feelings and psychological processes in others – in connection with increasing detachment from parents and other adults – can lead to a strong need for controlling feelings as well. Generally, in this stage of development mental perspectives develop on several levels of complexity. This also concerns the regulation of closeness vs. distance. Relationships are re-arranged, and processes pertaining to the origins of illness are formulated with increasing complexity. In friendships, intimate, reciprocal exchanges are especially important. In the cognitive realm, the ability to abstract and to think in terms of possibilities and hypotheses plays an important role. A refined sense of time is also observed, which will be the basis for long-term planning. Coping skills are increasingly characterized by a variety of differentiated strategies and their flexible use.

3. The Importance of the Developmental Context

The OPD-CA-2 is a resource-oriented diagnostic instrument. Accordingly, the comparison between normal and deviant development of children and adolescents will always depend on the age that patients achieve developmental tasks (accomplished by the defined age groups) as well as on the varying developmental contexts. Different developmental contexts can indicate deficits as well as strengths and resources in the child's development. Successful development in certain contexts can compensate for dysfunctional developments in other contexts or even demonstrate resilience. Conversely, developmental problems in only one area of life can bring about such distress as to require psychotherapeutic treatment. Here we see that the appropriate diagnosis of an individual is only possible if multiple developmental contexts are taken into account.

3.1 Family

Generally, parents are the first love objects in early childhood that significantly influence the development of the child. In addition, siblings present in the family will also have an early impact on development. All subsequent relationships are built upon these primary relationships or attachment experiences and attitudes, so that it is important that they provide a positive emotional relationship basis. Attachment is existentially important as it gives the child a secure base from which he or she can explore the world. Exploration is, in turn, a basic prerequisite of learning and cognitive development. This is also shown by studies of neglected children, who often have significant cognitive deficits (Seiffge-Krenke, 2009). Clinical sampling reveals frequent insecure attachment representations (Bakermans-Kranenburg & van IJzendoorn, 2009).

Adequate parental support of emotional regulation in the child increases resilience to developmental and other psychosocial risk factors. Most conducive to development is the authoritative, i.e., accepting and clearly structured, parenting style, which helps the child move towards emotional and social competence and autonomy (Baumrind, 1991).

The importance of the familial context for the development of children and adolescents is shown by the extreme opposite of support: Neglect and abuse as well as parental loss can have a tremendous impact on psychosocial development. For example, neglect and abuse in early childhood can lead to mental symptoms such as the loss of basic trust in parents and later in oneself. Insecure attachment qualities have a negative impact on future relationships and behavior towards one's own children (Nowotny, 2006). An increased developmental risk for children and adolescents can also arise from the somatic illness of one or both parents (Barkmann, Romer, Watson, & Schulte-Markwort, 2007). Equally serious can be the effects of parental mental illness on children and adolescents (Linderkamp, 2006). The loss of a parent or of both parents reduces the available resources dramatically.

Moreover, in the familial context, not only do parents influence their children, but children also influence their parents as well as the development of their siblings (Seiffge-Krenke & Pakalniskiene, 2011). The birth of a sibling can be a critical event for the older child and lead to a regressive process: The older child worries about losing the parental love and attention that he/she must now share with his/her siblings (Burchartz, 2012).

Besides the attachment to a primary caregiver, the gradually commencing individuation, the development of a social network, and the process of separation from the original family are significant developmental tasks. This separation manifests itself in increasing conflicts within the family, among other things.

3.2 Kindergarten, School

Nurseries and kindergartens can promote the development and consolidation of resilience factors such as realistic self-perception, the aptitude for self-regulation, and active coping strategies, if nursery school teachers and teachers support the successful accomplishment of developmental tasks (Bengel, Meinders-Lücking, & Rottmann, 2009).

In addition to the growth of knowledge and cognitive development, schools promote structural skills, such as cooperation, self-perception, self-control, empathy and helpfulness, appropriate assertiveness, and the ability to establish social contact. Failure to acquire these functions sufficiently can lead to various emotional and behavioral problems (Schreyer-Mehlhop, Petermann, Siener, & Petermann, 2011). An especially critical event seems to be the transition from elementary school to secondary school, which is marked by an increased strain with regards to performance and to social relationships (Ball, Lohaus, & Miebach, 2006; Winkler Metzke & Steinhausen, 2002).

3.3 Play, Leisure

The most important functions of play for the child's development are abreaction, recreation, practice in important types of performance, and recapitulation (Oerter & Montada, 2008). The study of 13 to 47 month-old children identified a development of play and therefore also social behavior beginning with playing in parallel with other children, proceeding to complementary and reciprocal play and finally leading to complex, social make-believe play. Children thus acquire the ability to play social roles with the use of metacommunication at the age of 3 and half years. In fact, social learning also takes place during play. Play also has a coping function: Problems typically tackled in play may be roughly grouped into developmental issues and relationship issues. Developmental issues pertain to power, control, the desire for separation and the establishment of boundaries. Relationship issues pertain to problems with significant others and wishful thinking about relationships with them (Oerter & Montada, 2008).

In middle childhood through adolescence, negotiation and overcoming conflicts within symmetrical relationships are an important stage in development, which can be attained through playing with others, among other ways. Children and adolescents without the opportunity to spend time with their peers cannot appropriately develop social skills and ego functions.

The developmental context of leisure promotes above all autonomy, self-determination, motivation, personal initiative, the ability to set goals, identity, social commitment, the development of moral guidelines, emotional regulation, social skills, and the development of social relationships (Caldwell & Witt, 2011). Adolescents are increasingly prone to risky behavior in leisure activities, which decreases in tendency with ageing, however (Raithel, 2004).

3.4 Peers, Friendships, Romantic Partners

Social support from peers and friends is an important protective factor for mental health and can also partially compensate for the lack of support from parents during adolescence (Schmitz & Wurm, 1999).

Peers

During childhood, peers are important attachment figures, as they enable symmetrical communication or interaction, which leads to the understanding of equality and fairness and contributes to the child's conceptualization of self. This has bearing on the development of social identity. As children of the same age are very similar to one another on the cognitive, moral, and emotional levels of development, they are a source of particularly intensive developmental impulses (Oerter & Montada, 2008).

All in all, peer groups enable children and adolescents to acquire nonfamilial experiences and bring about new or consolidate existing social skills. Peer groups also promote the development of basic ego functions such as perception, thinking and planning, as well as the control of drives. Social competence comprises developmental goals such as the ability to adopt perspectives, the recognition of the importance of friendships, the planning of appropriate problem-solving strategies for social interactions, the development of moral values and communication skills (Eisenberg & Harris, 1984), but also emotion regulation.

Adolescents spend much time with their friends and cliques. This serves the purpose of sharing and exchanging ideas on common interests, objectives and age-specific issues, and also provides an opportunity for talking about emotional and sexual subjects that are often not addressed by adolescents within the family in their endeavor to achieve autonomy.

Friendships

Even more important than belonging to a peer group are friendships. They can promote development even more powerfully and also carry greater weight in the case of maladaptive outcomes. Rejection by or loss of friends can have long-term effects, which even two years later may intensify internalizing symptoms (Hoza, Molina, Bukowski, & Sippola, 1995).

Childhood friendships develop during the preschool years through physical closeness and shared play activities. During middle childhood, developmental issues such as belonging and acceptance gain importance. Finally, during adolescence, friendships above all serve identity development (Parker & Gottman, 1989). Selman (1984) identifies four stages of friendship relations: Stage 0 in early childhood involves momentary physical interactions. Stage 1 in middle childhood concerns rather one-sided support. Stage 2 in middle childhood comprises fair-weather cooperation. Intimate exchanges occur during adolescence (Stage 3). Finally, a balance between autonomy and interdependence is attained in adulthood (Stage 4).

For girls, intimacy in friendships is especially important, being attained around two years earlier than boys (Seiffge-Krenke & Seiffge, 2005). For boys, shared activities have priority. Friendships during adolescence are generally characterized by great closeness and intimacy, and also serve as the prototypes for future romantic relationships (Connolly & Goldberg, 1999). In general, developmental disorders in the area of friends and peers can lead to serious interactional, but also interpersonal, problems.

Romantic Partners

Finally, the attainment of emotional independence from the peer group and friends is just as important as emotional independence from parents, and this independence usually culminates in a stable partnership. According to Seiffge-Krenke (2003), the ability to enter into a solid partnership develops through four different phases of personal attitudes toward romantic partners. The first initiation stage, at the age of about

12 to 14 years, coincides with pubertal development and, therefore, also with the development of sexual desires. In the second status phase, the focus moves away from the self towards one's attachments to others. During early and middle adolescence, peer networks play a special role, as they provide a context for getting to know potential partners.

Here the goal is to attain a high status through attachment to a peer group. In the third affection phase, adolescents deepen their relationships with romantic partners, the relationships become emotionally and sexually more fulfilling, and the partner becomes the centre of attention. Finally, the fourth bonding phase deepens the attained level of intimacy with the partner to include pragmatic and personal concerns. This phase usually occurs during the transition from adolescence to adulthood. The possibility of a long-term relationship and obligations to the partner become the object of inner reflection. The relationship is also evaluated according to pragmatic and emotional criteria.

3.5 Body, Body Concept, Illness, and Gender Role

Body and Body Concept

From the outset, the human body undergoes a development and maturation process that reaches a dramatic climax in adolescence through the development of sexual maturity. However, babies and toddlers already pass through important and momentous stages of physical development. Very important here is psychosomatic triangulation. The child takes possession of his/her body and experiences it as belonging to him-/herself, thereby overcoming the phase of his/her own body being part of the mother. As a result, until adolescence, when the child assumes full responsibility for his/her own body, the body plays the role of a third party in the triangulation between the child and his/her mother. Failure can lead to psychosomatic symptoms (Grieser, 2010).

Successful psychosomatic triangulation results in an initial, more stable, conception of one's body in late childhood. This also includes the child's sense of his or her gender.

Previous findings regarding satisfaction with one's own body reveal that the adolescents' body image is sex dependent: Girls have a more negative body image than boys, and their satisfaction with their bodies has a greater impact on their self-esteem. Female adolescents show greater attention to their bodies, greater dissatisfaction with their figures, a perception of inferior athletic skills, and a higher sense of body alienation (Roth, 2002).

Adolescents often undergo piercing to underscore their personality or identity, their aesthetic sensibilities, and their autonomy. Such staging of the body should not be considered *per se* as pathological. It becomes pathological if the staging must be constantly repeated in order to maintain a substitute identity.

Illness

The child's concept of illness is very much governed by a physical and mechanical perspective around the age of nine years. Pains are associated with exogenous factors. Only at the age of about twelve years are endogenous factors of pain integrated in the concept of illness. Pains can now be interpreted as sensations of the body, and as caused not only by external phenomena. Children first develop ideas of personal responsibility or of themselves as the causes of their illnesses, with the latter conceived as punishment or as a contagion. With progressive cognitive development, the concept comes to include general causes as well as psychological factors of illness (Siegal & Peterson, 1999; Williams & Binnie, 2002).

In the case of children with chronic physical illness, inadequate coping with illness increases the risk of behavioral and other mental disorders (Petermann & Walter, 2000).

Gender Role

By about the age of 6, children have for the most part adopted the cultural gender role standard concerning toys, activities, and professional roles, for example. For adolescents, the development of gender identity is an important task in the context of identity formation (Erikson, 1968). Feminine gender role identification is systematically associated with the coping style of rumination (obsessive worry). However, this coping style cannot be inferred solely from gender (Broderick & Korteland, 2002).

3.6 Social Networks, Culture, and Migration

Social Networks

The social network and social support are considered important factors in relationship to illness and health (Sarason, Sarason, & Pierce, 1990). As development progresses, the social network becomes increasingly important for attaining the various stages of development. For example, playmates of the same age are already important developmental aids in development in early childhood (see Section 3.3: *Play, Leisure*). The more autonomous children and adolescents become, the larger their social networks will generally also become (see Section 3.4: *Peers, Friends, Romantic Partners*). Most adolescents rate their social network as efficient and adequate. Adolescents with a higher level of schooling have larger social networks. There is no difference between boys and girls in terms of social network size, although the type of social support significantly differs between girls and boys (Frey & Röthlisberger, 1996).

Culture and Migration

Our socialization deeply roots us in our own culture. We can therefore understand the magnitude of the changes facing migrants when they leave their home countries for a host country with a different and alien culture. Migration-specific mental risks have been discussed from various points of view, such as the risk from re-interpreting one's own identity (Alamdar-Niemann, 1992). In the case of a vulnerable premigration personality structure, migration can lead to serious mental disorders. Internal and external protective factors facilitating the adaptation by children and adolescents when changing their places of residence are the high expectation of self-effectiveness, internal convictions of control, as well as an attractive appearance or athletic ability. The absence of these protective factors will therefore complicate adaptation, with the complication varying according to the degree of dissimilarity of the new cultural environment (Vernberg & Field, 1990). Changing to a different culture or ethnic group can be experienced as especially burdensome if the change occurs not voluntarily but for political reasons or out of poverty. For children and adolescents, this change means in particular the loss of their social network and therefore emotional and instrumental support, as well as the unemployment of their parents (Perrez, 2004).

Not infrequently, the parents of immigrant or refugee families will also be traumatized and develop mental disorders. These parents will then not serve as an optimal protective factor in the sense of a resource for their children in the new environment. In this regard, the transgenerational transmission of trauma to the offspring of immigrants is an important factor in development. There exists the phenomenon of reduced boundary formation between traumatized parents and their children (Kogan, 2003). Past and present intermingle, fantasy and reality merge into one another, and self and object are not differentiated in the parent-child relationship. These children may even become the guarantors of the intrapsychic stability of their traumatized parents and themselves assume a parental role for the latter (von der Stein, 2006).

4. Past Experience and Empirical Findings Related to the OPD-CA

Since its publication, the OPD-CA Manual (Arbeitskreis OPD-KJ, 2003) has been used for diagnosis and therapy planning by child and adolescent therapists in all settings of care. Various studies have tested interrater reliability as well as the empirical and clinical validity of the instrument, with satisfactory results obtained along all axes. An initial review by Weitkamp, Wiegand-Grefe, and Romer (2012) systematically took stock of the empirical findings on the OPD-CA. The main findings are presented below. Psychometric findings are available for each of the axes, and in several areas it was shown that some revisions were needed.

4.1 Interpersonal Relations Axis

For the *interpersonal relations* axis psychometric findings on construct validity and reliability are available (Fliedl & Katzenschläger, unpublished; Weber, v. Klitzing, Westhoff, Willemin, & Bürgin, unpublished, both cited in Weitkamp et al., 2012; Winter, Jelen, Pressel, Lenz, & Lehmkuhl, 2011). In the study by Winter and colleagues (2011), trained ward therapists conducted OPD-CA interviews with hospitalized patients according to an interview guide. On the basis of these 60 cases, factor analyses testing construct validity were conducted for the *interpersonal relations* axis. The factor analysis of the object-directed circle yielded a 2-factor solution. Factor 1 comprises the items for a positive affect, Factor 2 the items for control and a negative affect. The factor analysis for the subject-directed circle yielded a one-factor solution. A replication of these findings with a larger sample is pending. The internal consistency in two of the mentioned studies was satisfactory to good for both the constructed factors and the circles designed in the OPD-CA (Cronbach's α = .70 to .87; see Weitkamp et al., 2012). Interrater reliability was tested for agreement between three clinicians who independently of one another rated 20 video-recorded interviews with in-patients (Weber et al., unpublished, cited in Weitkamp et al., 2012). Agreement on the item level was moderate to very good, with the exception of the item *friendly directive*, which had a low level of agreement. The assessment of interaction patterns accompanying aggressive affects revealed on average a higher degree of agreement compared with affectively neutral and positively nuanced interaction patterns, which were evidently more difficult to distinguish from one another. Thus, very good agreement was achieved only in three out of six aggressively inclined items (*reproachfully deprecating, aggressive-hostile,* and *angry in contact*).

In summary, interrater agreement along the interpersonal relations axis was moderate to good and the internal consistency satisfactory, with factor solutions for construct validity being coherent in content.

4.2 Conflict Axis

Regarding the *conflict* axis, findings are available on criterion validity, clinical validity, and interrater reliability. In several studies, the conflict axis was systematically applied in the indication for and planning of treatment with in-patients and out-patients (Benecke et al., 2011; Seiffge-Krenke, 2012a; Seiffge-Krenke, Mayer, Rathgeber, & Sommer, 2013; Seiffge-Krenke, Mayer, & Winter, 2011; Winter, Jelen, Pressel, Lenz, & Lehmkuhl, 2011). To the extent reported, the conflicts of *dependency vs. autonomy, submission vs. control, need for care vs. autonomy, self-worth* were most often identified. On the other hand, *loyalty conflict, oedipal conflict,* and *identity conflict* were rarely seen as prominent. Significant differences between the studies have been found with respect to severe life stress (stressor-induced conflicts), which the study by Winter and colleagues (2011) indicated for 70.7 % of the in-patients, while the study by Benecke and colleagues (2011) found this condition in none of the healthy or mentally ill subjects.

The criterion validity of the *conflict* axis has been tested according to the connection of the significance of the individual conflicts with the patients' interpersonal problems (Inventory for Interpersonal Problems, IIP; Horowitz, 1999) and personality styles (Inventory for

Personality Styles and Disorders [Persönlichkeitsstil und -störung-sinventar], PSSI; Kuhl & Kazén, 1997). Since only conflicts K1 to K4 were considered significant, conflicts K5 to K7 were excluded from the calculations. This partly resulted in medium-sized correlations with the scales of the PSSI and the IIP. The authors emphasize the importance of the assessment of the prevailing processing mode (active/passive) for each conflict theme classified as present (Benecke et al., 2011). Clinical validity was assessed with a group comparison between conspicuously internalizing and externalizing in-patients. The patients were diagnosed by an independent clinician on the basis of the semi-structured Schedule for Affective-Disorders and Schizophrenia for School-Age Children (K-SADS; Chambers et al., 1985) and later underwent an OPD-CA interview by the respective ward therapists. Significant group differences were found in two conflict constellations. In line with a theory-based and plausible expectation, patients with internalizing disorder patterns (ICD-10 diagnoses) were diagnosed more frequently with a significant intrapsychic conflict of *need for care vs. autarky with passive processing mode*, which according to psychoanalytic ideas is seen as a typical depressive conflict pattern. On the other hand, patients with externalizing disorder patterns (ICD-10-diagnoses), were more often diagnosed with a significant intrapsychic conflict of *submission vs. control with active processing mode* (Winter et al., 2011) which, according to psychoanalytic ideas is considered a typical pattern of aggressive assertiveness against dysregulated fears of excessive control by the object in one's (anal) drive-related desires. Interrater reliability showed good to very good agreements (Benecke et al., 2011; Seiffge-Krenke et al., 2011; Stefini, Reich, Horn, Winkelmann, & Kronmüller, 2013). Seiffge-Krenke and her colleagues have, moreover, reported a tendency towards better interrater agreement among internalizing disorder patterns and older patients (i.e., adolescents).

The finding of only five of the eight defined conflicts playing a numerically significant role among the collected patient samples agrees with the empirical studies for the OPD-CA (see Winter et al., 2011). High interrater agreement was revealed for the conflict axis (Benecke et al., 2011). Regarding criterion validity, an exploratory approach found significant agreement with scales for personality styles and interpersonal conflicts. So far the clinical validity has been investigated only in two studies. Initial findings on the differentiation between internalizing and externalizing disorder patterns indicate the clinical validity of the conflict axis (Winter et al., 2011).

It is noteworthy that the study by Seiffge-Krenke and colleagues (2011), where trained students with no clinical training or experience acted as raters, obtained good interrater reliability for the *conflict* axis. This indicates a closely observed operationalization of this axis that necessitates interpretations to a greater degree than the other axes, given the complex and hypothesis-guided target of the operationalization, namely the (assumed) presence of unconscious intrapsychic conflicts.

4.3 Structure Axis

For the *structure* axis, psychometric findings on concordant and clinical validity, on construct validity, and on reliability are available (Benecke et al., 2011; Müller-Knapp, 2012; Seiffge-Krenke et al., 2011; Fliedl & Katzenschläger, unpublished, cited in Weitkamp et al., 2012; Weitkamp, Wiegand-Grefe, & Romer, 2013; Winter et al., 2011). The concordant validity was tested in the study by Benecke and colleagues (2011). They found high correlations of the items of the structural dimensions with the number of personality disorders. This sample of healthy and mentally ill children and adolescents thus showed a clear relationship between low structural integration and mental disorders of Axis II of the DSM (recorded with the SCID-II). On the other hand, the Global Assessment of Symptomatology showed no significant correlations with the structure axis. In addition, patients with a low-level structure manifested less pronounced empathy. The clinical validity was tested in the study by Winter and colleagues (2011). The comparison between patients with internalizing and externalizing disorder patterns showed a significant difference for the *control* dimension only, to the effect that, as expected, patients with externalizing abnormalities revealed a lower degree of integration along the control dimension. For the other dimensions and the overall value, no significant differences between the patients with externalizing and those with internalizing disorder patterns were found. Two studies with out-patients or hospitalized patients with mixed disorder patterns tested the construct validity of the structure axis. In both studies, the factor analysis consistently revealed a 2-factor solution, with the *control* structural dimension yielding one factor and the structural dimensions of *self and object perception* and *communication skills* together yielding the second factor, with good internal consistency in each case (Weitkamp et al., 2013; Winter et al., 2011). This underscores, first of all, that the theory-guided operationalization of the structural dimension *control* undertaken in the OPD-CA, compiling five individual items as an independent entity, represents a clinically valid construct. The revision of the *structure* axis submitted in the OPD-CA-2 takes into account the inadequate conceptual differentiation between particular items of this axis by rendering more precise item formulations and anchor examples. The interrater reliability of the structure axis varied among trained raters – partly good to very good (Benecke et al., 2011; Stefini et al., 2013) and partly rather moderate (Müller-Knapp, 2012). A study with trained psychology students showed slightly less agreement on the structure axis in the moderate range (Seiffge-Krenke et al., 2011). The internal consistency was satisfactory to good (Benecke et al., 2011; Fliedl & Katzenschläger, unpublished, cited in Weitkamp et al., 2012; Weitkamp et al., 2013).

A recent study showed that the structure axis can be used for differential indication and treatment planning for in-patients and out-patients, and that, in the case of patients with structural deficits, the OPD-CA affords diagnostically specific additional information (Seiffge-Krenke, Fliedl, & Katzenschläger, 2013a). Changes in the structural dimensions due to therapeutic treatment were also confirmed. Jelen-Mauboussin and colleagues (2013) moreover documented changes in the structural dimensions over time for a sample of child and adolescent psychiatric in-patients. Another in-patient sample revealed changes in ten of 18 items (Müller-Knapp, 2012), although these changes after several months of in-patient treatment were only partially representable along the structure axis.

In sum, it can be said that in the case of the structure axis, the two studies in which the particular raters had training in the OPD-CA Manual yielded moderate to very good interrater agreement, indicating that generally better interrater reliability will be obtained if the raters adhere as closely as possible to the Manual and to its specifications. It has been our experience with the *structure* axis in the many training seminars with clinicians that video-based sample ratings at the end of a training seminar yielded amazingly good agreement among the participants. Feedback from the trainees rates the subjective validity of this axis as especially good insofar as clinically observed structural abilities and deficits of patients can be described in a very differentiated way. Typically, participants in our seminars report that they let various known patients pass before their "clinical inner eye" before they give their rating for that particular patient. The construct validity of the structure axis was examined in a factor analysis, which yielded two factors, with one factor combining the dimensions of *self and object perception* and *communication skills*. The two-factor solution of the three dimensions suggested the obtainment of higher precision in the item operationalization. Concordant validity is supported by the agreement of a low structural level with the number of comorbid psychiatric diagnoses.

4.4 Prerequisites for Treatment Axis

Three different studies tested the clinical validity, the construct validity, and the reliability of the prerequisites for treatment axis (Fliedl & Katzenschläger, unpublished and cited in Weitkamp et al., 2012; Weitkamp et al., 2013; Winter et al., 2011). In addition, in a conference presentation, Winter and colleagues reported data for testing the predictive validity of the *prerequisites for treatment* axis (Winter et al., 2007), suggesting that these prerequisites allow the prediction of therapeutic outcome. The report found important predictors of better therapeutic outcome to be familial resources, peer relationships, higher motivation for treatment, better ability to form a therapeutic alliance, and lower mental and somatic impairment (Winter et al., 2007). Clinical validity was tested via group differences in the treatment prerequisites at the level of individual items between hospitalized patients with internalizing disorder patterns and those with externalizing disorder patterns (Winter et al., 2011). The following significant differences were found: As expected, based on their statements in interviews, patients with internalizing symptoms were rated higher with respect to *subjective mental impairment, motivation for change, specific motivation for therapy, insight into biopsychosocial interrelations*, and *gain from illness* as compared with patients with externalizing symptoms. Regarding resources, no significant group differences were found. The *construct validity* of the treatment prerequisites was tested in factor analyses of two independent samples (60 hospitalized patients and 171 out-patients, in each case with mixed disorder patterns) (Weitkamp et al., 2013; Winter et al., 2011). Both factor analyses consistently yielded a 3-factor solution corresponding to the predicted higher-level substantive categories: *subjective dimensions, resources*, and *specific prerequisites for treatment*. Only the item *extra-familial support*, was assigned in both factor analyses to the *specific prerequisites for treatment* dimension and not the given *resources* dimension, contrary to the division in the original OPD-CA Manual. In the factor analysis of Weitkamp and colleagues (2013), the item *insight into biopsychosocial interrelations* was assigned not to *specific prerequisites for treatment*, but to *subjective dimensions*, contrary to the division in the original OPD-CA. The *reliability* of the prerequisites for treatment varied between the dimensions. For the *subjective dimension* satisfactory internal consistencies were found (Cronbach's α between. 0.70 and 0.79), for *resources* and *prerequisites for treatment* the internal consistencies were low to some extent (Cronbach's α between 0.55 and 0.77).

In total, the construct validity of the *prerequisites for treatment* axis has been successfully tested in two independent studies. The factor analyses, for the most part, confirmed the dimensions defined in the Manual. Only in the case of *extra-familial support*, which according to its original definition refers to the knowledge and use of professional assistance and in the original OPD-CA manual was assigned to the dimension *resources*, do the two mutually independent factor analyses suggest an alternative assignment to the dimension *specific prerequisites for treatment* (Weitkamp et al., 2013; Winter et al., 2011). For this reason the OPD-CA-2 renames the original item, *extra-familial support*, as *utilization of the care system*, and includes it in the higher-order dimension *specific prerequisites for treatment*, in accordance with the results of the factor analyses. The internal consistency was satisfactory to low. As to clinical validity, differentiation consistent in substance between patients with internalizing and those with externalizing disorder patterns was obtained, as was the predictive capability for success in treatment with several aspects of the prerequisites for treatment (Winter et al., 2011). Compared with the *prerequisites for treatment and coping with illness* axis of the OPD for adults, the construct validation for the OPD-CA appears altogether more positive. For the corresponding Axis I of the OPD, *experience of illness and prerequisites for treatment*, an ambiguous factor structure has been reported so far, with 3-, 5-, and 6-factor solutions. On the other hand, the high clinical relevance of Axis I of the OPD has been stressed by the authors of several studies (Cierpka et al., 2007).

4.5 Conclusion

Given the number of studies conducted, the empirical validation of the OPD-CA lies well behind that of the OPD for adults. Nevertheless, the available findings to date point to success on the part of the authors of the original Manual in achieving a differentiated, reliable, and valid operationalization of the employed clinical constructs for interpersonal relations, conflict, structure, and prerequisites for treatment, which in the cases of structure and prerequisites for treatment seem to have an even better construct validity along the defined dimensions in comparison to the OPD for adults. Here the authors of the original OPD-CA Manual surely benefited from their past experience with the first OPD Manual for adults, and were able systematically to improve upon some of its weaknesses, already discernible in practical tests, to develop a conception of the axes of the OPD-CA with greater validity. The bandwidth and the methodological quality of the psychometric testing methods has not been fully exhausted yet for the OPD-CA. For example, reliability has been determined merely by analysing the internal consistency and interrater reliability. So far, there are no findings on retest reliability. Moreover, while the applied method of choice for testing construct validity has been factor analysis, this was in parts conducted on small samples. Reproduction of the results in further independent and larger samples would be the appropriate next step. It would also be relevant for the quality of the psychometric testing to incorporate, in a further step, confirmatory factor analyses. As a result, validity testing is primarily exploratory in character. For future studies, it would be desirable to explicate in advance expected relationships of the axes with other instruments or criteria in the form of hypotheses and to test such hypotheses systematically.

Ten years after the publication of the original OPD-CA Manual, the empirical stocktaking as to the reliability and validity of this instrument is on the whole encouraging, so that we may expect an altogether good validation capability for further studies. This present revision of the original Manual (OPD-CA-2) has attempted to systematically tackle the weaknesses revealed by the aforementioned studies by improving the conceptual and terminological precision of the particular item operationalizations, and we, therefore, may accordingly expect improvements in the reliability and validity as well.

5. Theoretical Conception of the Axes

5.1 Interpersonal Relations

In psychodynamic diagnostics, we assume that the patient's mental structure and the current intrapsychic conflicts will become visible in the relationship with the examiner. During psychotherapeutic treatment, the patient's internal mental conditions from which he or she is suffering form current relationship constellations ("transference neurosis"), relative to which certain internal responses (or counter-transference reactions) emerge in the therapist. This dynamic begins to develop from the outset of the initial contact between the patient and the therapist.

We therefore find already in the diagnostic process, in the way the patient initiates a relationship to the clinician, the core of the typical relationship constellations that psychodynamic diagnostic assessment aims at detecting. Capturing in operationalized form and as reliably as possible what is happening in the relationship as it develops is a demanding task, for the examiner him-/herself forms part of the relationship process, making it difficult to separate description from his/her own subjectivity. Operationalization of this important diagnostic level requires the examiner to describe what he/she observes in the patient as an offer of relationship and as relationship behavior, along with the examiner's own internal reaction to this behavior, in a way that is understandable to others. Only then will the subsequent diagnostic process be able to verify the extent to which what is happening and forming a constellation in the relationship expresses the conditions existing in the patient's internal world and is therefore diagnostically usable.

Unlike adults, children and often adolescents tend less to report about themselves and their relationship problems and more to incorporate these issues in their relationships with the examiner in the form of actions. These actions are either directly visible in the relationship itself or are revealed in play. Nowadays we understand these actions as a special form of expression of the child or adolescent that allows for direct diagnostic and therapeutic access to the patient. In assessing the relationship on the basis of the OPD-CA-2, we rely less on the typical relationship episodes reported by our patients and more on the direct formation of the relationship in the patient's contact with us. The relationship behavior is then coded from the participatory observation on the basis of the operationalization. Instead of confining ourselves to dysfunctional behavior, we also code positive relationship behavior, in the sense of resources.

In defining the interpersonal relations axis we were guided by the idea that relationships and their associated affects always represent "composite" modes of behavior and feeling. We often experience children who are willing to love us, and yet also feel in the diagnostic process the downside of this love, namely aggression and hatred. Children who from the outset are extremely concerned with their autonomy also let their desire for dependency and security be known, which they only feel compelled to ward off. These complex feelings can be represented by a circumplex model (see **Figure 1**) based on the circumplex model of the *Structural Analysis of Social Behavior* (SASB; Benjamin, 1974), since this model represents certain relationship constellations along opposite axes as complementary vectors of the same level. For example, if a child initially interacts with the therapist in an affectionate way only to attack him/her later, the ratio can be represented in terms of the existing ambivalent ways of how the relationship is handled.

An adequate relationship diagnosis for childhood and adolescence must take into account the different relationship levels of the child. For this reason, the interpersonal relations axis consists of different modules. Thus, the examiner is able to code the relationships according to the operationalization between the levels: child–examiner, child–father, child–mother, etc.. We suggest a stepwise approach, depending on which relationship appears most important to the examiner. Generally, we assume the child–examiner model will be used.

The basic reduction of the relationship levels to dyads is not to claim that children actually grow up only in dyadic constellations. The relationships also take form on triadic and polyadic levels.

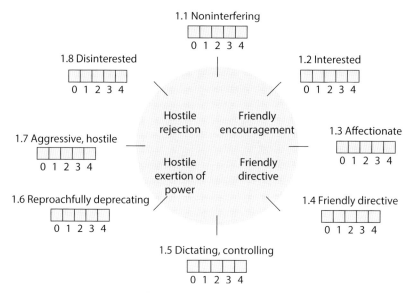

Figure 1. Circumplex model of interpersonal behavior in the case of the "object-directed OPD-CA-2 circle."

Theoretical Background

Representations and Interactions

The operationalized assessment of relationships based on observable interactions is part of the OPD-CA-2, presupposing as we do a significant connection between intrapsychic representations and interpersonal relationships.

Most likely the early interaction sequences will have a very simple structure compared with later ones. Owing to abstraction and compression processes, continuing reorganization and coregulation by the real objects, interaction representations are abstractions that never happened exactly as recalled.

The tendency to reactivate intrapsychic relationship representations in the external world brings about the phenomenon of transference. In any situation with external interactions (and especially, of course, in longer-term relationships), this transference will, therefore, tend to emerge with a specific emotional tone and/or ascribe particular importance to the actual development of the relationship between the two protagonists. The transference resembles a particular sort of "spectacles" that distort perceived colors and shapes to varying degrees.

As the interaction with the examiner develops, transference in this sense will include the unconscious parts of the child's or adolescent's offer of a relationship that are grounded in previous relationship experiences with significant attachment figures. Neither the examiner's clinical perception nor the observable level of interaction (in a video recording, for example) allows differentiation between the parts of this initial offer of a relationship to the examiner rooted in earlier relationship experiences and the parts developing exclusively and situationally from the interpersonal encounter. The child's or adolescent's relationship behavior and interactive behavior directed to the examiner are perceivable only as an overall phenomenon, referred to in ordinary clinical language as "spontaneous transference" or "spontaneous transference offer," in distinction from "therapeutic transference" in the narrow sense, in which the gradually discernible themes of the relationship can be seen as reactivations of previous relationship experiences. For reasons of phenomenological clarity, along the *interpersonal relations axis*, the concept of transference is avoided in the operationalization of the relationship behavior, and instead the observable interactive behavior is recorded in strictly descriptive terms.

Thus, the phenomenon of transference in the diagnostic or therapeutic setting is observable and describable in differentiated form. Given the intrapsychic experience, the real interaction itself modifies the relationship representations by the corresponding relationship partners to a greater or lesser extent. We may, therefore, speak of intrapsychic and interpersonal processes as loop-shaped and mutually interacting.

The younger children are, the less they will have been able to form representations of interactions that could, in turn, affect their current relationship behavior. As a consequence, their relationship formation can also be more reactively influenced by that of the interacting partner. Among children, in particular, therapists often also represent a "new object." Anna Freud (1965) describes this phenomenon in the child as a "hunger for experience," which exists alongside the repetition compulsion and is opposed to it in every way. Overall, it may be said that, in every stage of life, relationship behavior is determined by the offers of relationship from partners and by the transference to and curiosity about new experiences of relationships. The ratio between these three factors in relationship behavior can vary greatly given, for example, the degree of the psychopathology.

Dyads and Triads

We assume that the infant from the outset is capable of triadic or polyadic relationships (Bürgin, 1998a, 1998b; Fivaz-Depeursinge & Corboz-Warnery, 1999; von Klitzing, Simoni & Bürgin, 1999). More recent studies have shown that infants have triadic capabilities as of the third month of life. Even at this age they are able to share situationally changing emotions with both parents through eye contact and facial expression (Fivaz-Depeursinge, Favez, Lavanchy, de Noni, & Frascarolo, 2005; Fivaz-Depeursinge, Lavanchy-Scaiola, & Favez, 2010; von Klitzing, 1998).

The dyadic relationship is preferred because of its relatively simple structure. Being much more difficult to stabilize, triadic or polyadic forms readily decompose into multiple dyadic ones. In everyday life, the infant prefers dyadic relationship forms, as they require significantly less effort to be sustained over longer periods of time. The preference for one male or female partner remaining constant in a relationship is obvious, as only then is continuity possible in the development of intrapsychic relationship representations in the internal world. Many dyadic processes are characterized by attempts at changing mutual influence on the other party – owing to each other's own needs and specific desires to exert power – as invasiveness or respect for the other's independence develop.

Triadic and polyadic interactions are extremely stimulative, however, as they aid the child in the course of his/her development to understand and construct more complex forms of relationships up to the level of relationship networks. Triadic and polyadic relationships provide the child with significant relationship experiences that can compensate for deficits or disorders in the dyadic interaction. Especially children of mentally ill mothers are subject to disruptions of the dyadic interaction. In their studies, Tronick and Reck (2009) showed that the presence of postpartum depression in the mother is negatively associated with the quality of the dyadic mother–child interaction and with the child's cognitive as well as motor development. In shared play, depressed mothers exhibit less positive play behavior and less eye contact with their children. Moreover, they participate less in shared play and show greater boredom compared with nondepressed mothers (Tronick & Reck, 2009). Work by Field (1998) shows that infants and young children whose mothers suffered from postpartum depression identify in the presence of depressed mothers with their depressive emotions. This identification can be mitigated, however, if a nondepressive father (or other third party) is available with whom the child can maintain a relationship in which depressive emotions do not prevail. The presence of a nondepressed father who provides the infant or toddler with cognitive and motorically stimulating interactions may supplement a limited dyadic interaction and thereby constitute a significant protective factor for the development of the child.

According to Stern (1985), the subjective self begins to manifest itself between the 6th and 18th months of life. The child experiences that he/she has a mental life of his/her own, and discovers in the course of his/her further development that this is also true of the other real people in his/her relationship network. A shared subjective experience creates intersubjectivity and intermediary spaces with shared significances, even given the certainty that the feelings and intentions of other persons differ from the child's own.

With primary intersubjectivity, sharing occurs but not with communication about a third person. If the child succeeds in seeing him-/herself again in the living mirror image of the other party, nonfusional imitation and comparison will be possible. In the case of secondary intersubjectivity, both or more attachment figures exchange information about some other subject and metacommunication arises. Only if the real other can be ascribed an inner world of the same sort as the toddler's own, can the latter suppose that the other person can also have relationships with different objects and therefore with others.

The real objects are extremely important, as they persistently contribute to regulation and, therefore, as it were, directly intervene in the child's inner world. Mahler and Gosliner (1955) recognized that, for the child in the separation and differentiation phase of the second year of life, the third person serves as a powerful and even necessary support against the "re-engulfment of the ego into the whirlpool of the primary undifferentiated symbiotic stage" (Mahler & Gosliner, 1955, p. 210). In this regard, Abelin has stressed the father's ability to make him-/herself constantly and reliably available as a "third object" to the child in this process, and, thereby, enable the child to undergo separation from the maternal object in the first years of life and beyond (Abelin, 1971).

In a dyadic relationship, too, there always exists a virtual third person in the inner world of the other. Of course, it depends on the quality of the early object relations of the relationship partners whether this third person can be symbolically present and introduce an element of qualification into the directly experienced dyadic relationship between self and object, or whether the third person is excluded, as can be observed in the "fragmented triad" (see Göttken & von Klitzing, 2013, for a case study). Brickman defined the triangulation as "the process that locates perceptions of objects (including other persons) in the three-dimensional world or three-dimensional space" (Brickman, 1993, p. 908). Should the perception of self and the other exclude the third element, however, the relationship of subject to object will remain immediate and without qualification. Serious distortions of self- and object-perception may result.

The triadic competence of the parents, i.e., their ability even before the birth and afterwards to establish a relationship matrix with their child in which the third person is not excluded, is a precondition for a successful process of triangulation of the child. Parents who are able to establish a relationship matrix that excludes the third person neither in reality or symbolically will enable their child's process of development into triadic relationships. In this way they also enable the child sufficiently to separate him-/herself from the initially symbiotically experienced self–object unity with the mother – an important prerequisite for healthy mental development. The working group of von Klitzing and Bürgin (2005) showed that the triadic competence of parents during pregnancy is negatively associated with the number of externalizing problems of the child at the age of four years. The authors identified a low ability on the part of the parents to anticipate their future relationships triadically without excluding any of the three relationship partners from the triadic relationship constellation as a predictor for the number of externalizing problems of the child at preschool age (von Klitzing & Bürgin, 2005).

In the course of mental development, the dyadic as well as the triadic and polyadic interactions and representations of relationships – parallel to the ego development of the child with all his/her cognitive, affective, and motor skills and needs, and parallel to the offer of relationships in the external world – thus assume increasingly complex forms and significances as well as exhibit other intensities of emotional makeup and implementation in action.

The early pre-oedipal threesomeness or many-someness develops through the post-oedipal stages into adolescent and adult forms. Depending on the libidinal and aggressive cathexes, different dyadic relationship configurations will come to the fore or recede into the background. Depending on the affective closeness or distance, the relationship triangles or squares will be either symmetrically balanced or asymmetrically unbalanced.

The triadic constellations during the oedipal stage are still relatively unstable. The child alternates rapidly between libidinal and rivalry-type attitudes towards his/her parents, with one parent or the self being excluded (both in fantasy and in the real relationship constellations). In the latent-stage phase, the child's instinctual life quietens down, and he/she turns more to social-emotional and cognitive developmental tasks outside the familial relationship context. Ideally as a result of the oedipal stage, the child will have been able to establish a stable triadic relationship representation, in which flexible, reciprocal dyadic and triadic interactions with the parents (and, consequently, also with other relationship partners in and out of school) are possible. The establishment of such triadic competence on the part of the child depends largely on how much the child "can already recognize the significance of the father as a symbolic third person, or whether [the child] has still not experienced any qualification of his/her relationship to the maternal object by a third person (ideally by the father)" (Göttken & von Klitzing, 2013, p. 163, text translated by the editors). Detailed case material on stable and unstable familial triadic constellations has been presented elsewhere (see Göttken & von Klitzing, 2013).

Relationship Diagnostics

Psychoanalysis has a long tradition of the description and identification of interpersonal relationship patterns. Significant conscious or unconscious modes of experience and behavior in the handling of interpersonal relationships occur again and again (repetition compulsion and transference) and are, therefore, also in principle identifiable.

Most psychodynamically or interpersonally oriented psychotherapies as well as some methods of cognitive behavioral therapy view solidified and dysfunctional interpersonal relationship patterns as essential preconditions of psychogenic illnesses (Strupp & Binder, 1991). Such self-sustaining patterns arise from intrapsychic "schemata" developed over the person's life history, i.e., "traces" of relationship experiences are at issue. These schemata are continually confirmed or modified in relationship processes with other people. The theoretical basis of this view is provided by the psychoanalytic object relations theory, systems theory, and the interpersonal psychoanalytic psychotherapy of Sullivan (1953). Such internal schemata crystallize from redundant relationship experiences, in particular with the relevant attachment figures of childhood and adolescence. On the intrapsychic level of the child, they become internalized "self–object–affect schemata" (Kernberg, 1984; Stern, 1985). Here essential features are not only that the child identifies with the caregiver and the familial relationships and functions, but also that the child constructs, influences, and changes these relationships from the start. The child thus identifies with relationship patterns, to the construction of which he/she has herself contributed in a major way (Cierpka, 1992).

The child internalizes subjectively processed experiences in interpersonal relationships as a willingness to realize certain constellations of transference in the relationships with the interpersonal world (so-called "readiness for transference relationships"). Conflictual relationships with the relevant relationship partners can restrict the relationship experience and behavior to a considerable extent if these conflicts are not resolved in a developmentally appropriate way. In addition, occurrences of intrapsychic distortion can contribute to the emergence of maladaptive interactions in familial and other interpersonal relationship systems. For example, a child's developmentally appropriate expectations of affective attachment from the mother may be condemned to failure from the start due to the mother's depressive state, and lead to negative self-esteem on the child's part. Such relationships can be described as dysfunctional relationships.

The clinical importance of the diagnostic assessment of dysfunctional relationship behavior derives from the connection between interpersonal complications and the emergence and persistence of mental symptoms. Therapeutic efforts consequently focus on the representations of maladaptive, conflictual relationship patterns.

Psychodynamic diagnostics in child and adolescent psychiatry and psychotherapy examines how relationships are handled between the child and his or her parents and siblings as well as between the child and the examiner. Independently of the central concerns of identifying and describing dysfunctional patterns, the examiner should look for signs of resources in the patient's relationships.

Attempts to schematize the descriptions of typical patterns have led to problems explainable by the fact that different psychoanalysts have interpreted the observed phenomena in different ways (Seitz, 1966). These problems of consensus and interrater reliability can be minimized if the constructs under investigation are operationalized as closely as possible to observation (Thomä, Grünzig, Böckenförde, & Kächele, 1976).

On the one hand, the past two decades have seen increased scientific interest in relationships on the part of other, nonpsychoanalytic orientations of psychotherapy (e.g., cognitive behavioral therapy and systemic family therapy), on the other hand there has occurred a development of measurement methods attempting to capture interpersonal communication in a valid way. These methods differ in their complexity, their measurement levels, and the concomitant influence of subjective factors (see Luborsky & Crits-Christoph, 1990). A review by Schauenburg and Cierpka (1994) compiles those methods stemming from the psychoanalytic tradition. Following their description and assessment of numerous methods, the authors conclude that the *Structural Analysis of Social Behavior* (SASB; Benjamin, 1974, 1982, 1987, 1988, 1993; Tress, 1993) and the *Core Conflictual Relationship Theme* (CCRT; Luborsky & Crits-Christoph, 1990) are the methods that have been best researched and most often applied. "The relationship behavior and the resulting patterns of relationships should be formulated so as to identify above all the behavior […] observed by the examiner […] and described by the patient" (Arbeitskreis OPD, 1996, p. 53, text translated by the editors).

In addition to the current habitual relationship behavior exhibited in the examined situation, relationships to the main attachment figures must also be considered in the cases of children and adolescents.

The aim of the operationalized diagnostics of relationships is not to arrive at nosological diagnoses of relationships; rather, the identification of relationships should form part (one axis) of a multiaxial classification system. In its approach, it is most formally comparable to the diagnostic system *Zero to Three* developed in 1994 by the National Centre for Clinical Infant Programs (ZTT-DC: 0–3, Zero to Three, 2005), even if the theoretical assumptions are different.

Circumplex models of interpersonal behavior

The interpersonal circumplex models of relationship behavior (Benjamin, 1974; Kiesler, 1983; Leary, 1957) form the heuristic basis for the substantive classification of habitual behavior in relationships. These circumplex models have a long tradition in clinical psychology. They imply that in social relationships interaction partners base their respective relationship behavior on the definition of status and desired closeness. Common to these models is the depiction of the behavior on a circular surface (see Figure 1). Analysing the relationship behavior in terms of similarities and polarities, we arrive at an arrangement of the relationship patterns in a circle (Plutchik, 1997). This arrangement is definable in terms of two orthogonal and bipolar dimensions: Control (dominant/controlling vs. obedient/submissive) and affiliation (loving/attached vs. hostile/distanced). Qualities of interpersonal behavior can be determined as a ratio between these two basic dimensions, and thus as positions in the circular area they form. These circumplex models, and the measurement tools derived from them, have been well studied and validated within personality, social, and clinical psychology (Wiggins, 1991).

5.2 Conflict

In psychoanalytic theory, particularly in the illness model, intrapsychic conflicts play a central role as the causes of mental disorders (see Loch, 1986; Mentzos, 2005). For the conceptualization and operationalization of intrapsychic conflicts for childhood and adolescence, those psychoanalytic theories are of particular importance in their focus on the development and relationships. Here the object relationship theories (Kernberg, 1975; Mahler, Pine, & Bergmann, 1973; Winnicott, 1953, 1956, 1958), the results of family diagnostics (Cierpka, 2008) and family therapy (Stierlin, 1970) as well as the results of observations of infants and of infant research (Lichtenberg, 1983; Stern, 1985) deserve particular mentioning.

What Is an Intrapsychic Conflict?

Intrapsychic conflicts are unconscious intrapsychic collisions of opposing affects, bundles of motivations, ambitions, or behavioral tendencies, such as the fundamental desire to be cared for on the one hand and the fundamental desire to be self-sufficient, i.e., to take care of oneself, on the other. As defined in the OPD-CA-2, we regard psychodynamic conflicts as long-lasting if they persist for more than six months and are characterized by a child's or adolescent's established experiential patterns that repeatedly lead to similar behavioral patterns in corresponding situations without the child's or adolescent's awareness of this fact. These conflicts are dysfunctional, i.e., they hinder development and interfere with interpersonal relationships.

Long-lasting conflicts develop via internalization processes from early relationship experiences and conflictual episodes within the age-related radius of a child's or adolescent's important relationships. Intrapsychic conflicts pertain to issues that affect all children and adolescents, but not with the development limiting exclusivity meant here. Once internalized, these conflicts will influence future interactions and relationship episodes.

Long-lasting intrapsychic conflicts have two sides: On the one hand, they inhibit development by fixating a child's or adolescent's motivations and affects in different areas of life on a conflict theme and, thereby, restricting further developments. On the other hand, long-lasting conflicts are achievements of the ego, which has managed to process conflictual relationship episodes, even if, as noted, with restrictions and fixations. Long-lasting conflicts can thus develop into issues shaping the entire life history, giving it subjective sense. In most cases, intrapsychic conflicts are unconscious for the affected children and adolescents, but they can also occur at the preconscious or even conscious level. Such conflicts can be experienced as egodystonic or egosyntonic in terms of character pathology. However, among those children and adolescents presenting for diagnostic assessment and treatment, development-inhibiting, unconscious, and egodystonic aspects of long-lasting conflicts predominate.

The precondition for the occurrence of long-lasting intrapsychic conflicts is a mental structure in which self and object representations can be reliably differentiated. An intermediary space (Winnicott, 1971a) between self and object is available, that is, the child or adolescent has the ability to fantasize, to symbolize, and to play. The mental structures described are formed around the age of 24 months. However, long-lasting intrapsychic conflicts cannot develop before the Age Group 1 (3 to 5 years). In Age Group 0, these structural preconditions are not yet firmly established, although even at this stage forerunners of long-lasting intrapsychic conflicts can develop.

We assume that long-lasting intrapsychic conflicts develop in a sequence of stages. Through repetitive interaction processes cognitively and affectively complex internal patterns develop that are continually adjusted and expanded. The children's dispositions seem partially to determine whether an early, largely inflexible expression of conflict will arise or whether a pre-existing flexibility will also allow for corrections. We also need to suppose that intrapsychic constellations of conflicts will arise if the child's needs are acknowledged and satisfied by his or her important attachment figures, either inappropriately and inadequately or excessively.

How Are Intrapsychic Conflict, Structure, and Interpersonal Relations Related to One Another?

Conflict, structure, and interpersonal relations are not mutually independent constructs in the OPD-CA-2. Conflicts are determined by the underlying integration level of their structure and can be observed in characteristic relationship episodes. The formation of an intrapsychic conflict is modulated by the integration level of the mental structure. A fragmented, disintegrated mental structure prevents a focus on a conflict theme. Nor can any conflict theme be developed if the developmental preconditions are lacking.

What Kind of Intrapsychic Conflict Themes Are There?

The following describes the seven intrapsychic conflicts and their theoretical foundations. In each case the prominent affect can be helpful for the assessment.

Conflict: Closeness Versus Distance

The *closeness vs. distance* conflict was formerly called dependency vs. autonomy in an earlier version of the OPD-CA. The renaming underscores the difference from the previous conflict of dependency vs.

autonomy, which suggests a too mature theme. In contrast, the conflict of closeness vs. distance concerns the existential importance of attachment as well as the importance of emotional security, as described in the concepts of Margaret Mahler and colleagues (1973) and Edith Jacobson (1964). These ideas were later taken up in the attachment theory of Bowlby (1975). As attachment research (Fonagy & Target, 2003) and psychoanalytic infant research (Stern, 1985) have shown, the emotional availability of an attachment figure and the affective exchange are extremely important for the development of a child and form the basis for secure bonding. A healthy development enables the child to establish flexible and reciprocal relationships in which he or she can resolve the polarity of desires for closeness and distance. In the the conflict case, there are no secure attachments, with the consequence that, in relationships with significant others, the fear of closeness accompanied by excessive emotional independence will dominate in the active mode, while the fear of separation coupled with a search for close relationships will dominate in the passive mode. The typical prominent affect for this conflict development is therefore existential anxiety.

Conflict: Submission Versus Control

Control of self and others evolves with the increasing physical, emotional, and cognitive maturation of the child in interplay with noninterfering or contolling interactions with the parent or other caretakers. In connection with the description of obsessive-compulsive disorders and the anal triad, Sigmund Freud (1908/1959) very early on described the tendency of adult neurotics to control relationships. Like all developmental trajectories, the issue of submission vs. control runs through all stages of development, but reaches its first formative level at the ages of 2 to 5 years, when behavioral norms are increasingly internalized (A. Freud, 1936). The potential for conflict is more pronounced the more rigid or lax the familial and social rules are. Tensions occur in the first stage of the conflict in basic interpersonal form (submission in the passive mode vs. rebellion in the active mode), and in intrapsychic form only as cognitive maturation progresses and internal values and rules develop. Accordingly, different affects will occur depending on the stage of development. In interpersonal conflicts and precursors to conflicts, anger, rage, and fear predominate. After completion of internalization, complex affects like shame, guilt, and anxiety also come into play.

Conflict: Taking Care of Oneself Versus Being Cared For

The conflict of *taking care of oneself vs. being cared for* was formerly termed "need for care vs. autarky" in earlier versions of the OPD-CA; this renaming makes it even clearer, what the essential theme is. Theorists such as Winnicott (1971a) have described the early mother–child interaction in terms of the total dependence of the infant on the mother's care, and have spoken of a "primary maternal preoccupation" on the mother's part as an almost intuitive empathy for the child's needs. Balint (1952) has given a similar description, termed "primary love." In her famous essay *Envy and Gratitude*, Melanie Klein (1975) also elaborated the oral level and established its relationship to depression. Object-relation theorists like Bion (1963) also described the importance of incorporation by means of the "container-contained" model. Characteristic of this type of conflict is that the child–parent interaction is based on the experience of relationship security – although largely governed by either the claims to material and/or emotional care in the passive mode or by their rejection in the active mode – related to a striving for self-sufficiency. This focus of interaction, which initially predominates because of the total dependence of the child on care and, as a result, stands in the way of the child's independent development of needs, will be internalized as conflictual if this does not correspond to the parents' style of interaction and, further, if certain predispositions of the child fuel this conflict. The prominent affect typical for this conflict is dissatisfaction, the feeling of wanting more, not getting enough, and the fear of losing care, as well as feelings of depression in the face of excessive demands. Anger can arise in countertransference because of "clinginess."

Self-Worth Conflict

Winnicott (1956) described the holding function of the mother and the necessity of emotional mirroring for the child's feeling of self-worth. The consolation afforded by the transitional object (Winnicott, 1953) facilitates separation from the mother, mitigates the feelings of abandonment and constitutes an initial stage of autonomous self-worth regulation. Even if differently weighted, most theories of the origin of narcissistic disorders regard the frustration of the child's need for being loved and recognized (mirroring) in the context of a nonempathetic parent–child interaction as aetiologically significant for the emergence of a disorder in self-worth regulation (Blanck & Blanck, 1979; Kohut, 1971). Typical for these disorders are also correspondingly pathological self-aspects such as fantasies of diminutiveness or an aggrandized self. When parents use children as containers in Bion's sense or project self-aspects onto children, a false sense of self can develop in the child or adolescent.

During their development, children and adolescents increasingly learn to regulate their positive feelings of self-worth in an enduring way and less dependently on others. Should conflicts occur, self-aggrandizement emerges in the active mode and a collapse of self-esteem in the passive mode. The prominent affect is narcissistic rage and, given a decline in self-esteem, significantly noticeable shame.

Guilt Conflict

The guilt conflict was termed the "loyalty conflict" in an earlier version of the OPD-CA. The name was changed for the sake of a better distinction from loyalty conflicts following separation of the parents, which are not meant here. Enrolment in school provides children with sufficient (superego) demands and prohibitions (A. Freud, 1936). The internalization of these demands, norms, and values due to identification with the parents is the precondition for having feelings of guilt. Guilt conflicts in children and adolescents are governed by the endeavor to secure the relationship with the parents by all means (Fairbairn, 1952). Due to the necessity of existentially securing the relationship with the parents, children are willing to sacrifice their credibility and their sense of reality when it comes to protecting the parents or their parents' values and norms from outside attacks. Children and adolescents in whom this conflicting issue prevails in a dysfunctional and developmentally inhibiting way thus suffer extremely in the passive mode under (inappropriately) intense feelings of guilt towards the parents, or they inappropriately feel responsible for certain family issues. In the active mode, these feelings of guilt are fended off and the parents are accused for everything in an inappropriate form. Stierlin (1970) has described in detail the dynamics of parents and adolescents in the process of separation. In extra-familial relationships too, the children in the passive mode appear anxious and willing to make sacrifices, with an inappropriate assumption of guilt, and those in the active mode seem egotistic, transgressive, and reckless, with a refusal to accept guilt. The prominent affect is guilt, with the polarization of good vs. evil.

Oedipal Conflict

With regard to the conceptual background of the oedipal conflict, Sigmund Freud's discussion of the Oedipus complex (1905/1953) and his theory of infantile sexuality (1961), in which he explored the sexual orientation of the (male) child and the identification with the parent of opposite sex, are of historically lasting importance. In addition, Melanie Klein (1962) described the early stages of the Oedipus complex, in which she estimated the onset of triadic relationships as occurring sooner compared with S. Freud's theory. Later, Abelin (1971) and Rotmann (1978) again took up the idea of early triangulation. As the first important love objects, parents thus have a formative significance for children, while, conversely, children are important objects of love for their parents. The conflict discussed here centres on the satisfaction of erotic and sexual desires and on the tendencies and inhibitions standing in the way of these desires. In the active mode, oedipal issues are disproportionately stressed, while in the passive mode they are avoided. Inappropriate eroticization or excessive neutrality can therefore become noticeable as prominent affects.

In adolescence, a special dynamics arises from the fact that the physically mature genitals theoretically allow acting upon instinctual desires. Laufer and Laufer (1984) consider the integration of physically mature genitals in the body image and the entry into sexual relationships to be crucial steps in development. Their mastery promotes the progression of development and their failure results in the breakdown of development.

Identity Conflict

Identity formation is a life-long process, but according to Erikson (1959, 1982) preferentially develops during adolescence. For Blos (2001) too, adolescence plays a central role in identity formation. More recent conceptualizations (Seiffge-Krenke, 2012b) show that the process of re-assessment of old identifications and the integration of new identifications has extended through young adulthood. Mentzos (2005) differentiates primary conflicts in the individual developmental stages that lead to crises in the identity development of children and adolescents.

As these crises are overcome, new aspects of self-images arise (Erikson, 1959). Successful integration of the new aspects of self-images in the pre-existing self-image will be reflected at each stage of development in a subjective sense of continuity and coherence. This phenomenon is always associated with different significant object relations, i.e., there will exist numerous different identities appearing as coherent self-identities in the conflict-free case and as contradictory, confused self-images in conflictual cases. The active mode may involve an excessive adoption of changing identifications, and the passive mode disorientation and helplessness. Unlike identity diffusion (Foelsch et al., 2010), which is a structural problem, an identity conflict presupposes at least a moderately integrated structural level. The transgenerational problems in migration can compel the development of an identity conflict (Kohte-Meyer, 2006). An immigrant background may also contain the potential for identity development, however (Schepker & Toker, 2009).

How Do Intrapsychic Conflicts Differ From Forms of Severe Stress in Life and Everyday Conflicts?

Forms of severe stress in life must be distinguished from enduring intrapsychic conflicts. These severe forms of stress in life can lower the structural level, but also exacerbate the aforementioned intrapsychic conflicts or impair the person's ability to process them. Research on coping distinguishes between three different types of severe life stress: critical life events (such as the parents' divorce or unemployment), chronic stressors (such as chronic illness), and serious trauma such as rape or torture. Characteristically, these forms of stress are not very predictable and allow the child/adolescent little control over the event (Seiffge-Krenke & Lohaus, 2007). These severe forms of life stress place an enormous burden on children and adolescents, since in coping with these pressures they must rely on their own, developmentally based and possibly inadequate coping skills as well as on family resources. In addition, parents are particularly affected by the consequences of these stressors and may lack insight into their children's sensitivities. Generally, the effects will be more serious the less developed or integrated the child's mental structure and his or her capability for mature ego achievements (defence mechanisms) are. In addition – as already mentioned – traumatizing events may occur that even children and adolescents with well-integrated structures cannot appropriately process. Also worth noting, however, is that about a third of the children and adolescents who had been exposed to such stress as well as a small proportion of the children and adolescents subjected to traumatc experiences (see Egle, Joraschky, Lampe, Seiffge-Krenke, & Cierpka, 2015) developed no symptoms (so-called "invulnerables"), which is not to say that they enjoyed mentally healthy and undisturbed development. We can distinguish between current (dating back to less than six months) and previous severe life stress (dating back to more than six months) (see also Axis V of the Multi-Axial Classification Scheme, World Health Organisation, 1996). Children and adolescents are often presented to psychiatrists or psychotherapists because of current or previous severe stress in life, which, in turn, often aggravates intrapsychic conflicts, however.

Intrapsychic conflicts as well as severe stress in life may be differentiated from everyday conflicts, i.e., conflicts that occur in everyday life between parents and their children. They are mildly distressing, predictable (because frequent), and do not inhibit development, but generally promote autonomy. These everyday conflicts are not considered in the OPD-CA-2.

Overall Assessment

The intrapsychic conflicts described in the above sections can be identified and validated according to the operationalizations in the Manual (see Part 2: Manualization of the Axes, Chapter 8: *Conflict*). The individual conflicts are assessed according to importance: very important (3), moderately significant (2), of little significance (1), and absent (0). Two modalities are described pertaining to the processing of these long-lasting intrapsychic conflicts. For each conflict area a passive and an active mode of the conflict coping are distinguished from one another. The active mode is present when counterphobic defence and reaction formation prevail. In the passive mode, regressive defensive attitudes may dominate. While an active or passive mode is described in reference to prototypes, in clinical reality mixed types often occur. In the overall assessment up to two of the most important conflicts are identified, which will be considered as especially significant and reliably diagnosable. In addition, possible preceding and enduring, internalized conflicts of the parents should be considered.

5.3 Structure

The concept of mental structure (Rudolf, 1995) integrates the ideas of self-psychology (P. F. Kernberg, 1989; Kohut, 1971) and object relations theory (Mahler et al., 1973; Sullivan, 1953) towards a theorem of a repertoire of experiences and actions on the basis of interaction experiences. The intermediate space (Winnicott, 1965), allowing internally represented intentional action, should then also be explored. Findings from infant research (Stern, 1985), attachment research (Bowlby, 1980), research of emotions (Damasio, 1999; LeDoux, 1996), research of temperament, clinical developmental psychology (Oerter & Montada, 2008), and developmental psychopathology (Resch, 1999b) also have influence on the assessment of the child's personality development. Mental structure is understood as the result of a bidirectional interaction of innate dispositions and interactional experiences, leading to the formation of specific experiential and behavioral dispositions on the part of the child in interacting with his or her environment.

A description of the observable and perceptible behavior of children and adolescents is summarized in the OPD-CA-2 in terms of four dimensions. The three dimensions known from the OPD-CA have been modified with the addition of the *attachment* dimension. The OPD-CA had conceptualized attachment only inadequately and implicitly as the capacity for internalized communication. Central aspects were thereby not sufficiently represented. The addition of attachment as a separate dimension with several aspects should now allow a more accurate and differentiated representation of qualities or inadequacies of mental structural elements and abilities. Psychodynamic assessments must take into account the developmental age and refer to defined time frames in which a comparable developmental-psychological adaptive competence is to be expected (Resch et al., 1998).

This is significantly facilitated in the OPD-CA-2, since for all four structural assessment dimensions and in each age group particular abilities are described in the form of anchor-point descriptions, and are operationalized for each of the four structural levels (good integration, limited integration, poor integration, and disintegration). The general assessment scale we have so far employed (assessment of structural abilities according to the criteria of functionality, flexibility, variability, continuity, and the issue of support) has been replaced by a description of each individual structural level.

We assume that descriptions are possible of the qualitative differences between age groups as well as between the individual structural levels in a given age group. As in the OPD-CA, we have refrained from defining a "perfect structural level" (0) as provided for in the DSM-5, for example, since in our view such a level would be a theoretical phenomenon with little practical relevance. In difficult situations and life crises, temporarily suspending one's structural abilities is certainly a healthy reaction. In this event, we already deal with a good and not a perfect structural level. In order to describe similar phenomena on other structural levels we have introduced intermediate levels (1.5; 2.5; 3.5). They should rather describe the oscillation, at least occasionally, occurring between two structural levels than the exact interposition. The anchor-point descriptions now elaborated in the OPD-CA-2 for each structural level in each aspect and in each age group provide a significantly more detailed framework for assessments.

The assessment of the structure should always be resource-oriented and extend beyond the symptom, in view of the context-dependence of dysfunctional or functional modes of reaction. The assessment of the availability of dispositions to act should cover the preceding six months, and refer to the biographical context, in addition to the assessment of situational behavior within and outside the examination situation. The OPD-CA-2 has changed nothing on this point.

In the development and organization of the mental structure as a disposition of the individual, the OPD-CA-2 now considers the child's or adolescent's ability to cope with negative affects, the establishment of his/her impulse regulation and self-worth regulation as well as the institution of controlling instances (control dimension), his/her ability to experience him-/herself (coherence and self-perception) and others (object perception), and to differentiate him-/herself (self–object differentiation) from others (identity dimension). The third dimension of interpersonality deals with the question whether there is, inwardly, room for fantasizing, whether affects can be experienced (affective experience), whether contact can be established with the outside world (initiating emotional contact), and relationships can be developed (reciprocity). Here, the degree of empathy is crucial, as is the ability to break free of relationships (capacity to separate). The fourth dimension of attachment seeks to capture the internal working model by describing to what extent internal images of others and of relationships exist at all (internalization), in what way the attachment system can be regulated intrapsychically (secure internal base), to what extent the child or adolescent can tolerate situations of being alone (capacity to be alone) and can use attachment relationships in order to establish a sense of security and protection (use of attachment relationships).

The extent to which this subdivision of the OPD-CA-2 deviates in detail from that of the OPD-CA can be seen in **Table 1** and **Table 2** (see Chapter 9: *Structure*). Besides the addition of the *attachment* dimension, especially noteworthy is the subsumption of "self- perception and object perception" with its individual aspects from the OPD-CA under the concept of identity.

In our view, communication skills are now also described more accurately in the OPD-CA-2 in terms of interpersonality. All in all, the revision widens the richness of detail in structural abilities, with none of the abilities previously treated in the OPD-CA being dropped in terms of content.

Table 1. The structural dimensions of the previous version of the OPD-CA at a glance (Arbeitskreis OPD-KJ, 2003, 2007)

Control	Self-Perception and Object Perception	Communication Skills
Negative affect	Self-perception	Contact
Self-worth	Self–object differentiation	Decoding of others' affects
Impulse control	Object perception	Communicative function of own affects
Controlling instances	Empathy and object-related affects	Reciprocity
Conflict resolution		Internalized communication

Table 2. Structural dimensions of the OPD-CA-2 at a glance

Control	Identity	Interpersonailty	Attachment
Impulse control	Coherence	Fantasies	Access to attachment representations
Affect tolerance	Self-perception	Initiating emotional contact	Secure internal base
Controlling instances (conscience formation)	Self–object differentiation	Reciprocity	Capacity to be alone
Self-worth regulation	Object perception	Affective experience	Use of attachment relationships
	Belonging	Empathy	
		Capacity to separate	

Control

The *control* dimension concerns the ability to form a buffer against negative affects (displeasure, annoyance, disgruntlement, lack of enthusiasm). For this dimension, the conceptual terms have above all been adjusted in the OPD-CA-2 and affect tolerance (formerly "negative affect") and self-worth regulation (formerly "sense of self") are interpreted in a slightly broader sense. At Level 2 the child achieves a balance between the sides of his or her ambivalence and can then consciously experience, acknowledge, and communicate these sides. Initially, in general, (Age Level 1: 3 to 5 years) and, later on in a differentiated way, adapting to the situation (Age Levels 2 and 3: 6 to 18 years), the establishment of impulse control pertains to the ability to control impulses and to achieve a disactualization of what is experienced. Already in early childhood, the child should be able to modulate self-worth to a rudimentary extent and to restore it when it has been endangered. Later on (Age Levels 2 and 3: 6 to 18 years), this must be possible in a more differentiated way and without help. Parallel with moral development, a controlling instance must be established that can also be externally stabilized in early childhood (Age Level 1: 3 to 5 years). The ability to make moral judgements will then develop moving from knowing what is considered to be forbidden to general norms up to perceiving the complexity of moral issues within a framework shaped by society.

Identity

The dimension of Identity was formerly known in the OPD-CA as self- and object perception. Compared with the OPD-CA, we have added the aspects of *coherence* and *belonging* to this dimension and have moved empathy as a subsidiary aspect in the interpersonality dimension. In terms of development, this dimension pertains first to the ability to describe one's own person from external variables (external appearance, clothing, gender characteristics), then towards increasingly sophisticated attributions (skills, qualities) (*self-perception*) that also come to have an increasingly temporal and situational stability in experience (*coherence*). This process is similar to the experiencing of other persons (object perception), who may be initially perceived and described in terms of their external features, but with time become the recipients of increasingly differentiated attributions that also become perceptible and tangible as distinguished from self-perception (self– object differentiation).

Interpersonality

The dimension of *interpersonality* was formerly known in the OPD-CA as "communication skills". The primary change here is the integration of internalized communication of the OPD-CA in the subcategory *fantasies*. We have also added to this dimension the capacity to separate as a central partial aspect of how relationships are handled.

This dimension comprises the aspects *fantasies, initiating emotional contact, reciprocity, affective experience, empathy*, and the *capacity to separate*. *Fantasies* is the key element of internal communication. It allows experimentation and the establishment of a private protected space. The ability to appropriately *initiate contact* and express one's needs in an adequate and understandable way evolves and can be increasingly used for self and affect regulation. On the other hand, responsiveness to the other person's emotions leads already to an interest in a mutual dialog in Age Group 1 (3 to 5 years). Offers to play are accepted and further developed in playful dialogs. Communication with the child triggers in the other person an experience of adequate participation and manifests itself as *reciprocity*. From Age Group 1 (3 to 5 years) on, communication with the child (e.g., in the examination situation) leads to a sense of togetherness. Fine-tuning is possible. Negotiation between the child's wishes and those of the other party give rise to a third element. A jointly shaped work emerges from play. Sensitivity to others' feelings and interactive behavior are the other key elements of interpersonality. *Empathy* already begins to develop during early childhood and is refined over time. Finally, a child or adolescent should be *able to separate him-/herself* from relationships and, in the case of permanent loss, strip the emotional investment from the object.

Attachment

As already mentioned, a new dimension added is that of *attachment*. It comprises the aspects *access to attachment representations, secure internal base, capacity to be alone*, and the *use of attachment relationships*. The overall purpose of this dimension is to represent in its development and expression what Bowlby (1975) has conceptualized as an "internal working model". *Access to attachment representations (internalization)* begins with the relationship experiences with the primary attachment figures, who from the age of three through early childhood (Age Group 1: 3 to 5 years) should be available as security-providing mental representations of objects and relationships in some form. On this basis, these attachment representations should become differentiated and networked during middle childhood (Age Group 2: 6 to 12 years) and, finally, during adolescence (Age Group 3: 13 to 18 years), form a complete working model. While initially the existence of relationship representations is of interest, the category *secure internal base* pertains to the applicability of the available mental repertoire. The activation of the attachment system triggers a need for protection and security. During early childhood (Age Group 1), a child should be able to allow this activation as well as to bring about deactivation intrapsychically. Initially, the child needs to succeed only to a limited extent, depending on the intensity of the activation and only in the case of individual triggers (darkness, separation, etc.), without interactive aid. During middle childhood (Age Group 2), regulation should be possible even in the case of multiple triggers that do not activate the attachment system too intensely. During adolescence (Age Group 3), this regulation should practically always succeed as a temporary solution if no interactive regulation resources are available. Children should also be able at the age of three to occupy themselves alone, without becoming overwhelmed by their negative feelings. While this ability may be present during these early years only to a temporally very limited extent and only in familiar surroundings, it must evolve further, so that the adolescent will at least be able to tolerate longer periods of time in a foreign environment. Finally, the use of relationships to satisfy attachment needs is also important. That is, the child or adolescent should be able to develop a goal-adjusted partnership with an attachment figure.

5.4 Prerequisites for Treatment Axis

The axes described in the preceding sections, namely *relationship*, *conflict* and *structure*, operationalized explicitly psychodynamic constructs intended to represent the phenomenology and internal dynamics of disorder patterns, with the emphasis on interaction. In addition, a series of other important aspects also have to be integrated in the diagnostic process, in particular concerning the indication for and planning of treatment. They are summarized in the *prerequisites for treatment* axis. The differential indication for psychotherapy in childhood and adolescence is always embedded in general psychopathological, psychopharmacological, social-psychiatric, and family-therapeutic perspectives. The *prerequisites for treatment* axis serves as an important bridge between these perspectives. It pertains primarily to aspects significant for the indication and planning of psychotherapy. The assessment of this axis should also lead to considerations of a multimodal approach and/or relative contraindications or to further differential-indication considerations, for example, to initiate educational or pharmacological interventions. The items defined in this axis, which are mainly derived from clinical-pragmatic considerations, are divided into the three categories: *subjective dimensions*, *resources,* and *specific prerequisites for treatment*. They are largely mutually independent in their theoretical conception, a fact that distinguishes this axis clearly from the others (the modifications in the grouping of the items compared with the first and second editions of this Manual were informed by factor-analytic examinations of this axis [Weitkamp et al., 2012; Winter et al., 2011]). Our conceptualization of the items avoids overlaps with the multiaxial psychiatric or psychosomatic diagnostics of the multiaxial classification scheme (MAS) of the ICD-10, which, in any case, should be applied as an indispensable basic standard assessment, independently of any particular psychotherapeutic approach. This led to, among other things, more consistent orientation on patients' subjective experiences compared with the OPD for adults. For example, in the OPD the severity of impairment from a symptomatology is to be assessed objectively, which in the multiaxial diagnostics of children and adolescents according to MAS/ICD-10 already occurs along Axis VI (General Psychosocial Functional Level).

The subjective experience of illness and the associated coping with that illness make up an important element in the evaluation of the specific psychotherapeutic indication in different settings. They are operationalized in the *subjective dimensions* items. In the realm of subjective dimensions, patients' perspectives and modes of experience unfold in the patients' own words, before they are abstracted and translated by interpretation into a professional perspective. Psychodynamic diagnostic assessment is explicitly oriented to the child's or adolescent's subjectivity. Only a subsequent step establishes connections to and dissonances with objectively or interpretively found results. In clinical routine, it is not always easy to accept the child's subjectivity and establish diagnostic intersubjectivity. In this regard, the *prerequisites for treatment* axis is a prototypical example of the connection between psychodynamic operationalization and normative dimensions.

The evaluation of the patient's impairment in the OPD-CA-2 is left up to his or her subjective assessment and only in a subsequent step checked against the examiner's objectivized diagnostic assessments. The subjective illness theory is of the utmost importance for the compliance with, adherence to, and development of a shared definition of problems and of the corresponding treatment contract, especially in childhood and in the family context. Sociocultural characteristics must also be identified and assessed as to their relevance to the treatment planning process. The OPD-CA-2 differentiates the patient's motivations for therapy into two items; namely, the motivation for change with regard to reported symptoms or issues and the specific motivation for therapy in relationship-oriented psychodynamic or psychoanalytic therapy in the narrower sense, as this motivation emerges from the diagnostic dialog. Some patients show a seemingly high motivation for change, but are not yet ready or able to accept and persevere with a specific psychotherapy.

Resources play a central role in treatment planning and are operationalized and assessed in the OPD-CA-2. A basic resource orientation is therefore presupposed as a therapeutic attitude on the examiner's part. Specifically assessed are the subjectively experienced support from friends, family, and the extended social environment, in line with the social support construct established in research on risk and protective factors for mental health problems. Added as an individual resource is the reported sense of present and potential self-efficacy based on the psychoanalytic construct of ego strength. Concepts like compliance or adherence which, while regularly used, are often imprecisely defined, were moved in the OPD-CA-2 to the item of Ability to form a therapeutic working alliance.

6. Diagnostic Assessment and the OPD-CA-2 Interview

6.1 Diagnostic Assessment

In each psychodynamic diagnostic investigation the examiner is a participating observer in interaction with the patient. The scenic unfolding of the relationship between patient and examiner as well as the examiner's affective participation and resonance enters into the diagnostic assessment. In the OPD-CA, the categories of the diagnostic assessment are operationalized as far as possible on the basis of observed phenomena.

Generally, the examination room must be equipped according to the age of the child or adolescent. The different age groups must be taken into account. Also with intellectual impairment, the real age is of primary importance. The time frame should be about 60 minutes for Age Group 3 (13 to 18 years), about 30 minutes for children of Age Group 2 (6 to 12 years), with the subsequent possibility of continuing the diagnosic investigation with play materials (Sceno Test, von Staabs, 1964; story completion, Weber & Stadelmann, 2011; MacArthur Story Stem Battery [MSSB], Bretherton & Oppenheim, 2003; Squiggle Game, Winnicott, 1971b). In the case of small and pre-school children (Age Group 1: 3 to 5 years), the diagnostic investigation should primarily rely on play materials. The initiative for playing should be left to the child; the interviewer's active participation should be a response to the child's offer of play.

Owing to the actual dependencies and age-dependent limitations on children's and adolescents' perceptions, important attachment figures must be included in the examination. The core of the diagnostic assessment lies in the interview, play, and, where appropriate, projective techniques, with the relative importance of the interview and play depending on the patient's age.

In the case of children and adolescents, the focus of the diagnostic assessment depends on the age group:

- In Age Group 1 (3 to 5 years), observation of behavior and interactions as well as playful communication stand in the foreground; induced playful narratives can also be used here.
- In Age Group 2 (6 to 12 years), transitions from communication during play to conversation will be more frequent. In addition, narratives induced through story completion, the squiggle technique or the Sceno Test are very informative.
- In Age Group 3 (13 to 18 years), verbal communication becomes increasingly important, although play can still have importance. Also important is behavioral observation, however.

The following discusses some relevant aspects of the diagnostic assessment.

Appearance and Behavior

- In his/her appearance and behavior, the child displays his/her noticeable problems (e.g., anxiety) without being able to name them.
- It becomes clear from his/her appearance whether the child is in a good or possibly neglected state.
- The adolescent states his/her value orientation through his/her appearance (e.g., clothes, hairstyle, etc.).
- How does a child move about in the therapist's room?
- Does the child show hyperactive behavior or does he/she hide behind his/her mother?
- Does the child need regulations from others in controlling his/her behavior?
- Does the adolescent's actions show what he/she thinks of adults, is he/she distrustful or communicative?

Interaction Observation

In particular, with a young child it is important to obtain a picture of the interaction between the mother and child or father and child.

- What does the attachment behavior look like?
- Does the child show an interest in exploration or does he/she remain tied to the mother in a way inappropriate for his/her age?
- Does the child show interest in the playthings in the therapist's room?
- Is the child able to establish contact with the therapist?
- Does the child have to check back with his/her mother?

Observations in Free Play

The child or adolescent reveals his or her subjective reality through play. Active participation by the examiner is useful if the patient needs help in choosing and arranging the form of play.

- Does the child show an interest in the toys?
- Does the child create any playful scenes?
- Does the child have to be restricted in his/her activities?
- Does the child have fantasy, can he/she communicate through play or does his/her play remain chaotic, without any intelligible meaning?

Children in Age Group 1 begin with concrete play, which becomes symbolic play in pre-school age. From the age of six years (Age Group 2), role play has priority; among adolescents (Age Group 3) play has only a minor role – communication occurs rather through action.

Playful Enactment in the Sceno

The Sceno box (von Staabs, 1964) has proven to be a successful component of the diagnostic assessment. The child is asked to build something that just occurs to him/her or is going through his/her mind. Here we can distinguish between the content of the game, the ability for fantasy, the length of play, and the arrangement of play. The arrangement of play may reveal central conflicts, such as that of taking care of oneself vs. being cared for. The findings may reveal structural difficulties pertaining to the ability to exert control and the ability for fantasy, object perception, or affect tolerance, for example, which are important for the diagnosic investigation of the structure axis (Streeck-Fischer, 1999). Play also provides information about how relationships are handled.

Another aid in diagnostic assessment is story completion. Here the McArthur Story Stem Battery (Bretherton & Oppenheim, 2003) is suitable, which can also be used in a modified form in structural diagnostics (Weber & Stadelmann, 2011). Children are confronted with the beginnings of stories about everyday conflictual situations in the family and with peers. The continuations can point to the children's thoughts and feelings. These investigative methods provide access to the cognitive and emotional development of children. The methods were developed for children from three years and up.

Analysis of the stories can shed light on hidden conflicts as well as on the different structural levels. Here the dimensions of control, identity, interpersonality, and attachment can become visible. In a case study, Weber and Stadelmann (2011) have illustrated these application criteria. Focussing on the attachment dimension allows use of the Attachment Story Completion Task (ASCT) by Bretherton and colleagues (2011).

Previous History Provided by Others

Interviews with the parents or other attachment figures are important not only in the case of children in Age Groups 1 (3 to 5 years) and 2 (6 to 12 years), but also with adolescents (Age Group 3) who have significant mentalization impairments or pronounced reality testing disorders, for example. Here the extent of the disorder can be made clear only with the aid of external anamnestic data. In addition, children and adolescents tending towards primarily adaptive behavior will often be unable to communicate or will avoid communicating the extent of their problems. External anamnestic data are necessary for obtaining a complete picture of the child's or adolescent's problems and those of the parents.

The OPD-CA-2 does not provide a standardization of the investigative procedure. The basic ideas of the individual axes serve rather as a guide for interviews and play.

- All sections of the diagnostic assessment can provide information on dysfunctional relationship patterns and on the actual psychosocial living conditions of a patient.
- The second part of the examination should, in particular, yield information about repetitive intrapsychic conflicts governing experi-

ence, behavior, and multiple areas of life, as well as information on the level of integration of the mental structure as a holistic arrangement of dispositions available to the child or adolescent.

- The third part provides the examiner with information on the parental figures' intrapsychic conflicts and mental structures, which constitute important conditions for the development of children and adolescents.

6.2 OPD-CA-2 – The Interview

In the past, the OPD-CA Task Force has provided few specific details on conducting interviews. Because of the high demand for such information, we explain the basic considerations of the OPD-CA-2 interview in more detail, giving a specific account of the course of the interview and an interview guide is provided in Appendix A.

The special ability of the OPD-CA interview lies, on the one hand, in generating sufficient material for the assessment along the four axes with the aid of a rather exploratory interview attitude. The advantage of such an approach is that the psychodynamic assessment can be verified by the patient's utterances and in this way operationalized. It should be kept in mind that the responses to the questions posed are self-assessments which may also be governed by rationalizations and self-deception (Mertens, 2012). On the other hand, enough leeway must be given to the scenic material with the aid of a basic relationship-dynamic attitude (Diederichs-Paeschke et al., 2011; Windaus, 2012; Winnicott, 1971b). The perception of one's own subjectivity is of central importance for scenic understanding, given the examiner's internal response or resonance and the lead affect they experience. The examiner him-/herself is an observing participant in a scenic dialog and cannot remove him-/herself from what is going on in the relationship. Scenic understanding involves the perception of images, fantasies, dreams, and physical feelings, which can only come about through the "flow of impressions from the preconscious and unconscious" (Mertens, 2012, p. 186, text translated by the editors). On the other hand, the therapist's assessments may become subjectively nuanced to the detriment of him/her understanding the child or adolescent correctly. Use of the

OPD-CA at this point can improve diagnostic quality (Rudolf, 2012). All in all, we assume that the quality of psychodynamic diagnosis will be greatest when both scenic understanding as well as the exploratory interview technique are applied for the diagnostic assessment with varying degrees of emphasis on the child or adolescent and the questions asked.

For an assessment of all OPD-CA axes, the histories of the parents and/or other attachment figures are usually indispensable, while we recommend acquiring the external anamneses of the attachment figures beforehand. Special ethnic and social features of the families must be considered in particular. The interview with the child or adolescent remains the core of the diagnostic assessment, however (Arbeitskreis OPD-KJ, 2003).

OPD-CA-2 – Interview Procedure

Each examiner is, of course, free to decide how much preference to give the exploratory interview technique or a more open approach focussed on scenic understanding for the collection of information and hypotheses, in order to carry out the OPD-CA. This preference will certainly also depend on the purpose for which the interview is conducted. In the research context, a more structured approach is necessary for obtaining findings, while in clinical contexts a more open-ended dialog may be preferred. Experienced psychotherapists can retain their usual interview technique for performing the OPD-CA assessment. The point is not to learn a new interview technique, but rather to provide space for the constructs of the OPD-CA in the interview.

Generally, we recommend a moderately structured approach with children and adolescents taking into account the psychodynamic aspects, with guiding questions in line with the interview guide (see Appendix A). By a "moderately structured approach" we mean giving priority to the subjects and interactions initiated by the child or adolescent, but also asking the child or adolescent guiding questions and giving him or her space to respond to these questions and/or to respond behaviorally. The focus should lie on scenic understanding, which assumes that children and adolescents present their histories not only in words, but also through arranging an interactional process. To this extent, self-reflection of the countertransference with the resulting hypothesis formation plays an important role. **Figure 2** shows which interview technique when emphasized can obtain information for which axes of the OPD-CA.

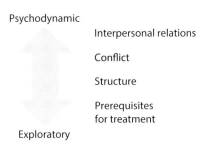

Psychodynamic

Interpersonal relations

Conflict

Structure

Prerequisites
for treatment

Exploratory

Figure 2. Interview techniques for the different axes.

For example, the more structured approach allows the exploration of the degree of the symptoms, while a more open-ended dialog allows the child to communicate his or her inner, unconscious experiences. Relationship-dynamic aspects can be considered on the basis of the child's interaction with the examiner and the latter's internal resonance. Depending on the possibility for the child to contribute to a question or subject, the interview should be less structured if the child provides detailed accounts and more structured if the child is reticent. In accordance with Dührssen (1981) and Erikson (1959), the OPD-CA defines the following important aspects of life for children and adolescents: family, peers, kindergarten/school/vocational training, body/illness, culture/migration. These areas should be given special consideration when conducting interviews.

Phases of the Interview (Modified According to Diederichs-Paeschke et al., 2011)

Initial Scene

The start of the interview is preceded by welcoming the patient and initial contact. Of great importance is that the therapist consciously perceives the scenic and situational information contained in these initial moments and brings to mind his or her own emotional reactions and resonances (Köpp, 2002). At this point, the therapist can observe the patient's taking leave of the attachment figures as well as his/her body posture, facial expressions, and gestures. In line with the OPD-CA, we can derive hypotheses for all the axes: The information whether the child and the parents appear on time for the appointment can be employed for the *prerequisites for treatment* axis (ability to form alliances). The observation of how the child behaves towards the examiner can be taken into consideration for the *interpersonal relations* axis (interested – disinterested). Information is also provided for the *structure* (inter-personality – emotional contact) axis and for the *conflict* axis (closeness vs. distance).

Opening Phase

As children are generally not familiar with interviews, the purpose and time frame of the interview should be carefully explained before starting. In doing so, the interviewer should also introduce him-/herself by name and state his/her function. Mentioning confidentiality is important, especially with adolescents.

Depending on the context, a more structured approach focussing on the *prerequisites for treatment* axis may be suitable at the beginning of the interview, i.e., the focus lies on the current mental or somatic symptomatology as well as on severity and *level of suffering*. In this regard, the *subjective illness theory* and triggering situations are of particular importance. Questions can then be asked about the general *motivation for change*, the *specific motivation for therapy*, and *intra-psychic resources*. A less structured approach is also conceivable at the beginning and a funnelled, increasingly more structured approach as the dialog progresses.

Main Phase

This phase of the interview focusses at first on the current life situation (school) and *relationships with peers* (resources). Stories about relationship episodes with peers (structure and conflict) may be used for generating material. The current family situation, *familial resources*, and relationship episodes within the family (structure and conflict) then become important. It should also be worked out how the symptom that was the reason for presentation can be understood in the context of the patient's life history. The symptom should also be viewed in the patient's interaction with the most important attachment figures.

The assessment of the item *utilization of the psychosocial care system* should be obtained primarily from the anamnestic discussions with the parents. Questions about the mental structure in reference to *identity* and *control* can then be asked as part of the exploratory interview technique. At this point, questions about intrapsychic conflicts can also be asked and their significance for the existing symptomatology worked out. It is also important to establish affect-logical relationships of meaning between apparently irrational experiential and behavioral patterns.

Childhood memories and dreams should also be considered. The Three Wishes Task can also often bring new aspects to light. At this point of the interview, the patient's activity of association should be stimulated and the transition to a less structured dialog enabled. This will support the development of the relationship between child and examiner as well as aid the latter's observation, reflection, and hypothesis formation. The focus on scenic understanding increasingly gives leeway to the unconscious and sheds additional light on the *structure* and *conflict* axes. The observable behavior should also be entered into the *interpersonal relations* axis.

During this in-depth phase, information about all OPD-CA axes is to be obtained: The description of contacts with peers and intrafamilial relationships yields information for the *prerequisites for treatment* axis (resources from family and peers). The observation of how relationships are handled in the interview provides information for the *interpersonal relations* axis. The dialog situation itself as well as the description of the relationship episodes indicates more important aspects for the *structure* axis (*interpersonality* and *attachment*). Information about the conflict dynamics can be obtained from the description of self-perception and of the relationship episodes as well as from the observation of the dynamics of the relationship with the examiner. In addition, guiding interview questions for approaching individual conflicts are provided in Appendix A.

Final Phase and Leave-Taking

The child should be prepared at an early stage for the end of the dialog. By now the child has emotionally opened up. Sensitive handling of this situation requires a basic appreciative attitude towards the child. Towards the end of the dialog, increasingly structured interviewing is desirable. A summary of the dialog and a clear agreement with the child or adolescent and the attachment figure on the further procedure conclude the interview. Contact with the attachment figure as well as the patient's leave-taking of the examiner (body posture, eye contact, facial expressions, and gestures) provides valuable information for all axes, namely when assessing the *interpersonal relations* axis (affectionate treatment – aggressive-hostile), the *conflict* axis (closeness vs. distance), the *structure* axis (interpersonality) and the *prerequisites for treatment* axis (ability to form working alliances).

Reflection and Evaluation

During the interview the patient's lifeworld ("Lebenswelt") is revealed through the consideration of the interviewer's own inner experiences. Special attention should be given to information gaps. Following this clarification, the patient is confronted with his or her typical modes of behavior. The obtained findings allow the formation of psychodynamic hypotheses and their confirmation or falsification in trial interpretations. If the patient can engage in this form of work (clarification/confrontation/interpretation), a high level of specific motivation for psychotherapy in terms of the ability for insight may be assumed.

Documentation and Diagnostic Formulation

A protocol or video can serve as the basis for the diagnostic evaluation. The assessment can be made alone or through exchanges with experienced consultants, which can be used as a quality circle. The OPD-CA-2 Manual should form the basis for the diagnostic assessment. A thorough knowledge and use of the Manual is a prerequisite for the reliability of the assessment. The overall clinical assessment occurs in a review of all findings from the interview (dialog or play, depending on the age group) and the external anamneses. Written documentation summarizing the findings in terms of mental structure, conflict dynamics, and handling of relationships, including assessment of the prognosis with particular consideration of the prerequisites for treatment, is recommended.

Sheets for the diagnostic assessment can be found in Appendix B.

Interview Guide

The interview guide (modified according to the Arbeitsgruppe OPD-KJ-Institut für Psychotherapie Berlin, 2009; Rathgeber, Sommer, &

Seiffge-Krenke, 2009; Winter, 2004) is reproduced in Appendix A. The first part of the interview guide contains general aspects regarding suggestions for conducting the dialog during the interview phases. The dynamics and suggested formulations for the different interview situations are described: Helpful information for the interview is provided, from initiation of contact in the light of possible refusals and pauses through to a deepening of the dialog to concluding the interview. The second part of the guide contains aspects with sample questions specifically corresponding to the axes of *conflict, structure*, and *prerequisites for treatment*. These questions are not intended as a template for conducting a structured interview, but rather as in-depth questions that may be useful in the course of an interview. Behavioral observations and internal resonances are also included.

Part 2: Manualization of the Axes

7. First Axis: Interpersonal Relations

The concept presented here takes the categories described by the OPD Task Force (2001) as its starting point, which refer to the interpersonal positions in the patient's habitual relationship behavior. The OPD-CA-2 has deemed far-reaching modifications to be necessary.

The following premises hold:

1. Relationships and the form they take depend on the age and level of development.
2. Relationships with the (primary) attachment figures are greatly significant, so that dyadic relationships can be described.
3. The description of the categories should be functional and not limited to maladaptive patterns; the identification of resources is useful.
4. The relationship patterns are formulated so as to take into account observable or verbally described experiences and behavior. There is also the possibility of describing symbolically presented material from play or projective procedures if this material can be validated by the history of the child or by the child him-/herself.

7.1 Circumplex Model of the OPD-CA-2

An especially important foundation for the circumplex model of the OPD-CA-2 is the structural analysis of social behavior (SASB, Benjamin, 1974; Tress, 1993). This analysis assesses the relationship behavior on three different levels – pertaining to the directionality of the interaction – namely, the transitive level, the intransitive level, and the intrapsychic (self-referential) level.

On the basis of the SASB model, the OPD-CA-2 assesses the dyadic interpersonal relationship behavior on two levels:

1. Transitive level: The *object-directed circle* describes the communication directed at the interaction partner (the patient behaves towards …).
2. Intransitive level: The *subject-directed circle* describes the reaction to a message from the interaction partner or utterances referring to the emotional state triggered by the interaction partner (the patient's reaction to the examiner …).

The examiner generally endeavors to keep his/her relationship behavior under control, even in the face of negative or very positive affects. As his/her internal response to the patient or the family is an important diagnostic tool, the examiner should also assess his/her experience or his/her own impulses and affects as the *examiner's internal response* for the transitive and intransitive levels with subject-directed and object-directed circles.

On the intrapsychic level (*self-referential circle*), the OPD-CA-2 investigates how the patient deals with him-/herself. For each of these three circles the degree of affiliation (affectionate friendliness vs. hostility) and the degree of influence (allowing independence or being independent vs. exerting control or submitting to control) are determined.

7.2 Operationalization

The general rules of diagnostic assessment apply.

Sources of Information

1. Central to the assessment are the observable relationships in the examination situation. The issue is how the child or adolescent and possibly the parents or other relevant attachment figures directly and currently handle relationships between one another and with the examiner.
2. In addition to the observable behavioral level, the modes of experience, and reactions of the examiner (his or her internal resonance) to the offer of relationship by the child or adolescent and the presenting family group can be drawn on in the assessment. By "internal response" or "resonance" we mean specific reactions, impulses,

feelings, or inner experiences on the part of the examiner triggered by the particular interviewee or interactional couple or family. The examiner is aware of these specific responses, which are accessible to him/her and directly observable or perceivable within him-/herself. This corresponds to a very wide definition of countertransference. As psychoanalysis defines countertransference in different ways, however, we employ the concept of "internal resonance" in operationalizing what is going on in the relationship. The examiner must critically ask him-/herself whether phenomena pertaining to his/her own transference may also be involved instead of a specific response when, for example, he/she perceives him-/herself as adopting a dismissive or benevolent stance towards a person. Such a transference-related dismissive or benevolent attitude would affect the observable interactions and their assessments by the examiners.

Besides the observed interaction, the examiner's information about his/her internal resonance provides important details about how relationships are handled. The examiner can compare his/her observed internal resonance to a parent, for example, with how others, such as the child, behave towards that person.

While correspondences may exist, responses can also run contrary to these interactions, so that the latter must be put in a relative perspective.

3. Depending on their age, children's own reports of relationship experiences and stories in which the child or adolescent verbally expresses him-/herself about his/her relationships with significant others can be included when applying the OPD-CA-2. Also included are reports by the parents or other significant relationship persons about important or frequently recurring relationship experiences with the child or adolescent.

4. As another data source for assessing the interpersonal relations axis, the relationship configurations of symbolic figures from scenes of play, projective examination procedures, graphic or other means of expression are used in the assessment if their significance is supported by different sources, the anamnestic material, and the relationship experiences of the child or adolescent. An evident association must therefore exist.

Unlike adults, children and also often adolescents tend to report less about themselves and their relationship problems directly and instead bring these issues directly into the relationship with the examiner. In assessments of the interpersonal relations axis of the OPD-CA-2, we therefore rely less on the patients narratives of some of their typical relationship episodes and more on how the patient directly and immediately develops such typical relationship episodes with the examiner or with significant attachment figures. As participating observers, we then attempt to operationalize what is immediately happening in the relationship. Instead of confining ourselves to dysfunctional behavior, we also code positive relationship behavior, in the sense of resources. We have decided to pursue this line because, in view of the rapid development during childhood and adolescence, dysfunctional and functional forms of behavior are sometimes difficult to differentiate and because the therapeutic process is based specifically on functional aspects of the ego.

Assessment Scales

The dyadic and self-referential circumplex models plot the degree of affiliation along the horizontal axis vs. the degree of influence along the vertical axis.

In the circle, eight loci are separately defined with a description and allocation digit via the degree of affiliation (affectionate friendliness vs. hostility) and influence (allowing independence or being independent vs. exerting control or submitting to control). The examiner bases his/ her assessment of the eight items initially on the given frequency of the behavior to be investigated. In particular, he/she determines whether the behavior or internal response is *absent* (0), *rarely present* (1), *moderately present* (2), *often present* (3), or *very often present* (4). Sometimes the item can be better assessed according to its intensity than its frequency if, for example, the examiner notices that while only isolated actions occur, they still govern the situation. The designations are then: *absent* (0), *somewhat present* (1), *moderately present* (2) *strongly present* (3), or *very strongly present* (4).

Example: During a half-hour examination, an adolescent experiences aggressive impulses towards the examiner on two occasions and threatens that the examiner is about to get a nasty surprise. If only the frequency of such aggressive impulses were to be considered, the adolescent would be insufficiently assessed as aggressive, so that the examiner here rates not the duration but the degree of aggressiveness and assigns the adolescent a "4."

Depending on the examination situation and the clinical question, various numbers of relationships (e.g., child with mother, mother with child, and child with the examiner, examiner's internal response to the mother and to the child, in each case both subject-directed and object-directed) can be assessed on the dyadic level (anamnestic, observed, symbolized).

The relationship behavior is assessed on the dyadic level with the object-directed circle (Appendix B.1) and with the subject-directed circle (Appendix B.2).

- The object-directed circle describes the communication directed at the interaction partner. Here it is described how influence is exerted on the interaction partner or how a qualifying statement is made about that person.
- Example: The mother acts towards her child reproachfully and deprecatingly.
- The subject-directed circle describes the reaction to a message from the interaction partner or to utterances relating merely to the child's own state of mind.
- Example: The child seems sullen and withdrawn in his or her relationship to the examiner.

The examiner's subjective experience (impulses, emotions, etc.) in relation to the patient (the examiner's internal response) provides an additional source of relevant information and can therefore, as the examiner's internal response, be assessed with Assessment Sheet B for the subject-directed (Appendix B.3) and object-directed (Appendix B.4) circles.

On the intrapsychic level (self-referential circle, Assessment Sheet C: Appendix B.5), the person makes him-/herself the subject of a qualifying statement. The person treats him-/herself in a praising or controlling manner as with a third party. Example: An adolescent exhibits auto-aggressive behavior.

In the following we give instructions for each assessment level (A, B, C) with their respective circles.

7.3 Assessment Level A: Dyads

Introduction

For each item we assess whether the relationship formation described there is observable and, if so, to what extent.

The assessments should not be based on average patients with the particular disorder (as in: "For an autistic person the patient shows quite an amount of interest") or on the rater's horizon of clinical experience ("Compared with my other patients she is very affectionate"). The description of an item corresponds to a gestalt-like unit and cannot be seen as simply the sum of the two qualities: For example, 1.4 *friendly directive* means being both friendly and directive. If someone is friendly, but does not provide directions, a "0" should be coded.

In the object-directed circle, it is assessed how the person under study (such as the child) deals with the other person (such as the examiner); that is, how the subject actively shapes the relationship to the other party. In contrast, the subject-directed circle represents the reaction to the other party's construction of the relationship or to aspects of self-regulation and of the internal relationship that, however, also develops with the relationship to the other. The issue is therefore "well-being with…"

The examples described for each item have been formulated so that the behavior and experience in each case occur very often or are very pronounced and are to be assigned a "4." Lower frequencies or weaker forms per observation period are consequently rated lower (0 = *absent*, 1 = *rarely/somewhat present*, 2 = *moderately present*, 3 = *often/strongly present*). If the rater is not the same as the interviewer, the interviewer can also be assessed. Depending on the setting and role, the interviewer will generally be rated less high for some items (such as "enjoys contact," "acts aggressively").

To prevent the Manual from becoming too comprehensive, with few exceptions, we have limited the examples to observable relationship behavior in examination situations, and they can be extended to symbolized scenes in play or to the described relationship behavior in particular dyads. Anchor-point descriptions for each age level are then listed in tables.

Comments on and Examples of the Individual Items
Object-Directed Circle

1.1 *Noninterfering*

In this attitude, the person allows the other party to do whatever he or she wishes to do at the moment. *Noninterfering* is understood as giving the other person space. A concurrent positive or negative affect towards the interactional partner does not play any role in the assessment of this item. For example, should a child show indifference to all questions asked about him-/herself without having any influence on the examiner, the child is said to be noninterfering. A persistently active refusal to cooperate and a permanent desire to determine things oneself would mean the absence of noninterfering, and the rater would assign a $0 = absent$.

The behavior of a child who lets the examiner ask whatever he/she pleases, but barely responds to the questions, is characterized as partly noninterfering and as partly dictating and controlling, since the examiner may also allow him-/herself to be halted in his/her intention to ask questions.

1.2 *Interested*

Corresponding to its position in the circumplex model, this item is characterized by a combination of noninterference and positive affects towards the dialog partner. This also includes listening to differing opinions, paying attention to the other person, and/or acknowledging the other person's intentions and points of view. In an interview, friendly attentiveness towards the other person's utterances and activities shows "interest." The aforementioned phenomena can also be observed on the basis of gaze, posture, and voice. Interest is also evident when, for example, the child's behavior encourages the examiner to continure with the questions in a similar fashion. The child's being difficult during the interview by, for example, constantly running away and keeping at a spatial distance would indicate a low level of interest and therefore be rated lower in the coding. In this case, the examiner would not be very encouraged to continue with his/her current offer of dialog.

1.3 *Affectionate*

This item can be alternatively described as amicable concern about the other person's emotional state, to which interest and friendliness belong. The assessment of an initial interview will seldom assign the child a very high rating, as his/her relationship to the interviewer will generally be less well defined than with a parent. A child who approaches the examiner through facial expressions and gestures (smiling, seeking physical closeness in the case of younger children) and co-operates well with the examiner, is behaving affectionately and the rating must reflect the degree of this behavior.

1.4 Friendly Directive

Corresponding to its position in the circumplex model, this item is characterized by a combination of control and a positive affect towards the dialog partner. Events are steered in a particular direction (accompanied by an existing positive affect) or a friendly influence is exerted on the other person, regardless of whether a verbal dialog or action is concerned. Caring, giving advice, and a mode of behavior that is stimulating to others are also included here. An adult who shows his/her expectations to the child in a friendly and supportive way, and then structures the situation accordingly, is friendly and directive.

1.5 Dictating, Controlling

This refers to the following modes of behavior: The person takes the lead in the dialog, dominates the conversation, controls or restricts the interlocutor's actions. Or the person wants to stipulate to the other what he or she has to do. A concurrent positive or negative affect towards the interlocutor plays no role in the assessment of this item.

1.6 Reproachfully Deprecating

Corresponding to its position in the circumplex model, this item is characterized by a combination of control and a negative affect towards the interlocutor. In older children, adolescents, and adults, attention should be given to whether the language, facial expressions or behavioral responses indicate reproachful, accusatory, and deprecating tendencies. An examiner who speaks to a child in a combination of incredulous amazement and implicit criticism or the like – "What, you didn't know this?" – or repeatedly expresses critical distance by frowning is exhibiting a negatively emotional, controlling form of behavior towards the child to be coded as *reproachfully deprecating*. Among younger children the designation within the inner circle, namely "hostile exertion of power," i.e., exerting power with a recognisably negative affect, is a more appropriate description. An example is a toddler who tells his mother "Stupid, go away!" and in this way tries to determine the mother's actions.

1.7 Aggressive, Hostile

Aggressive behavior in the form of rejection, verbal or physical aggressiveness, or exploitation of the other's weaknesses is meant here. If strongly pronounced with a deliberate and intentional component, a 4 is assigned. In the case of a child who, for example, "stonewalls" the interviewer, this item should be rated only if aggressiveness is clearly observable either verbally or behaviorally. Annoyed looks, grumbling, and the like are included according to the intensity of affective expression. Slightly aggressive behavior occurs when, for example, the examiner seems impatient without cause or when an examiner expresses annoyance or displeasure towards the child through facial expressions or tone of voice.

1.8 Disinterested

Corresponding to its position in the circumplex model, this item is characterized by a combination of noninterference and a negative affect towards the interlocutor – the person cold-shoulders the other, takes no notice of him/her, neglects his/her needs, pays no attention to him/her, or does not respond to his/her difficulties, even if he/she needs that person the most.

Subject-Directed Circle

2.1 Acting on One's Own Impulses

This refers to fully independent behavior, e.g., the child does what he/she wants regardless of the attachment figure. As with the other items, the assessment is based on observable facts (behavior, language, facial expressions). A concurrent positive or negative affect towards the interlocutor plays no role in the assessment of this item.

For example, a toddler who is both exploring his/her environment and is keyed to the examiner (social referencing), will be rated in the middle, since the child both contributes his/her own impulses to the interaction and lets him-/herself be guided by the other's impulses.

2.2 Open and Unbiased

Corresponding to its position in the circumplex model, this item is characterized by a combination of acting on one's own impulses and a positive affect towards the interlocutor. Here the person shows openness or refers to his/her own desires and feelings in a friendly way. For example, a child who already begins an initial interview by providing very personal information about him-/herself, such as about his/her family, his/her relationships, and his/her fears, indicates a high degree of openness and impartiality. In such a case, an examiner will usually receive less high ratings because of the setting. But such behavior will also be observable to the examiner, if, for instance, he/she openly addresses his/her positive response to the patient or amicably expresses his/her own feelings in brief utterances (an astonished "Yes!" or a regretful "Oh!").

2.3 Happy in Contact

In the other's presence, the person feels well, is visibly relaxed, and enjoys the nearness to the other. For example, should a child suddenly blossom in play with the examiner, this change in behavior must have occured in connection with the examiner. For a high rating, the pleasure must definitely be related to the contact with the other person; the pleasure itself cannot be simply coded if the child enjoys something else.

2.4 Trusting and Well-Adapted

Corresponding to its position in the circumplex model, this item is characterized by a combination of "complying with external impulses to act" and a "positive affect towards the interlocutor". At issue is trustful reliance on the other person, imitation or willing obedience, or joyful adoption of the other's initiative. In an initial interview, this would consist in a friendly "going along" on the part of the child, who, for example, agrees without hesitation with the examiner and the latter's desires and adapts to the situation.

2.5 Submissive

By this we mean adaptive, obedient, and submissive behavior towards the interlocutor. A concurrent positive or negative affect towards the interlocutor plays no role in the assessment of this item. In an initial dialog, we have in mind, for example, the pronounced adaptation and subordination to the examiner's undertaking and desires.

2.6 Dissatisfied, Compliant

Corresponding to its position in the circumplex model, this item is characterized by a combination of "compliance with external impulses to act" and a "negative affect towards the interlocutor". Adaptation and subordination are combined with a negative affect, as in the case of a depressive girl who answers only in monosyllables, but whose facial expressions when she discontentedly makes a face also indicate a certain degree of dissatisfaction. Compliance combined with resentment or testiness is an instance of being dissatisfied-compliant.

2.7 Angry, Anxious in Contact

This comprises all existing negative affects towards the interlocutor, such as anger, annoyance, anxiety, and distrust. If a person is sceptical about the other's statements, and appears tense and distrustful, the rating depends on the degree of such behavior. Aversion by the child can be a sign of anger. If, on the other hand, the child becomes angry and, for example, it becomes evident that he/she is angry not with the examiner but, say, his/her father, about whom he/she happens to be speaking, then anger in contact is not indicated.

2.8 Sullen and Withdrawn

Corresponding to its position in the circumplex model, this item is characterized by a combination of "acting on one's own impulses" and a "negative affect towards the interlocutor." The item comprises inaccessible and stand-offish behavior accompanied by anxiety, defiance, anger, or existing unhappiness; nonresponsiveness to the other's offers of a relationship, accompanied by negative affects also belongs here.

Anchor-Point Descriptions for Age Group 1 (3 to 5 Years) With a High Rating (4)	
Object-Directed Circle	
1.1 Noninterfering	During the entire observation period, a toddler lets his/her father build a castle from pieces of wood without wanting to take part or contributing own ideas.
1.2 Interested	A three-year child likes having his/her mother read a book aloud, constantly asks questions and continues listening to his mother despite his sibling's interesting offers of play.
1.3 Affectionate	During the observation sequence, a three-year-old child often displays how much he/she likes his/her mother, lovingly stroking her hair and enthusiastically showing her his/her discoveries.
1.4 Friendly directive	A preschool child constantly tries to carry out ideas in free play with the examiner in a friendly way and with clear instructions, e.g., "Okay, now – you play the cow that would be great!"
1.5 Dictating, controlling	A preschool child plays with the examiner and leaves her no openings to contribute her own ideas; the examiner must precisely implement the child's plans or otherwise be corrected immediately.
1.6 Reproachfully deprecating	A pre-schooler prevails over his mother and demands in a loud tone of voice that she build him a tower, which he then inevitably topples. The child threatens to bite her real hard if she doesn't do it. If the mother is too slow in putting together the building blocks, the child yells "Faster!"
1.7 Aggressive, hostile	A pre-schooler repeatedly hits his mother, giving her looks of hatred, and resists all her attempts to calm him down.
1.8 Disinterested	A pre-schooler consistently ignores the examiner's attempts to enter into contact with him, and looks away when the examiner offers him play materials.
Subject-Directed Circle	
2.1 Acting on one's own impulses	During initial examination, a four-year-old child constantly plays with the heater and cannot be dissuaded from his actions.
2.2 Open and unbiased	A four-year-old child tries to charm his mother into playing a sign game.
2.3 Happy in contact	A five-year-old child is full of joy when sitting on his mother's lap.

2.4 Trusting and well-adapted	A four-year-old child shows great motivation in following his father's playing instructions.
2.5 Submissive	A three-year-old child, visibly tired, follows his two siblings' ideas for play during the entire observation period.
2.6 Dissatisfied, compliant	A kindergarten child often complains and whines about a memory game played with his father, but nevertheless complies with his father's directions and continues playing when the latter insists on another round.
2.7 Angry, anxious in contact	A kindergarten child responds to initial questions by the examiner with great anxiety and tension, getting up and crawling under the table. Nor do the examiner's subsequent attempts at contact succeed in defusing the situation.
2.8 Sullen and withdrawn	Just as the mother begins to change the tower of building bricks that she and her toddler are building, the child runs away annoyed. The child begins to play with the dolls, continues to appear to be annoyed, and is unable to accept the offers of contact from the mother.

Anchor-Point Descriptions for Age Group 2 (6 to 12 Years) With a High Rating (4)	
Object-Directed Circle	
1.1 Noninterfering	During the entire initial interview, a schoolchild puts up with the many unpleasant things reported about him by his mother, and during subsequent questioning by the examiner does not resist providing information about himself. In such a case, a high rating (4) would be assigned in the dyad with the mother and in that with the examiner.
1.2 Interested	During an initial interview, a schoolchild consistently and visibly exerts himself to answer complex and not easily understandable questions.
1.3 Affectionate	In family situations a schoolchild is very affectionate with his younger brother, taking him on his lap, caressing and cuddling him, and initiating play with the toy telephone, to the toddler's delight.
1.4 Friendly directive	A schoolchild spontaneously and very precisely explains to the examiner his difficult family situation, and on sensing that the examiner does not follow despite her attempts to understand, again patiently explains what he's been trying to say.

1.5 Dictating, controlling	A schoolchild immediately interrupts the examiner during questioning and persistently insists that he won't be answering any questions and that the examiner should just let him play with the Gameboy.
1.6 Reproachfully deprecating	A schoolchild is continually irritated by the examiner and complains to him/her about the stupid questions being asked – it's all rubbish.
1.7 Aggressive, hostile	A schoolchild repeatedly throws the drawing materials from the table and repeatedly and violently kicks the shins of the examiner also sitting at the table.
1.8 Disinterested	A schoolchild makes no eye contact with the examiner and looks away during questioning.
Subject-Directed Circle	
2.1 Acting on one's own impulses	A child who is very restless during the initial examination, refuses to sit down at the table, and constantly takes toys from the toy cabinet, although the examiner offers other games to play.
2.2 Open and unbiased	During the initial interview, a child often speaks spontaneously of his experiences and asks the examiner to address these matters with the child's parents.
2.3 Happy in contact	A child radiates with his entire face while building castles together with the attachment figure.
2.4 Trusting and well-adapted	A schoolchild readily provides information, even if asked difficult questions by the examiner.
2.5 Submissive	In an initial interview, a schoolchild immediately accepts the examiner's suggestions without further reflection. The child immediately answers all questions without spontaneously reporting anything about himself or expressing wishes of his own.
2.6 Dissatisfied-compliant	A schoolchild's facial expressions clearly indicate protest and annoyance when asked questions by the examiner, but the child then backs down and answers the questions anyway.
2.7 Angry, anxious in contact	A schoolchild quickly reacts to the examiner and his/her questions with irritation, stands up several times in anger and says he's had it.
2.8 Sullen and withdrawn	A schoolchild is grumpily withdrawn in the initial interview and refuses to answer any questions.

Anchor-Point Descriptions for Age Group 3 (13 to 18 years) With a High Rating (4)	
Object-Directed Circle	
1.1 Noninterfering	During an initial interview, an adolescent openly answers all the examiner's questions, and his answers refer precisely to the questions asked, without proposing any other issues.
1.2 Interested	An adolescent sympathetically answers all the examiner's questions, so that the latter can address very personal matters and need not be shy about asking the adolescent for details.
1.3 Affectionate	An adolescent cooperates very well with the examiner, drops his otherwise characteristically brusque manner, and expresses his gratitude that his problems are getting so much attention.
1.4 Friendly directive	In the course of the dialog, through much dedication and humour, an adolescent brings his therapist to accept or share his suggestions and views despite the examiner's initial scepticism.
1.5 Dictating, controlling	An adolescent responds to all questions from the examiner by stating that they concern his private affairs, are none of the examiner's business, and, therefore, that he does not want to say anything, without justifying this attitude. He repeatedly asks how long he still has to sit here.
1.6 Reproachfully deprecating	An adolescent is constantly making derogatory statements about the examiner's clothing, appearance, and profession, and tells the examiner several times that he finds the questions all ridiculous. The adolescent comments in a derogatory manner on all the points of view and positions expressed by the examiner: "Only a shrink could say such things," "Typical – that was to be expected."
1.7 Aggressive, hostile	An adolescent massively abuses the examiner with foul language and threatens to have his friends "take care of her."
1.8 Disinterested	An adolescent acts totally bored during the interview, repeatedly looks at his watch or mostly turns away and looks out the window.
Subject-Directed Circle	
2.1 Acting on one's own impulses	During an initial interview an adolescent spontaneously relates his experiences of the past week in detail and does not respond to questions.

2.2 Open and unbiased	In an initial interview an adolescent is not afraid to talk about his personal feelings and experiences; among other things he speaks spontaneously about his sexual experiences and his anxieties about them.
2.3 Happy in contact	An adolescent in-patient greatly enjoys the affection shown by his parents in a family conference, and is very pleased about their questions about his care as an in-patient.
2.4 Trusting and well-adapted	An adolescent in-patient noticeably shows a high level of co-operation when the ward physician suggests a certain course of medication. The adolescent asks few questions and is of the opinion that he's so far had good experiences with the clinic and trusts in the physician's suggestions.
2.5 Submissive	An adolescent always gives comprehensive answers to detailed questions for the purpose of a forensic report.
2.6 Dissatisfied, compliant	An adolescent mostly rolls his/her eyes when asked questions by the examiner, or asks whether this is all really necessary, but then irritably answers the questions anyway.
2.7 Angry, anxious in contact	An adolescent reacts with loud cries to his father's announcement in a family conference that he will forbid his son having any contact with the son's delinquent friends in the future – the son says he won't stand for it. At the same time, the adolescent pounds on the table with his fists.
2.8 Sullen and withdrawn	An adolescent responds annoyed to the examiner's questions and offers no information about him-/herself.

Anchor-Point Descriptions for Adults With a High Rating (4)	
Object-Directed Circle	
1.1 Noninterfering	A mother imposes no limits on an unruly child and allows the child to mess up his entire playroom. In a discussion with the physician treating their son, the parents of an adolescent take no initiative in influencing the dialog and express no wishes or ideas of their own on how to deal with the situation. They leave the matter of how to proceed further entirely up to the examiner.
1.2 Interested	An examiner is very responsive to the child, even if the latter is pursuing other interests than the examiner's, and encourages the child to continue with his spontaneous drawing.

1.3 Affectionate	A mother notices the tired state and exhausted whining of her two-and-a-half-year-old son, takes him into her arms, manages to calm him down, and then looks at a picture book with him until he falls asleep. In an initial interview, the parents consistently show friendliness and concern towards their adolescent daughter, although she tries to provoke and annoy them.
1.4 Friendly directive	An examiner directs the child firmly and yet amicably towards the issues the examiner considers important. Even when the child wants to do something else, the examiner sticks to his plan and manages to motivate the child to cooperate further.
1.5 Dictating, controlling	In a familial situation, a mother imposes her ideas and plans on the adolescent, and determines the subsequent dialog as the most self-evident thing in the world.
1.6 Reproachfully deprecating	A father prohibits the child in an irritated tone from continuing to play with the ball, and says to the child repeatedly: "You know you're no good at playing ball."
1.7 Aggressive, hostile	During the entire initial interview, a mother interrupts in a loud and excited tone the child's remarks and severely criticises his desires to have contact with his estranged father.
1.8 Disinterested	A mother avoids contact with the child and does not try to get through to him. She does not respond to the child's remarks directed at her and is obviously elsewhere with her thoughts. Nor does she take any notice of the child's later offers to play. In an initial interview with the adolescent and his father, the father takes no notice of his son, ignores the son's remarks, and talks constantly about his own occupational concerns.
Subject-Directed Circle	
2.1 Acting on one's own impulses	An examiner remains rigid in her scheme of questioning, even after the child repeatedly wants to bring up other important issues or desires a different sequence.
2.2 Open and unbiased	A mother talks openly with her two adolescents about her physical illness and her corresponding sensations, which visibly makes her feel relieved.
2.3 Happy in contact	In contact with the child, the examiner is completely relaxed, is delighted over the child's drawings and very pleased when the child wants to give her one of the drawings.

2.4 Trusting and well-adapted	Without concern and in a good mood, the examiner leaves the arrangement of the play situation up to the child and does not pursue her own goals and objectives.
2.5 Submissive	An examiner complies with the child's wishes or initiatives without restrictions, does not reveal any intentions of her own, asks no questions, and takes no initiatives of her own for exploration.
2.6 Dissatisfied, compliant	During the entire time, a father very reluctantly joins his child in the card game the child brought along to the session, and continually displays his annoyance through his facial expressions.
2.7 Angry, anxious in contact	A father becomes very angry at his son's criticism of the father's manner of child-raising and displays extreme agitation through his loud tone of voice. Nor does the father calm down during the subsequent dialog.
2.8 Sullen and withdrawn	A mother reacts gruffly to the play wishes of her child and doesn't respond to the spontaneous comments of the child. She is completely occupied with going through the rules of a game that she has chosen herself.

7.4 Assessment Level B: The Examiner's Internal Response

The interaction with the patient, the shared dialog, the content of play, and the typical scenes trigger the examiner's own emotional reactions. Given self-awareness and supervised reflection, these reactions provide valuable information for diagnoses and treatment planning. From a psychodynamic perspective, the examiner's controlled and reflected reactions may be regarded as a central source of information, especially about relationship-related issues.

The assessment incorporates not only countertransference in the classical sense (Heimann, 1950; Racker, 1959), but also the examiner's directly perceivable emotions and irritations as well as indifferent affective states. According to the circumplex model, impulses may be considered which are agreeable and positively inclined as well as aggressive or fluctuating, depending on their severity.

For better differentiation of the interactions in a multi-person system, the examiner's internal responses can be represented on several levels:

on the one hand, in reference to the child or adolescent, on the other hand in reference to the parents or caregiver, respectively, but also in reference to the relationship between these persons and to the mother–child or father–child dyad.

Comments on and Examples of the Individual Items

The descriptions for each item have been formulated so that the behavior and experience in each case occurs very often or is very pronounced and is to be assigned a "4." Lower frequencies or weaker forms per observation period are accordingly to be rated lower (0 = *absent*, 1 = *rarely/ somewhat present*, 2 = *moderately present*, 3 = *often/strongly present*).

Anchor-Point Descriptions of the Examiner's Internal Response	
Object-Directed Circle	
1.1 Noninterfering	The examiner notices that no structuring impulses generated by the patient or other persons emerge within her and she thinks it best not to interfere with the child's play or the patient's narratives.
1.2 Friendly, interested	During the interaction, the examiner develops a very strong desire to understand her interlocutor; there develops in her a benevolent interest and she wishes to register the described issues in all their relevant nuances.
1.3 Feeling affection	On receiving information or when thinking about the patient and/or his family, the examiner becomes very touched in a positive way, and she feels a great deal of sympathy towards the patient. During the hour, clearly positive affective states predominate, as does an openness to what the patient has to say and sympathy for the patient.
1.4 Friendly directive	The examiner has a strong sense of having to help. She notices how quickly she offers well-meaning explanations and tips, quickly expresses friendly suggestions and encourages the patient to respond to the therapist's ideas. The examiner develops a sense of having to make suggestions, of the necessity for activation. This can occur verbally or during play.
1.5 Dictating, controlling	The examiner feels increasing pressured to intervene in a structuring way, frequently and promptly. The examiner also notices how she does not give the patient space, quickly interrupts him, and directs the dialog in a very definite manner.

1.6 Reproachfully deprecating	It is very difficult for the examiner to leave the patient's verbal and nonverbal communications uncommented. There develops in the examiner a very strong annoyance with the patient, along with a possibly increasing and pressing desire for action-guiding intervention. There develop pronounced, disgruntled feelings about the patient's abilities, motivation, and attitude.
1.7 Aggressive	A possibly irritated and at least latently aggressive underlying attitude leads to sharp, pointed, and, in particular cases, even ironically denigrating or reprimanding interventions by the examiner or to her internally distancing herself from the patient's problems.
1.8 Disinterested, averted	During contact with the patient, the therapist notices distinct fatigue on her part and a growing disinterest (not stress) caused by the patient's remarks. Nor can dramatic subjects activate the examiner, and she develops a relative indifference towards the patient's suffering. The examiner becomes tired, with her thoughts possibly wandering off to other subjects.
Subject-Directed Circle	
2.1 Independent	An inner freedom in forming hypotheses, admitting positive as well as negative impulses, feelings and thoughts, plus an openness towards the results of her own endeavours govern the examiner's self-experience. The examiner experiences herself as a free, autonomous, and creative co-organizer of the interaction, with no fear of resistance.
2.2 Open and unbiased	Spontaneous, open, and unbiased utterances and feelings are easily possible and shape the interaction depending on their prevalence. The examiner's own ideas can largely be brought into the interactions without internal censorship and control.
2.3 Feeling appreciated and comfortable	The examiner notes how much she feels appreciated in talking with the patient and how well she feels in the relationship with the patient, how pleased she is with the course of the hour, how much she enjoys the situation, and how difficult it is for her to terminate the dialog.
2.4 Trustingly accompanying	The examiner has the distinct feeling of being able to enter, with full trust, in the play initiated by the child, or notices in the dialog with an adolescent how she attentively listens to his narratives in a positive mood. The examiner is confident of a positive development in this case.

2.5 Compliant	The examiner experiences how she quickly responds to the patient's needs, desires, and ideas and how she loses sight of her own points of view. She notices how she totally abandons structuring the dialog and no longer makes use of clarifications, confrontations, and expressions of her own ideas.
2.6 Dissatisfied, feeling under pressure	The examiner has the feeling that she constantly has to justify herself and quickly gives in, perceiving her own negative emotions, such as self-doubt, doubt about the patient, and rejection of her own procedure. She is dissatisfied with herself, the course of the hour, and the patient.
2.7 Feeling ignored and sensing own antipathy	Aggressiveness, destructive ideas, and deprecation of the patient and his problems create a mood and attitude on the part of the examiner characterised by anger and sullenness. Aversive impulses to the extent of feeling disgust, desiring that the patient break off contact, or, at least, that the session end prematurely, govern the examiner's interaction and self-experience.
2.8 Sullen and withdrawn	Although the examiner is actively listening or participating in play, she experiences a strong sense of indifference or lack of desire. The problems appear minor or irrelevant or too alien to be important in the shared relationship. In extreme cases, the examiner pursues her own ideas and thoughts, is emotionally detached from the patient, listless and irritable, or wants to have nothing at all to do with this patient.

7.5 Assessment Level C: Self-Referential Circle

The central focus of the self-referential circle is the intrapsychic situation and not – as in the object-directed or subject-directed circle – interaction. This self-referential focus of observation considers how the person makes him-/herself the subject of a qualifying statement, i.e., as to how he/she deals with him-/herself. It is to be judged from the position of an outsider, so to speak, how someone deals with him-/herself – with praise or punishment, for example. The formulated items pertain to children and adolescents.

The remarks made in the Section 7.3, Assessment Level A: Dyads apply here too: The description of an item corresponds to a gestalt-like unit; the orientation refers to the average expected behavior of persons of this age in view of the contextual variables.

Given the intrapsychic focus, it is especially important to keep in mind that the assessment is geared to observable conditions or modes of behavior (behavior, language, facial expressions, etc.). The observed behavior is to be coded as such and not, say, hypotheses regarding the intrapsychic phenomena underlying behavior, such as (blocked) drive impulses.

Comments on and Examples of the Individual Items

The descriptions for each item have been formulated so that the behavior and experience in each case occurs very often or is very pronounced and is to be assigned a "4." Lower frequencies or lower intensities per observation period accordingly receive lower ratings (0 = *absent*, 1 = *rarely/somewhat present*, 2 = *moderately present*, 3 = *often/strongly present*).

Anchor-Point Descriptions	
Self-Referential Circle	
1. Free and carefree	The child is easy-going and his behavior is spontaneous. The child makes use of certain opportunities and disregards others. It may also be the case that the child does not avail himself of certain opportunities or situations or does not take into account consequences. A child will receive a high rating who (in the initial interview) talks openly about himself and his problems, but without being greatly concerned about himself and his problems (does not care about the issues).
2. Content with one-self	The observation of nonverbal signals is important here. The child seems in harmony with himself and balanced. Many positive expressions of feelings occur. This item is assigned a high rating if the child displays great pleasure in succeeding at something and is not worried about failure.
3. Finding pleasure	The child enjoys the situation and has fun. The child looks for what pleases him or is good for him. A child would receive a high rating here who joyfully immerses himself in play, as would also a child who clearly shows pleasure or enthusiasm in contact with another person. The interaction itself is considered elsewhere (see Assessment Level A).

4. Caring for oneself	The aspect of concern with and caring for one's own well-being is primary here. Indications of a certain degree of effort are particularly to be found in nonverbal responses. This item is rated high if the child very often does or has to do something in order to feel comfortable.
5. Controlling oneself	This item is rated high if the child very heavily controls himself in the situation. The child strictly attends to complying with norms and rules, and tries to do the right thing. A low rating will occur if the child makes little effort to limit and regulate his impulses, emotions, and actions.
6. Self-reproaching	This item is rated high if the child generally thinks of his own utterances and own modes of behavior in a self-critical and negative way. This characteristic is revealed in nonverbal expressions, particularly facial expressions. The child directs his anger against himself. Besides reproaches, self-doubt and self-deprecations also occur.
7. Self-tormenting	This item is rated high if the child directs aggression against himself. The child disregards his basic needs and overstrains and exhausts himself. Verbally clear self-deprecations and massive self-reproaches or self-blaming occur, along with nonverbal auto-aggressive behavior. If the child is always quick to feel that he is a victim, a high coding will also result.
8. Self-neglecting	This item is rated high if the child is not concerned with how he feels and how he is doing. The child endangers himself through carelessness and lack of caution. He disregards his appearance to the outside world and the perceptions of others. Aspects of clothing and personal hygiene among older children or adolescents may be indicative.

7.6 Specific Information for the Diagnostic Assessment

The interpersonal relations axis of the OPD-CA-2 can be applied both in clinical practice and in scientific research projects. As children and adolescents in practice are hardly ever examined alone and in separation from their familial and other relationship environments, a large number of relationship constellations can be assessed. As four scales are applied to each dyadic relationship (an object-oriented and a subject-directed circle for each of the relationship partners), and as the examiner's internal responses and the self-reflective circles can all be assessed, the number of scales seems unmanageable.

For clinical practice, these scales should be modularly applied; that is, the examiner should assess that part of the relationship structure that is applicable in accordance with the examination constellation. A minimum standard for clinical diagnostic assessment is the examination of the child and his/her two parents. Added would be the examiner's internal response to the child, the father, the mother, and the family as a whole, as well as the self-reflective circles for the child, father, and mother. This basic clinical module could then be amended depending on any roles played by siblings or other important relationship persons such as grandparents, etc. The clinician thus selects the relationship axes that he/she turned to in his/her examination.

The situation is different with applications in scientific research projects. Here the choice and design of the modules would have to be tailored to the project as well as standardized. Each examined person and each examined family would then have to be assessed according to a standardized set of scales. Only then could one arrive at comparable results suitable for statistical evaluation. Another special feature arises in connection with research: If examinations are recorded on video, persons other than the examiner may view the video and make assessments (raters). Such outside observers will then have additional options: They can assess the examiner's internal responses by identifying with the examiner. In this case, they estimate how they would feel in place of the examiner. But they could also assess the examiner's relationship with the various persons, such as the child and parents, "objectively," i.e., from the outside. In the clinical setting, this type of observational assessment could also be assigned to the supervisor.

8. Second Axis: Conflict

As described in Section 5.2 on the *Theoretical Concept of the Axes – Conflict*, the conflicts in question are lasting psychodynamic conflicts that repeatedly lead to similar behavioral patterns without awareness on the person's part. These conflicts are dysfunctional, i.e., they hinder the child or adolescent's development. They contain conflicting perspectives and actions whose integration is not successful and which tie up the child's or adolescent's defensive activities. Accordingly, we distinguish between a passive and an active mode. The active mode is present when counterphobic defence and reaction formation prevail. In the passive mode, regressive defensive attitudes dominate. While prototypes correspond to the identification of an active or passive mode, in clinical reality mixed types often occur.

As already described, certain structural conditions are required for the formation of conflicts. No conflict theme can develop in a fragmented, disintegrated mental structure. A conflict theme will develop very differently depending on the age group, so that the manualization is operationalized depending on the three age groups. We must assume that lasting intrapsychic conflicts will develop when the needs of a child's significant attachment figures are perceived and satisfied inappropriately, inadequately, or excessively. We assume that lasting internal conflicts are diagnosable at Age group 1; forerunners of conflicts may already be present earlier.

For the diagnostics of the OPD-CA-2, the following issues pertaining to intrapsychic conflicts are relevant:

- Closeness vs. distance
- Submission vs. control
- Taking care of oneself vs. being cared for
- Self-worth conflict

- Guilt conflict
- Oedipal conflict
- Identity conflict

The following describes the operationalization of each conflict theme, differentiated according to the three age groups. In each case, we compare the active and the passive modes with one another for better clarity. As it is crucial whether the conflict pervades in various areas of life or pertains only to a few such areas, we formulate anchor-point descriptions according to the following areas of life: family, peers, kindergarten, school, and body and illness. Should some areas be free of conflicts, this should be viewed as a resource and be utilized in the therapy. In addition, we illustrate each of the various intrapsychic conflicts with a case vignette, with one of the two processing modes. The Assessment Sheet for Conflict can be found in Appendix B.6.

8.1 Closeness Versus Distance

Attachment and relationships are of fundamental importance for the development of children and adolescents. The opposing strivings – on the one hand, for emotional closeness and a symbiotic relationship, and, on the other hand, for the development of emotional independence and distance – are reconciled in the course of a healthy development, allowing the establishment of flexible, mutual, and lasting relationships.

In a closeness–distance conflict, this integration of the opposing positions has not succeeded. Attachments are not secure. Instead, there is an existential fear of a closeness that would entirely monopolize the self, or of emotional distance/separation/being alone; this fear governs the experiences and behavior of these children and adolescents. For example, children and adolescents on the "borderline level" (see structure axis: low integration), cannot endure being either "too close" or "too far."

A closeness–distance conflict as a life-determining issue should only be diagnosed in cases where it towers over all other conflicts and where its identification is evident. This conflict does not exist if the children and adolescents are amenable to relationships with varying closeness and distance. An essential feature of this conflict is the development

Conflict

of a relationship pattern governed by fear that is triggered by closeness or distance. In connection with precursors for this conflict, the parents and social conditions should be considered as having a role in causing disruptions in the striving for closeness and distance during the earlier stages of development.

Clinical Anchor-Point Descriptions	
Passive Mode	**Active Mode**
The passive mode is characterized by a fear of isolation and loneliness. In children and adolescents this fear motivates a search for close long-term relationships, so that their own (distance) desires are perceived only insufficiently. Setting one's boundaries, having an opinion of one's own, and a clearly outlined appearance are difficult for these children and adolescents because they are afraid of losing the object. During the examination, these children and adolescents thus often convey a very undifferentiated image and seem immature for their age. At the centre of self-perception lie helplessness, the feeling of not being able to be alone, and later the longing for an exclusive, close friendship in order to ward off anxiety. Countertransference is characterized by concern and compassion, given the dependency of these children and adolescents. The prominent affect is anxiety triggered by separation and distance.	The active mode is characterized by a fear of intimacy and of being smothered. The result is a constant quest for distance and the emergence of an exaggerated emotional independence. The child's or adolescent's own needs for support and tenderness are suppressed. In their self-perception, these children and adolescents describe themselves as independent of others and as active. Their slogan could be: "I need no one – it's best if I rely only on myself". Rarely do they feel the desire for more closeness. For the younger children, contact with peers presents less of a threat from emotional intimacy and may, therefore, also seem largely unproblematic. In the examination, these children present themselves as pseudoindependent and aloof. Countertransference is characterized by concern, perplexity, and helplessness, an attitude preserving their aloofness and apparent emotional independence. The prominent affect is anxiety triggered by closeness.

Age Group 1 (3 to 5 Years)

Strong reactions are displayed in separation and in the presence of strangers, and can take the form of clinginess, protests against or anxiety over separations, or withdrawal and pseudoindependence, amongst others. Important is the parental attitude toward the regulation of closeness vs. distance of the child (e.g., overprotective and anxious or disinterested, neglectful).

Areas of Life

Family

Within the *family*, these children are often well behaved and sociable. The developmental steps usually observed in this age group, such as the increasing ability to cope with separation from the parents, the exploration of the world, and the integration of third parties, are conspicuously delayed. New demands (staying alone at home, beginning kindergarten) cause separation anxiety and a predisposition to somatization.

In the *family*, these children stand out at an early stage because of their independence and an attitude preserving their emotional aloofness ("I don't know what's going on in my child's head"). They are withdrawn and may fend off physical intimacy.

Peers

In contact with their *peers*, these children stand out with their reticence and clingy behavior. They give the impression of a lack of independence and, as a rule, usually get others to help them. This may be accompanied by a pronounced orientation towards adult attachment figures.

Contact with *peers* is hardly sought, but it is less threatening than relationships with adults. The children have difficulty in dealing with other children; the fear of closeness and dependency can affect the playful, free integration in children's groups.

Kindergarten

In *kindergarten*, these children often appear heavily burdened by the separation from their parents and become overwhelmed when it comes to acting independently. They are overly adjusted and fit slowly into the group. Adult attachment figures are the targets of their pronounced desires for closeness and attachment.

In *kindergarten,* children exhibit remarkably little stress from separation from their parents. In contrast to the family, here children have the possibility of admitting needs for closeness more casually, as these relationships are less exclusive. Generally, these children will fall back on playing with things that they alone can use.

Body/Illness

Illness not related to a separation from attachment figures is often accompanied by severe regression and includes a high secondary gain from illness. *Physical* symptoms may be discovered in order to compel closeness from attachment figures. Longer illness-related separations from attachment figures present an especially severe burden.

Owing to the usually increased attention from attachment figures, *illness* and related *bodily* suffering can bring about the child's loss of a sense of his/her own independence and can be accompanied by increased withdrawal and "suffering in silence." Depending on the severity of the conflict, trivialization or denial of the associated limitations may be observed.

Conflict

Age Group 2 (6 to 12 Years)

Centred on emotional closeness vs. distance, the conflict can be well described in terms of how relationships are conducted. In school, as a newly developing locus of achievement, children in active mode find the opportunity to compensate for past relationships that were formed only reticently and superficially, and to prove their independence. In the passive mode, entering school and assuming new (personal) responsibilities tends rather to intensify conflicts.

Areas of Life	
Family	
These children often need parental support inappropriate for their age and organize their days around participation in family activities or spending time together with the significant attachment figure (for example: going shopping with their mothers, despite offers of play from peers, which are looked down upon as "too boring"). Owing to the decreasing contact with peers, the children's claim on parents to meet their needs for closeness grows.	Often these children are distinguished in their *family* lives by emotional and social withdrawal and by their apparent emotional indifference. Attachment figures feel they do not know what is going on with their children, and find that their children are not taking part in family activities.
Peers	
These children seem cautious and insecure in their search for a relationship with their *peers*. Age-inappropriate and intensive desires for attachment in the search for securely experienced relationships with peers and adults are apparent. The majority of these children adapt themselves so as not to jeopardize the fulfilment of their desires for closeness and so as to avoid being alone.	These children show little interest in spending time with *peers*, and tend to be loners. For example, they may prefer individual sports to team sports. Attempts to promote the children's social contact by having them join clubs, for example, often fail. Generally such children can play well by themselves.
School	
These children are often described as well-behaved, overly adjusted *pupils,* and are often praised for their (supposedly) distinctly good social behavior in group work and with set tasks. Younger children show a strong rapport with the	Depending on their aptitude structure, these children will discover *school* as an achievement area for themselves, and are motivated and ambitious. This sector compensates for the merely superficial relationships with classmates and

homeroom teacher. A refusal to go to school may occur due to separation anxiety from the parents.

deficient participation in group activities. Difficulties may arise from demands for cooperation and teamwork.

Body/Illness

Illnesses afford the opportunity for regression and acting out intensified desires for intimacy. Physical suffering may be discovered as a way to compel closeness from attachment figures. An anxiously attentive perception of the *body* and its functions may develop (somatization tendencies).

Illness means too much intimacy from others and therefore a restriction of emotional independence. These children try to deny or hide their need for help from themselves and from others. Restrictions from physical suffering are ignored, as they threaten to intensify dependency and intimacy. They become rather negligent in handling their own physical needs.

Age Group 3 (13 to 18 Years)

The increasing ability for self-reflection leads to dealing intensively with the issue of closeness vs. distance in regard to other people. To meet their needs for sexuality and intimacy, so urgent during puberty, adolescents find themselves compelled to enter into relationships with others. Experiences of separation in relationships with friends and romantic partners often trigger acute symptoms. However, it must also be kept in mind that separation from the parents will intensify the conflict.

Areas of Life

Family

Within the *family* the adolescents behave quite childishly and accept no offers to explore the world on their own. They remain a mummy's boy or girl ("stay-at-homes") and the existence of conflicts has to be denied so as not to jeopardize relationship intimacy. In extreme cases, these adolescents will feel sad about growing older (no longer being a child and dependent) and try to preserve the family relationship through manipulation (e.g., illness or self-endangerment).

These adolescents seek a quick solution for the desired distance from the *family*, which can lead to acting dangerously ("taking flight"). The forced effort to develop an exaggerated emotional and existential independence is striking and often causes the parents to feel concerned.

Peers

The initiation of new friendships may be postponed, as they would mean distancing oneself from the parents. During further development, these adolescents associate with an exclusive, close *friendship partnership* the fulfilment of their insatiable longing for intimacy and are frightened by their partners or friends striving towards autonomy.

In their relationships with *peers*, they strive for a position of distinct, distance-preserving independence. Under the impact of puberty-related changes, these adolescents tend to seek contact with *peers* and, at the same time, experience intimacy as both dangerous and smothering. They experience friends' and partners' desires for a relationship as threatening.

School/Vocation

These adolescents usually have a subordinated role in the classroom or in a job, without the accompaniment of vocational or scholastic inadequacy. Connectedness is more important to them than individual achievement. As they often do not perceive and assert their own needs, they are notable for their distinctly good social behavior. Change of school or completion of *schooling* and the resulting separation from relationships present a special burden. Decreasing motivation and declining performance may occur, in order to postpone the end of school and therefore separation from the parents.

School or *vocational training* is the site of achievement rather than of social encounters. Cooperation and group work are difficult for these adolescents. They are achievement-oriented and ambitious, or often commit themselves to a particular field. They have problems with teamwork, and the performance level they attain is a way to become independent of others.

Body/Illness

Adolescents can discover their body and sexuality as an opportunity for satisfying the longing for intimacy. In *illnesses* these adolescents see the opportunity for justifiable dependency. Regression and stagnation of the recovery process are the result. The invalid role is, therefore, gladly accepted and can be used to obtain parental care, attention, and intimacy. An anxious fixation on body processes may occur at the same time.

The *body* with its sexual needs can be experienced as threatening, for it questions the notion of emotional independence ("I don't need anyone"). *Illness* and physical needs in general also pose a threat to independence. The adolescent may seek to ward off this threat by showing a lack of insight into the illness and by trivializing the severity of the symptoms. Offers of help from physicians or parents are rejected as interfering. Physical performance, on the other hand, may serve to demonstrate the adolescent's own strength and independence.

Conflict

Closeness Versus Distance – Active Mode

Case Vignette: Janine, Age 16 Years

Janine, 16 years old, comes to the initial session accompanied by her mother. The reason given for this session is that Janine lost ten kilograms last year and now weighs only 42 kg, with a physical height of 1.63 metres. The weight loss began at the time her mother entered a new relationship, which led to their moving. While the mother moved into her new partner's home, Janine has since inhabited a small apartment with a separate entrance in the same building. As a result, the mother and daughter see little of one another, so that the weight loss went unnoticed for a long time. Janine resisted going to the session, even signalling to the therapist that she doesn't understand the fuss about her weight – she feels fine. If absolutely necessary, she'll put on some weight again, but she doesn't need therapy for this.

Janine is attending high school with a fluctuating, but overall satisfactory, performance. She describes herself as a loner, with no close friends among the girls in her class. Still, she says she gets along with everyone quite well. The last class trip was an unpleasant experience, as everyone else got along with one another very well and she felt somehow like an outsider.

According to the daughter, the mother has already had a number of relationships, none of which has worked out. These relationships have even involved moving to a small neighboring town and a change of school. She has usually gotten along with her mother's new partners. The main thing for her has been that they don't "play dad" and leave her alone. The mother separated from Janine's biological father when Janine was three years old. He lives abroad, and Janine can visit him only during holidays. Sometimes she has lived with her mother alone, between relationships as it were, but even in the past her mother was often with her new partner of the time for days on end, and Janine had to take care of herself.

Her desire to lose weight became more urgent after the class trip. During the initial sessions, Janine appears expectant and hesitant. She talks rather unemotionally about her mother's relationship break-ups. While Janine's accounts move the therapist to want to take care of her, he feels kept at a distance by her cool manner.

The mother describes Janine as a child who is easy to care for. The relationship with the father was never good. He often worked abroad and, after Janine's third birthday simply, remained there. The mother admits that so far she has not been lucky with new relationships, so that she has been unable to offer Janine a "ideal family life." She has often asked herself whether this lack may have been stressful for Janine. Sometimes she'd been quite amazed how quickly Janine could adapt to a new living situation and a new relationship. Sometimes she hasn't been able to even guess at what's going through her daughter's mind. The child has never given the impression of suffering from the moves or changes of school, however. On the contrary, the teachers of the new schools have always come up to her and remarked on how independent and mature her daughter was.

8.2 Submission Versus Control

Given the experienced security of relationships and the increasing internalization of behavioral norms, this basic conflict focusses on *obedience and submission vs. control and rebellion.* For this conflict, behavioral norms, i.e., family-related, school-related, and social rules and, therefore, the submission to these rules or rebellion against them are very important. The potential for conflict is more pronounced the more rigid or lax (coddling) the familial and social rules are.

Primarily interpersonal tensions (submission vs. rebellion) develop in the first age group, with an intrapsychic conflict (spontaneity vs. rigidity) emerging only with increasing maturity. Different affects will accordingly be found depending on the stage of development. In interpersonal conflicts and precursors to conflicts anger, rage and fear predominate. With the development of the superego, involving the coding of behavioral norms, and with the ability for internalizing the conflict, children and adolescents develop more mature emotions like anxiety, shame, and guilt. During the preliminary stages of this conflict, special attention must be given to whether the parents' behavior exhibits distinct indulgence or an extremely controlling attitude because of their own internal conflicts.

Clinical Anchor-Point Descriptions	
Passive Mode	Active Mode
These children and adolescents seem overly compliant, withdrawn, and controlled. They are well-behaved and generally follow the adults' demands unquestioningly. Owing to their low profile, they run the risk of becoming "forgotten." Resistance is exhibited at most in forms of behavior like dawdling, forgetfulness, carelessness, etc. Their self-perception is dominated by the feeling of not being able to be effective. During the interview they are compliant, contribute few ideas of their own, and try to please the examiner. The prominent affects are fear and anxiety. Countertransference can give rise to feelings of perplexity, and impotence, as well as a tendency towards activating and controlling the child or adolescent.	Here we find children and adolescents who constantly protest and rebel against restrictions, obligations, and control. They seem impatiently demanding. Other people are supposed to submit and bend to their wishes; the insistence on getting their own way can go to the extreme of defiant aggression. During the interview they try to dominate, dictate, and exercise power. Their self-perception is dominated by the idea of constantly having to assert themselves and establish order. The prominent affects are defiance, anger, and resentment. Countertransference can give rise to feelings of anger as well as the desire to placate the child or adolescent.

Conflict

Age Group 1 (3 to 5 Years)

To a certain extent these children can choose to submit or to assert themselves in conflicts. A predominance of the passive mode must be considered as rather disadvantageous for this age.

Indicating an internalized, development-inhibiting conflict in the passive mode is fearful, submissive, and overly adaptive or defiant behavior. In the active mode, frequent and pronounced conflicts come to the fore, as does the attempt to control others and have them at one's disposal.

Areas of Life	
Family	
There exists a *family tradition* of strict, orderly hierarchy and tranquillity. The child is expected to function and – even contrary to his/her own desires – fit into this mould.	In their *family relationships,* these children stand out with their defiantly aggressive individualism and the desire to have everything done as they see fit. These children try to have their parents at their beck and call. The lack of clear-cut roles (between the parents and children) leads to power struggles. Within the families, rigid rules prevail or arbitrariness not constrained by any order.
Peers	
Among their *peers* the children seem docile and submissive, and accordingly show less initiative. Noteworthy is their inability to say "no." They show resistance indirectly through passive behavior like hesitation, dawdling, and obstinacy.	Relationships with *peers* are characterized by the endeavor to dominate, control, and organize shared activities as they desire. They show little flexibility in negotiating compromises.
Kindergarten	
In *kindergarten* and in other social activities they play a subordinate role, and appear passive and compliant. As they passively undermine demands through hesitation, dawdling, and refusals, they intensify the angry responses and controlling behavior of adults.	In *kindergarten* the children play the role of "decision-makers". They have difficulty in tolerating suggestions from other children or in submitting to them. The themes of play also concern power, control, and subjugation. These children comply only with demands compatible with their own ideas.

Body/Illness

Illnesses are docilely accepted, but symptoms and *bodily functions* are closely observed and controlled.	In dealing with their *bodies* and with *illness*, these children engage in fierce struggles against care-related parental demands (brushing teeth, clothing), with considerable opposition to parental instructions.

Age Group 2 (6 to 12 Years)

A requirement related to beginning school, namely a flexible reaction to different systems of values and rules (family, school, kindergarten), intensifies conflicts of the type "control vs. submission". Added are academic performance requirements. Children in passive mode tend to adapt well in school and to submit to its rules. Failure anxieties and/ or dawdling over homework may lead to vehement disputes with the parents. Children in active mode tend to be know-it-all's and involve parents and teachers in power struggles. Achievement can be exploited or even actively refused in the effort to dominate others. The main affects are anger and rage, but also fear of failure and shame.

Areas of Life	
Family	
These children have basically adopted the *family values* of a strict, orderly conservative hierarchy, but exhibit passive resistance in the form of dawdling and forgetfulness.	The internalized values and rules lead within the *family* to constant tension, struggles, and a know-it-all manner, up to the point of creating a distance between the generations.
Peers	
The children submit to their *peers* and enter into close dual relationships, which they shape according to their conflict patterns. Again, they subordinate themselves and exhibit resistance merely in a passive form.	As the conflict is internalized and cognitive maturity increases, the forms of behavior manifest themselves both interpersonally and intrapsychically. There is a constant know-it-all attitude, rules and norms are themselves set but not questioned, and *friends* are sought who will complement this behavior.
School	
In *school,* these children have difficulty in asserting themselves. They go back and forth in trying to make decisions for	Entry into *school* creates difficulties. Suggestions from adults and peers and their authority are accepted only reluctantly

fear of specifying anything and exercising power. Factual requirements are either docilely implemented or compliance is passively refused.

or not at all. Factual performance may be exploited in the endeavor to dominate and control others.

Body/Illness

Illness is endured docilely as a fate to which one must submit. The child feels at the mercy of his/her own *body*; feelings of guilt and shame can arise because of failures of the body.

The *body* can be exploited for performance in sports. Loss of physical strength due to *illness* is not accepted. The child protests against supportive and controlling interventions from parents or physicians, and defiantly rejects these measures.

Age Group 3 (13 to 18 Years)

Pubertal development intensifies intrapsychic conflicts. Adolescents in passive mode pliantly submit to existing rules and feel impotent. Adolescents in active mode intensify their struggles and their rebellion against the prevailing rules in all social areas and exercise power.

Areas of Life	
Family	
Typical adolescent conflicts within the *family* involving the negotiation of new rules do not take place. The families seem calm and orderly, but also boring. The child's own wishes and views are subordinated or suppressed.	Within the *family*, the child intensifies his/her efforts for control and dominance in the course of pubertal development. There is a constant struggle with the parents over rules and order that the child perceives as externally determined. General rules are not accepted, nor does the child question his/her own rules, but takes them for granted.
Peers	
These adolescents enter into firm dyadic relationships with *peers*, in which they adapt and subordinate themselves. Excessive conformity with group norms may occur.	Among their *peers* these adolescents aspire to leadership roles and seek friends whom they will be able to dominate and rule over. Power is important to them, and they take care not to lose control of their feelings. Antisocial, egosyntonically experienced actions may occur.

Conflict

School/Vocation

In *school and vocational training* these adolescents have difficulty in developing their own ideas and perspectives. They adapt to the demands of school and work without criticism, or passively resist through refusal, for example.	*School and work* have a high priority. Their content is exploited in the striving for power and dominance, but is especially conflictual because of the discrepancy between the initially available role (student, trainee) and the aspired role (instructor, boss).

Body/Illness

The *body*, with its developing sexuality, tends to be experienced as frightening; these adolescents experience themselves as impotently at the mercy of their bodies. Sexual relationships are shunned for fear of being overwhelmed or they are adapted to the conventions of the family of origin. *Illness* can provide relief through regressive aspects, but also trigger feelings of shame if the body fails in doing what it is supposed to do.	These adolescents enter into sexual relationships in the pursuit of dominance and power, but they may also become anxious over the loss of control and avoid them. *Illnesses* that jeopardize the adolescent's own claims to power and control over his/her *body*, as well as medical procedures requiring an increased level of compliance, may be denied or refused for fear of regression and the loss of control.

Submission Versus Control – Active Mode

Case Vignette: Mira, Age 6 Years

Six-year-old Mira is presented shortly after starting school because she is "overly attached to her mother." Each evening the mother has to bring Mira to bed and can never be by herself or go out alone with her father. If the mother tries to do so, the daughter screams and cries and/or vomits and wets her pants. According to the mother, Mira engages the parents in extensive discussions about trifles such as clothing or body care, always thinking she knows better than her mother and always wanting to have the last word. In these situations, she becomes very aggressive towards her mother and has great difficulty accepting limits. It is easier for her to get along with her father, but also with him there are altercations, with both "insisting on being right." Mira is one of the best students in the school she has been attending for several weeks now, and she has quickly assumed a leadership role within her class thanks to her creative ideas. However, there are also conflicts with classmates and teachers when it comes to subordination or giving in.

The patient arrives at the first session holding her father's hand. From the preliminary information, the therapist had expected a pale, shy, petulant, or bashful child, and was prepared for a complicated separation situation. Instead, the therapist finds a "blond angel," a very pretty little girl who, although pale and anxious, seems quite interested and expectant. The girl takes leave of her father in the waiting room and unhesitatingly accompanies the therapist into the treatment room. Here she spontaneously turns to the hand puppets, giving particular attention to the policeman and the princess. Asked for the reason of her visit, she first talks about a male classmate who had been her friend in kindergarten, but now only plays with the boys and constantly annoys her. That makes her sad but also angry. She then talks about her fears and about dragons, crocodiles, and snakes that are in her room, so that she has to call for her mother. Only she can calm her down. Her father scolds her, which is why she prefers her mother a bit more. From the family background, we learn that the patient's mother lost her own mother at the age of 12, and that she subsequently grew up together with the father and the "unloved" stepmother. Mira's father has broken off contact with his mentally ill mother, whom he had experienced as unpredictable, arbitrary, and neglectful. Mira is an only child who is very much loved, cared for, and encouraged by her parents. The mother coddles her daughter for fear of losing her affection, while the father is chummier and, in conflictual situations, arbitrary and unpredictable, which makes the patient feel insecure, anxious, and defensive.

The therapist feels called upon to protect and defend the patient against the father. In addition, the therapist is surprised about the patient's openness and wonders why she paints such a negative picture of the father, although she clearly gets along with him well. Are her dreams an expression of an unresolved oedipal conflict? But why the bossiness, tantrums, and panic? The subsequent trial sessions reveal an unconscious inner conflict between the desire to break away from the close relationship with the mother and the fear of losing the mother, and possibly also fear of the mother's revenge. As long as Mira maintains control, the object is safe for her; anything else would mean submission, placing her at the mercy of the object and its arbitrariness. The therapist is fascinated by Mira and begins to acquire her affection, but also feels scepticism and cautiousness in anticipation of a tantrum if she does not do what the patient wants.

8.3 Taking Care of Oneself Versus Being Cared For

Taking care of oneself vs. being cared for refers to the basic need of children and adolescents to obtain something, be assured of affection, or to give something. The objects of care can be material or immaterial – anything serving life-sustaining development. This axis then refers not only to orality (drive theory), but also caring affection (caring actions and tactility) as well as the offer of an interactive exchange.

The process in which children and adolescents take over the role of caring for themselves is a long one. Healthy development includes uniting the desires of being cared for, being able to take care of oneself, and taking care of others.

This conflict presupposes that children and adolescents are basically open to relationships, while the matter of relationships itself is greatly characterized by or restricted to the issue of "taking care of oneself vs. being cared for." The distinction from the conflict of "closeness vs. distance" can be difficult, as both motivational systems exist from the outset of development and overlap with one another. While the conflict of closeness vs. distance concerns existential anxiety and the dependence on the relationship itself, the conflict of *taking care of oneself vs. being cared for* focuses on having and receiving or giving as the themes governing the development of the relationship.

In the conflict of *taking care of oneself vs. being cared for*, self-perception is governed by a sense of inadequacy and of not having received enough care. Coping varies between striving to have others compensate for this inadequacy (passive) and accepting this inadequacy, suppressing one's own needs for care, and acting out caring for others (active). Even if a deep-seated discontent remains perceptible, the self-sufficient pole allows vicarious participation in caring as a giver and the feeling of not being dependent on care from others. In the passive mode, everything that is obtainable is greedily taken. Receiving material things is equated with care. Dissatisfaction with what one gets remains.

Depending on the child's disposition, conflicts can arise if the parents create conflictual relationships (land-of-plenty behavior or neglectful behavior) given their own lasting conflicts about "taking care of oneself vs. being cared for," or conflicts may arise because of extraordinary stress on the parents (illness, intensive problems with the partner, financial insecurity), resulting in inadequate care for the child or adolescent over a longer period of time.

Clinical Anchor-Point Descriptions	
Passive Mode	Active Mode
The experience of the self always contains the desire to be cared for. These children and adolescents hardly endure restrictions on care. They are demanding ("a lot and right away") and appear clingy. A feeling of "it's exhausting being with this child" arises. The adolescent fights his/her struggle by making claims and by refusing to develop so as to take care of him-/herself. Prominent affects are grief and the fear of losing care, not	These children appear modest and self-sufficient. Interactions clearly show the children's willingness not to make any claims on care: "I can take care of myself." They willingly yield, but initially also clearly indicate their desires. While they initially feel this lack in their experience of themselves, later on they industriously and constantly care for others. These adolescents strive unduly to take care of themselves, but may also reveal

getting enough care, or getting the wrong care. The examiner's countertransference or internal response gives rise to irritability and anger due to the insatiable avidity. Experiences of loss often trigger the appearance of symptoms.

extreme dedication and a willingness to make sacrifices for others. They overextend themselves and are prone to depressive slumps if their behavior is not acknowledged or if their own desires for care become too strong. Disappointment results in dominant affects such as dissatisfaction, irritability, and fear of their own greed. Countertransference in the examiner is driven by concern because of the patient's self-sacrificing attitude and because of compassion. The ulterior wish for care may become noticeable, usually accompanied with dissatisfaction over what is actually obtained. Experiences of loss and sustained excessive demands may trigger the symptoms.

Age Group 1 (3 to 5 Years)

Beginning kindergarten, conflicts with children and adults outside the familial caring structure reveal the child's being pulled back and forth between the poles of experience: wanting to be cared for more and suppressing his/her own desires and caring for others.

Areas of Life	
Family	
Demanding behavior and fear of loss of any kind associated with intense desires for care govern *family* relationships. The struggle with siblings over receiving care may lead to feelings of envy, rivalry, and discrimination and weigh heavily on the relationships.	Within the *family*, the children have adapted to the scarcity of care and to the fear of greedy impulses, which they may lose again in their relationships to other adults, however, within which they may appear starved. Older children may defer their own claims to care in favor of their younger siblings.
Peers	
The children show little interest in their *peers*. They are erratic and unreliable playmates, as any reciprocal togetherness will provoke their claims to care. They want special treatment, i.e., to get more than the other children, and take away other children's possessions when the latter are unattended.	In their relationships with *peers*, the efforts of these children in caring for themselves tend to be affirmed and recognized through their attitude of gladly giving. These children have a very ambivalent attitude towards possession. They feel the allure of ownership, but cannot really enjoy it for fear of their own greed.

Kindergarten

In *kindergarten* the children are demanding and challenging. They are nagging children who are not satisfied with what they get ("He's got more!"). As the other children do not meet their needs for care, they turn to adults, who usually also cannot satisfy them.

In *kindergarten* the children stand out by their attitude of "giving gladly." At this age, however, the opposite, namely letting oneself be overly cared for, is still possible. In play they clearly show their desires for care. While self-care is forcibly developed, these children have a propensity for impulsive outbreaks crossing boundaries, if their needs for care become too great.

Body/Illness

These children appear particularly self-pitying and nurture their *illnesses* in order to obtain the increased level of care for as long as possible.

When the children fall ill, they are still able to have themselves regressively cared for in unfamiliar surroundings. In their home environment, however, they show discontent, have an urge for activity, and tend to deny their *illness*.

Age Group 2 (6 to 12 Years)

Beginning school confronts children with the challenge of performing, actively participating, and meeting the age-related expectations of their impulse control and their ability to postpone the satisfaction of needs. Possession plays an increasingly important role, and yet everything that is available is either not enough or wrong. Social relations in school or friendships lead to conflicts that place their demands or defence against these demands at the centre of the particular relationship.

Areas of Life

Family

They enjoy being at home. They often demand and experience undue support from the *family*, which reinforces their dependency and can lead to blackmailing behavior ("little tyrants"). Parents may become annoyed and give up, and try to pacify the child through materialistic forms of care.

The children are firmly anchored in the *family's* framework of care. They often care for their younger siblings, support their parents, and seem self-reliant. They sacrifice themselves for the sake of their families, but sometimes still reveal a vulnerability whose denial can lead to a tense attitude.

Peers

They seek *peers* who do not present any danger of refusal. They appear covetous and try to obtain others' possessions without giving in return. In play, they are not willing to show commitment. Appearing insatiable and exploitative, they tend to turn others away.

With *peers* and friends these children are popular playmates or are perceived as pleasant since they make no claims on care. The children cannot show themselves with their possessions and are extremely modest. They display no envy when others show off their possessions. Nevertheless, greediness is observed with these children.

School

School presents them with the difficulty of giving, namely achieving things, instead of simply receiving the type of care they desire. They appear clingy, complaining ("Help me with my homework!"), and not very active.

They are well prepared for the situation of *scholastic* performance, where they are allowed to give of themselves. Because of their modesty, they are often described as socially oriented and adapted. In performance they show a great willingness to overextend themselves, and they can show themselves presumptuous when others insist on their own needs for care.

Body/Illness

While the *invalid role* is readily accepted, the experienced care only briefly fulfils the longing for unlimited care, and discontent ensues. The child also attends to his/her *bodily* needs as long as they lead to increased "being cared for." Towards themselves, the children are not actively caring, and no nurturing treatment of their own bodies develops.

An *illness* is hard to endure for children in this age group. They show themselves dissatisfied with everything and cannot admit the provision of care. At the same time, they signal neediness and insatiability. *Physical* needs are not perceived, since they usually lead to increased care and re-activate the anxiety over hitherto suppressed desires for care.

Age Group 3 (13 to 18 Years)

Pubertal development intensifies conflicts, which especially leads adolescents with a passive coping mode to avoid separation from the caring objects. Adolescents with an active processing mode become independent with altruistic and ascetic features at an accelerated pace.

Relationships are formed along the lines of "wanting to keep" and/or "having to hand over."

Areas of Life

Family

Within the *family,* the adolescents develop depressive and resigned moods. They suffer in silence as an unnameable inadequacy is constantly present. They can avoid separation from the care-providing objects in the secret hope of still getting something from the parents.

The adolescents are committed to *family* life owing to their attitudes of taking care of themselves and of self-sufficiency. They can take care of their siblings or parents, but do not want themselves to become a burden to anyone. At the same time, they tend to become independent earlier ("Thanks, but I can take care of myself"). In replacement of the family, they then participate in associations caring for others.

Peers

In their relationships with *peers,* they have a limited ability to explore new ways of living and forms of relationships. Others tend to be perceived and experienced as possessions, so that parasitic relationships increasingly govern life. In leisure activities and play they stand out because they always want to get so much from others. In romantic relationships, too, an acquisitive, exploitative form of behavior is noticeable ("I'll get it somewhere else").

In their relationships with *peers,* the adolescents show themselves to be unpretentious and easy to handle. The adolescents consider possessions as something to be despised, a belief they express in ascetically oriented ideologies that conceal the defence against the desires for care and security. Possession of this ideology is a substitute for renunciation. While the adolescents are respected people, they can also be easily exploited because of their total self-sufficiency.

School/Vocation

The relationships and performances in *school,* such as the beginning of *working life,* make neediness so great as to create passively defiant attitudes and a withdrawal to the domestic hearth, as well as the complaint that others are receiving more or are preferred by the boss or teacher. They seek a group that will meet their claims on care.

In *school and at work,* these adolescents behave altruistically towards their schoolmates or adults. They are dedicated when taking part in socially caring activities, and draw visible satisfaction from them. In these commitments, they tend to show a slightly irritable tension that reveals their own demands. They are popular with teachers and trainers, since they usually show themselves willing to do things for others.

Conflict

Body/Illness

Illness usually means the "justified" acting out of all desires for care, however far-ranging, and is associated with a distinct level of regression. They are demanding and discontented patients whose active co-operation in treatment is often wanting. The body is an opportunity to receive greater care and to show others what is needed. They do not provide for themselves. At most, they attempt to compensate for the perceived inadequacy with excessive eating or with addictive substances. Sexuality sometimes provides the opportunity of experiencing care in a compensatory way, which can extend to "sexual hunger." There is a strong desire to retain the partner providing care.

These adolescents cannot accept the invalid role and being cared for. Aid from others is rejected. The latent desires for being cared for often express themselves in discontent with what is actually offered and in complaining. The adolescent's own body is expected to function, and is normally not cared for. In sexuality, the desire for being cared for (hidden and usually associated with little joy) can be acted out.

Conflict: Taking Care of Oneself Versus Being Cared For – Active Mode

Case Vignette: Michelle, Age 14 Years

Fourteen-year-old Michelle comes to the first session accompanied by both parents. She reports hesitantly and often bashfully, whilst looking down at the floor, that she suffers from bulimia. About a year ago she started vomiting after meals. The trigger was a remark her father had made about her figure during a seaside holiday. Prior to this event, she had also been thinking about losing weight, however. Despite a rheumatic illness, she performs competitively in track and field athletics and, having gained some weight, has been achieving fewer good results in competitions. Comparing herself with the other girls in her class, she also feels unattractive. While they are already interested in boys, she wants none of that yet. Keeping her problem a secret from her parents has weighed heavily on her. About three weeks ago she broke down and tearfully confided first in her mother. She now wants to do everything possible to become healthy again.

Her parents proudly report that Michelle has been quite successful in track and field. Because of her rheumatism, this pursuit had been recommended to her at the time by her physiotherapist. She has always been a very well-behaved child.

Because of a birth defect, her four-year-younger brother is physically challenged and has always demanded much attention and support from the parents. Very early on, Michelle began taking care of her own needs, and has always been very independent. At school and at home, there have never been conflicts or disputes, the parents say; on the contrary, Michelle has always conscientiously performed her physiotherapy, done her homework, and also looked after her little brother as best she could.

Michelle herself reports in a later interview that during the past year she somewhat lost the joy in living. Neither her sports activities nor her academic successes could satisfy her any longer. She has felt dissatisfied with everything. At first she tried to compensate for this dissatisfaction through greater dedication, but she no longer finds pleasure in these things. The desire to lose weight then became increasingly stronger; at first she even attained a good weight loss of about four kilograms, but then the cravings for food had come. She kept gulping down larger amounts of food, which she then regurgitated. She's become very ashamed of herself for burdening her parents with worry. Last week the pressure became too great, however, so that she opened up to her mother and now wants actively to work on the problem.

The therapist initially feels a strong sympathy with the young patient, who apparently all her life has set aside her needs and never wanted to be a burden to anyone. In further conversation, the young patient also "provides" the therapist with active cooperation and an openness to talk.

Later on, the patient can admit that she pursued sports and good performance at school primarily in order to please her parents and give them some relief given their trouble with her younger disabled brother.

8.4 Self-Worth Conflict

Regulation of the feeling of self-worth is of fundamental importance for the well-being of children and adolescents and depends on the narcissistic input from others. Insults, failures, the absence of accustomed affection and attention, but also the confrontation with personal limitations (as in the case of a failure or an illness) can call self-worth into question.

Owing to the increased self-perception and the limited ability to invest in a relationship, a long-lasting, conflictual impairment of self-esteem always accompanies a disruption of interpersonal relationships.

During their development, children and adolescents increasingly learn to regulate their positive feeling of self-worth in an enduring way and less dependently on others. At issue here are children and adolescents whose efforts to regulate their feelings of self-worth are excessively strong, in some particular way unsuccessful or clearly conflict-ridden. Their experiences and behavior are governed largely by their own sense of worth and oscillate between the poles of "low vs. exaggerated self-esteem" and "low vs. exaggerated object value" ("I'm nothing – others can do everything"). Experiences of hurt feelings or feeling slighted are often found to be the triggers.

As most children and adolescents coming for treatment often have low self-esteem, a self-worth conflict can be diagnosed only if the deterioration of self-esteem is very pronounced and the polar tension is evident.

Clinical Anchor-Point Descriptions	
Passive Mode	**Active Mode**
These children and adolescents are distinguished by a clear lack or breakdown of self-esteem. This leads to a high level of insecurity and the fear of being slighted again. These children and adolescents evade critical (competitive) situations to avoid feared exposure, but remain in the background, making comparisons. The importance of an evaluation, of "being better or worse than others," always remains a noticeable concern. Self-perception is governed by the feeling of worthlessness and of not receiving any respect. Blame may be secretly placed on others. In countertransference, the examiner feels concern and compassion, as well as the desire to support the patient. The prominent affect is a clearly perceptible sense of shame.	If this mode prevails, reaction formations will dominate as attempts to deal with a feared or real crisis of self-esteem. There results grandiose overconfidence (also in fantasy) that need not conform to social norms (e.g., delinquency). Despite their initial appearance of confidence, these children and adolescents are governed by a latent insecurity as to their own importance and worth. With age, the urge to constantly prove themselves governs their contact with other people. The feeling of being under-appreciated and the belief in their own specialness dominate their self-perception in subsequent stages of development. Countertransference can give rise to feelings of smallness, incompetence, and deprecation in the examiner. The importance of an evaluation, of "being better or worse than others," always remains a noticeable concern: Prominent affects are anger and irritability (narcissistic rage). Their slogan could be: "I am a special child/teenager, have a right to be admired, and the rules do not apply to me." Experiences of hurt or feeling slighted are often found to be the triggers.

Age Group 1 (3 to 5 Years)

Partial independence of self-worth regulation and the growing ability to endure the limits of one's own possibilities as well as criticisms from peers and adults are developed. Difficult are all situations in which the children see the preservation of their grandiose self-images threatened by their confrontation with reality.

Areas of Life

Family

Out of fear of failure, these children avoid tasks or want to accomplish everything in a task right away. They are ashamed of their age-related difficulties in acquiring new skills, and typically place excessive demands on themselves. In extreme cases, they will even refuse to confide their self-doubts to anyone in their *family*, and they feel inferior compared with their siblings.

Within the *family*, these children are very sensitive to criticism, want to attain everything at once and cannot endure frustration. Besides their high demands, these children have a striking tendency to abandon efforts immediately if they do not achieve quick success. As a rule, they demand praise for even routine tasks. Tantrums are frequent.

Peers

These children encounter their *peers* with the feeling of being unable to sustain contact, given the uncertainty about their own value. They do not assert their interests from fear of exposure and of being rejected.

These children often try to dominate contact with their *peers* in play ("The others are there so that I can have fun"), and they cannot come to terms with limits set by their playmates' desires. They are cheeky and know everything better. They show a lack of understanding when things do not go their way, and not infrequently try to get their way by force (hitting, biting, scratching, etc.). Tantrums are frequent.

Kindergarten

The children have difficulty fitting into their *kindergarten group*. They seem insecure and suspicious. Desires for recognition become evident. They compare themselves with the other children, who are admired and envied. They are poor losers in games and avoid such activities ("Don't feel like it").

Striking is their endeavor to become the centre of the *kindergarten group*. Integration is difficult because of the lack of empathy and the unwillingness to fit in and to share. These children may be poor losers and respond to frustration with rage, deprecation, and escape into fantasies of grandeur. They demand a special role and the constant attention of attachment figures. Owing to their self-absorption, they exhibit a strong inhibition about playing and show little creativity during their free time, behavior they rationalize by claims of boredom. They prematurely end games with rules in the face of imminent defeat (knock over playing pieces, turning over the playing cards, etc.).

Body/Illness

These children may experience limitations from *illness* as something "earned" given their "worthlessness." They accordingly fit easily into the role of invalid, including the attribution of scapegoat in the family.	Limitations from *illness* may pose a threat to their sense of grandeur and lead to a crisis of self-esteem. The children may also deny the severity of their symptoms and resist treatment.

Age Group 2 (6 to 12 Years)

Regulation of the feeling of self-worth becomes increasingly successful, but is subject to the age-related fluctuations of self-aggrandizement and self-deprecation relative to others (self-worth vs. object value).

Areas of Life

Family

Within the *family*, these children avoid dealing with new requirements and competitive situations. There exists a strong sibling rivalry and a low tolerance of frustration. Self-deprecation is frequent. Within the family they may experience the role of "black sheep," for example.	Within the *family*, there occur uncontrollable tantrums if the desire for affirmation is not satisfied. Aggressive behavior is directed against siblings and parents, who are blamed for failure. These children are very sensitive to criticism and in extreme cases may not accept assistance or instructions. They have unreasonable claims about and ideas of their own aptitude, and immediately break off their efforts if quick success is not forthcoming.

Peers

They are cautious and hesitant in their encounters with *peers*, whom they cannot imagine as wanting them for friends. They do not dare assert their own demands. They admire and envy other children for the recognition the latter enjoy.	They always strive for a special role and want to be the best boy or girl. As a rule, they have many contacts, but few close friendships, among their *peers* due to a lack of willingness to handle others' criticisms and claims. Clothes, toys (status symbols) may serve as an "assurance" of self-esteem. These children are poor losers in games with rules. They react with narcissistic rage, quit the game prematurely, invent new rules or comment on the 'unfairness' of how the game is being played.

Conflict

School

The children constantly compare themselves (secretly) with their classmates and are jealous of their success. Fears of being unable to perform as demanded or of being laughed at by others and complaints about unfair treatment by teachers characterize the *school situation*. Fear of exposure and their ambition motivate them to do their homework, so that they may indeed achieve a good performance, which can at best satisfy them only briefly.

In *school* they will overestimate their own performance. Because of their intense emotional reactions to their own ignorance, learning disorders and difficulties in participating in the learning process will occur. In case of failure, tasks are not performed to their completion and are denigrated. These children have difficulty in keeping to the class rules, which they experience as evaluative. If they are to perform, they focus on results in order to compare themselves against others.

Body/Illness

Their attitude towards their *bodies* is also governed by a feeling of inadequacy, and they seek to conceal their bodies, as is expressed mostly in their *posture* (e.g., drooping shoulders, eyes directed to the floor). When ill, these children appear in need of aid, but are also self-deprecating ("serves me right").

The older children may perceive their *bodies* as a means for gaining attention, and place them at the focus of their self-absorption. Limitations from illness may pose a threat to their sense of self-worth and lead to a crisis of self-esteem. The children may also deny the severity of their symptoms and resist treatment.

Age Group 3 (13 to 18 Years)

The intense engagement with self-image issues occurring in Age Group 3 forcefully brings about the comparison of "self-worth vs. object value". The adolescent's dwelling upon him-/herself, including the image he/she has of his/her own body, makes relationship formation difficult.

Areas of Life

Family

Within the *family*, their constant self-depreciation is noticeable, and they may use it to establish their status as a "black sheep." Given their sense of worthlessness, these adolescents may make the *family* responsible for their own failures ("poor conditions, no money, no education").

The adolescents may use the status of their *families* to stabilize their sense of self-worth: "We're special". As a rule, these adolescents call for admiration and a special status, without being willing to make their own contribution to family life. They may also blame the *family* for their own setbacks and feelings of hurt or being slighted.

Peers

These adolescents prefer relationships with *peers* in which they are not confronted with the feelings of their own worthlessness. They believe they have not earned appreciation from others.

Fantasies of grandeur and grandiose behavior may very well appeal to *peers*. These adolescents may have a charismatic appearance that creates a good standing in their peer group, but which hardly allows closer friendships. Important above all is affirmation by others, a need that can lie behind rapidly changing relationships or the break-off of relationships for the sake of narcissistic affirmation ("fickleness"). In the absence of narcissistic affirmation, the relationships are often impaired by emotionally excessive reactions (narcissistic rage, strong deprecation of others).

School/Vocation

Comparisons with classmates are constantly being made. In *school or vocational training,* these adolescents almost never attain the (excessively high) levels of performance they seek, although they are strongly motivated. To mitigate their strong feelings of inferiority, they attribute their "failure" to circumstances and feel wrongly evaluated. Such slights (exposure, poor marks) will trigger the symptoms.

These adolescents appear arrogant in *school or vocational training,* and tend to see themselves as "colleagues" of their teachers. As a rule, they significantly overestimate their aptitudes. In addition to a strong sense of rivalry and their striving to excel, only achievements demonstrating their superiority over others count. Little perseverance and intrinsic pleasure lead to frequent changes of interests, even during recreation.

Body/Illness

Entry into sexual relationships is made difficult by the concern about physical imperfections. The *body* is concealed in shame. These adolescents often readily assume the *role of invalid* and may feel affirmed in their perspective of inadequacy ("serves me right"), or they may attribute failures in other areas to their physical symptoms ("If I didn't have a stomach ache, I could go to school and get good grades").

They may perceive their *bodies* as a means to obtain admiration, and they spend a great deal of time caring for their bodies as part of their excessive preoccupations with themselves. Fixation on the body and the use of appearance (drive to be thin, extreme sports, body-building) as a means to impress others may result. Possession as a status symbol supports self-esteem. Entry into sexual relationships also serves self-appreciation. Limitations from *illness* may pose a threat to their sense of grandeur and lead to a crisis of self-esteem. Serious illness may therefore be trivialized. Mental neediness hardly fits into the narcissistically exaggerated self-concept, and help may be hard to accept.

Self-Worth Conflict – Active Mode

Case Vignette: Maximilian, Age 7 Years

Maximilian, seven years old, comes to the initial session accompanied by his parents. Maximilian makes no eye contact and expresses through his altogether sullen, dismissive posture that he is not in agreement with the conversation being conducted. He initially responds to the therapist's questions with just a nod or shake of the head. His mother follows the initial scene with some concern, while the father leans back and begins his description, interrupting the examiner. The father is actually not convinced that Maximilian needs a therapist. The school has exerted pressure and the teacher cannot handle him and his way of thinking – maybe she's overwhelmed. The father has done some research, and found that, in any case, a test for giftedness should be performed.

It is also reported that until recently the family was living abroad because of the father's occupation. There Maximilian attended a private kindergarten and a German private school during the first grade. According to the father, while life abroad meant separation from relatives and friends, there were also many amenities, such as servants, a chauffeur, etc. Because of a career change and so that the son could attend primary school in Germany, the family has now returned.

After Maximilian began attending school in Germany, somewhat reluctantly, a "misunderstanding" led to a confrontation with his homeroom teacher, who had pointed out a mistake he made. Since then, he has not uttered a word in class and after the subsequent weekend he refused to go to school at all. The school thereupon urgently advised the family to contact the therapist's practice.

Whilst the mother responds to questions by discussing in more detail the school situation and the teacher's initial observations, Maximilian becomes increasingly restless, finally jumping up in anger, kicking the table leg and leaving the room, absolutely refusing to continue the first session. In a subsequent session with the parents alone, they report as pre-history that Maximilian had always had particularly close contact with the father, who was often away from home because of work. The family moved abroad when Maximilian was two years old. Following the birth of his three-year-younger brother, Maximilian began acting extremely jealous at home. The mother reports that she had very much looked forward to the younger sibling, as she had always had the feeling of not being able to penetrate the alliance between father and son.

Maximilian has always been very impatient with himself. For example, either he was able to perform a new task ably right away or he would never try it again. He learned to ride a bicycle and to swim only because of pressure from the parents, and with many outbursts of anger. Even today he is a poor loser with a total loss of control whenever he loses a game, and is becoming excessively ambitious in sporting competitions. Solid friendships were also reportedly not the case at kindergarten age. While Maximilian has always been respected, in the group he was a bit solitary, domineering, and something of a know-it-all.

A play period with the examiner and Maximilian one week later underscored the issue of self-esteem. Maximilian has little joy in doing things with others or in constructing play scenarios. For him winning is important, and he turns nearly all offers of play into a competition. The examiner himself feels drawn into a competitive situation. Maximilian's noticeably increased sensitivity to slights leads the examiner to handle him "with kid gloves," while also reacting with annoyance to expressed "delusions of grandeur" ("I can play the game much better than you").

8.5 Guilt Conflict

Feelings of guilt arise when a person injures or offends another, either on purpose or accidentally, and stands in the way of the other person's needs or violates his/her rights. Such conflicts of conscience or conflicts related to the superego and loyalty are closely connected with egoistic or pro-social tendencies, and may concern not only actual offences and encroachment on others, but also violations of internalized norms and values. A precondition is that the child or adolescent has developed such internalized norms.

Children in Age Group 2 (6 to 12 years) have sufficiently internalized obligations and prohibitions along the lines of socially desired pro-object tendencies when starting school. These children give priority to the internalized relationships with their parents, to their values and norms, and, therefore, to the protection of this relationship with and loyalty to the parents. They transgress pro-social obligations and prohibitions despite their knowledge of right from wrong when it comes to safeguarding the existentially important relationship with the parents. Their guilt conflict is thus governed by the striving to secure the relationship with the parents. Preserving family loyalty can become so important as to distort reality. These children and adolescents are willing to sacrifice their credibility and their sense of reality when it comes to protecting the parents or their parents' values and norms from outside attacks.

A guilt conflict is therefore characterized by a permanently distorted perception of reality and guilt, particularly in relationships with the parents or in warding off the parents, while nonfamily relationships may be relatively free of conflict. Frequently associated with this conflict are inappropriate feelings of guilt and defensive measures taken against this guilt.

The distinction from self-worth conflicts can be difficult. Taking into account the prevailing affect is of great use here. While guilt conflicts mainly concern feelings of guilt, the issue of self-worth pertains primarily to shame (or to defence against it). Not so much right and wrong are the issue (as is the case with guilt), but rather strength and weakness, big and small.

Clinical Anchor-Point Descriptions	
Passive Mode	**Active Mode**
These children and adolescents are characterized by exaggerated ties of loyalty to their families. They may exhibit inconspicuously realistic relationship behavior towards people outside the family, as long as these relationships do not affect attachment to the family. Regarding the family and its interests, they are quite willing to make amends in exaggerated form, to the extent of even setting aside their own primary interests. They give the impression of having taken heavy blame on themselves, so that atonement is possible only through self-sacrifice, and they exhibit, to a certain extent, a masochistic and self-punishing processing mode. The prominent affect consists of feelings of guilt, with fear of punishment and sadness also possibly being observed. Countertransference gives rise to compassion and the endeavor to counteract the patient's tendencies towards self-punishment.	These children and adolescents stand out with their accusatory, deprecating remarks and modes of behavior regarding matters of the family. Despite the appearance of disloyalty, this behavior is loyal from a psychodynamic point of view, for it represents the attempt to get rid of the culpable feelings of loyalty. This basic attitude of constantly making remarks ranging from the critical to the accusatory also governs relationships outside the family. These children and adolescents, therefore, seem to act beyond the social framework and to be self-centred. Despite this behavior, there clearly exists an ability for attachment, even if in a negative way. The avoidance of loyalty and the shared responsibility for the welfare of others is so decisive that these children and adolescents often appear amoral and conscienceless. Prominent affects are anger at parents or others, and among the adolescents a cynical attitude. Countertransference may give rise to the temptation to confront the child or adolescent with his/her "amoral" behavior.

Age Group 1 (3 to 5 Years)

This age group increasingly internalizes inner values and norms from the most important relationships. During the "defiance phase," prosocial vs. egotistical tendencies become acute for the first time and the first feelings of guilt arise.

Areas of Life	
Family	
Within the *family*, the children with a developing passive mode stand out by their forced ego development and by their willingness, for example, to help their parents or siblings or relatives to an extent going beyond what is usual for this age.	Children inclined more to an active mode appear within the *family* dissatisfied, defiant, and with little attachment to the parents.

Age Group 2 (6 to 12 Years)

The development of internalized values and norms (superego) extends more and more beyond the primary relationships, and discrepancies between the constellation of values of the parents and of the social environment may increasingly occur. Depending on the level of development, feelings of guilt will be experienced and integrated, or suffered or denied.

Areas of Life	
Family	
Within the *family*, they are willing children ready to sacrifice themselves. They hardly make any demands, but are always ready to pursue parental and familial interests. They experience problems within the *family* (death, divorce, illness) in terms of their culpability and feel remorse over what they could have done "better" and how they could have prevented the problems arising ("If I hadn't behaved so badly, my mother wouldn't have gotten sick".	To the *family*, they stand out by representing how much better off the other children are. Parents and siblings try to please them, but always feel their efforts are inadequate, since they meet with no success, or they respond to the child in the same way ("You're to blame").
Peers	
In their relationships with *peers*, they are willingly accepted and, given their readiness to help others, used and exploited by the others.	As within the family, in their *relationships with peers*, they are full of accusations and claim their constant innocence to others.

School

In *school*, they show a high level of performance, as they work conscientiously and a great deal. They stand out by their readiness to support others in everyday school life.	In *school* they meet performance requirements with a plethora of accusations about impossible demands and circumstances that make learning difficult, and they do not see their own share in this difficulty.

Body/Illness

Illnesses can greatly disquiet them, as they are kept from helping others and being there for others. They want to become healthy again quickly and do not follow the sort of behavior necessary for recovery.	When *ill*, they become accusing and reproachful because not better attention was paid to them, which is why they've become ill, in their view. This accusation is aimed particularly at the parents, who accordingly perceive themselves as inadequate and to blame for their child's illness.

Age Group 3 (13 to 18 Years)

The development of inner values and standards (superego) provisionally concludes in the interplay with identity acquisition and more and more resembles the conflict conditions of an adult. The incipient detachment from the parents can be accompanied by the development of guilt issues, such as guilt about autonomy.

Areas of Life

Family

In their *families*, they act as helpers and supporters for all family problems ("I'd do anything for my parents"). They do not succeed in distancing themselves as would be typical for their age, or do so only to a limited extent. As a result, they are unduly bound to and utilized in their *families*; they give the impression of having to do penance and make amends. This can lead to parentification or to the adoption of a "scapegoat role" for family problems.	Within the *family*, these young people exhibit self-righteous behavior. A negativistic attitude and a tendency to place blame on others govern their interactions within the *family* ("Because of you …"). They also make accusations about the *family* to outsiders. They cannot admit to their own share in matters that are not right.

Conflict

Peers

In their relations with their *peers*, these adolescents are reticent and undemanding. When they are asked or someone needs help they become available and show attentiveness and self-sacrificing helpfulness. Relationships with the opposite sex may be foregone out of loyalty to parents; in close *friendship relationships* they often display an "altruistic relinquishment" ("I'm happy for you!").

In relationships with *peers*, they are always dissatisfied and legalistic, so that others are always to blame. They are constantly accusing, which makes them isolated in their peer group. *Partner relationships* are actively sought, but may be burdened by their denied loyalty to their parents; they often make their *partners* feel guilty and they behave accusingly.

School/Vocation

In *school* or at *work*, they endear themselves through diligent helpfulness and through their availability in times of crisis, at the same time feeling that they have not done things properly ("My mistake"). Slumps in performance and work may also occur if they are not in demand despite their availability or if they are blamed for mistakes, which they readily admit to. Autonomy guilt can also lead to a refusal to perform or decline in performance in order to postpone separation from the parents.

In *school* or at *work*, they always blame external conditions for their difficulties or the bad intentions of others for thwarting their success. For this too, they tend to see the reason as lying in discrimination and insinuate that others are in their debt.

Body/Illness

When *ill* they experience their neediness only to a limited extent, and they experience appropriate care more as a burden of debt which they will have to repay ("I don't want to become a burden to you"). For this reason they pay little attention to bodily concerns – including sexual interests.

Illness seems to them the result of bad desires or the wrongdoing of others. They regard caregivers as doing everything basically wrong and not really helping.

Guilt Conflict – Passive Mode

Case Vignette: Katharina, Age 15 Years

Fifteen-year-old Katharina experienced, at the age of eleven years, the sudden death of her best friend of the same age, and saw a behavioral therapist for bereavement counselling over a long period of time. Following a holiday trip last summer, which Katharina spent for the first time with a friend and without her parents, she began to suffer from nightmares nearly every night in which she met her dead friend.

At the initial session, the very worried mother appears with her daughter, who seems a bit fatigued, but who, with her red cheeks, sparkling eyes, and likeable "baby fat," gives an impression of great liveliness. Katharina reports that she has difficulty falling asleep, wakes up in a panic, and then usually remains awake until dawn. At school (10th Grade, junior high school) she can barely concentrate because she feels so tired, and her parents are now worried that her academic performance will begin to decline. Before the trip to Spain, which was great ("just partying"), she had dreamt of her friend only occasionally, but now she has the same dream each night: She sees all the members of her family asleep, goes into the backyard and encounters her friend, who is then suddenly torn away from her. One night four years ago, Katharina took leave of her very happy and adventurous friend, with whom Katharina had often played outdoors, and the next morning the friend was dead.

In a private conversation with the adolescent (in a low-cut T-shirt), the therapist learns that the church community and the strictly Catholic high school have done a lot in helping her work through the mourning process, which in fact has been going on for an overly long period of time, and has still not reached its end. Katharina also fantasizes in school that her friend is sitting next to her. She is afraid that she could forget the sound of the friend's voice. At present, Katharina says she is worried about another friend, who is anorexic, and she is afraid that this friend could also die. She does a lot with friends, but there are sometimes conflicts with Katharina's parents. She always has to be home very early. Asked about a boyfriend, she replies that she wants to concentrate on school, and that she can do without relationships for the next few years. In the trial sessions she yawns repeatedly, as if she had to make clear that she's having a hard time, whereas the atmosphere is one of a newly kindled optimism and joy, with anger also mixed in. Striking is how much she idealizes her parents and endeavors to maintain the role of the little, well-behaved daughter. Katharina is generally very socially oriented, belongs to the school first aid service and is very active in the church.

Katharina was born as a latecomer, after three siblings, when the parents were "over the worst of childrearing." The mother was treated for depression during the pregnancy, and had much fear of the childbirth. On her account, she was not depressed post-partum, only very exhausted. She describes the infant and toddler periods as unremarkable, although Katharina has always been a very anxious child. Last year, the sister (9 years older) moved out, which caused Katharina much suffering. Since that time, Katharina has developed very rapidly, even to the point of being overwhelmed; she also has problems with her body ("too curvy"). Asked about her own childhood, the mother says that she herself "had a lot of energy, and would have liked to have kicked up her heels, if people would have let her." Katharina's father also reports having had old parents who were very strict.

Katharina lives in a family that imposes high moral demands on themselves and on others and whose rigid superego keeps everything impulsive in check. The internalized commandments of the Catholic Church, with its vengeful God demanding penance, confirm and strengthen the high ego ideal of the family members. Katharina is confronted by a mother who herself fends off or was not allowed to act out drive-related tendencies and possibly also reacts with depression for this reason. The deceased girlfriend seems to have served as an ally for Katharina; both were "wild" girls who would leave their safe haven to play "in the open air." At the beginning of puberty and of the breakaway from parental ideals, she now experiences the sudden death of her girlfriend, which she unconsciously perceives as a punishment and warning. Her initial reaction is heightened social commitment. Only when at the age of fifteen she once again has a good time with a girlfriend far away from the parents does the superego's prohibitions kick in. Breaking away and development are punishable by death – the girlfriend's death appears as a warning. How much of a role is played by unconscious envy in the mother towards the daughter's blossoming into life can only be conjectured at present. During the further course of therapy, Katharina tries to make the therapist a "confidant and ally", with the latter swinging back and forth between seduction fantasies and feelings of guilt towards the parents in countertransference.

8.6 Oedipal Conflict

The oedipal conflict as an internalized, lasting conflict moves between the poles of satisfying erotic and sexual desires on the one hand and fending them off on the other. Despite today's children receiving a more liberal upbringing and socialization, this conflict continues to have broad clinical importance today. As the first important love objects, parents acquire a formative significance for children, while, conversely, children are important objects of love for their parents. Sexual motives closely interlaced with other motives enter into the children's relationships with their parents and in parents' relationships with their children and have to be integrated. The oedipal constellation presupposes the real or imagined presence of three persons, who are held in a field of tension between appreciation, rivalry, and eroticism. In contrast to the self-worth conflict, the oedipal conflict concerns not the recognition of "value," but recognition as a boy/man or girl/woman. The aim is to win over the other person through particular physical attractiveness, to outdo rivals and to feel pleasure, or to fend off all these aspects.

In terms of developmental level, an internalized, lasting oedipal conflict can be diagnosed more accurately at the start of puberty, when the oedipal conflict must be finally resolved. Precursors of this internalized conflict can already be found after conclusion of the oedipal phase. During latency, such conflicts can also be interpreted as precursors, with the tendency towards developmental impairment. During adolescence, the internalized, permanent quality of this conflict – including its supression – can be clearly diagnosed. In this age group there arises a special dynamic from the fact that the physically mature genitals theoretically allow acting upon instinctual desires.

Clinical Anchor-Point Descriptions	
Passive Mode	**Active Mode**
At issue are children and adolescents who lack the sort of sexual curiosity befitting their age. They dress conspicuously unattractively or try to conceal themselves through their physical appearance by enshrouding themselves in clothing, for example. These children and adolescents cannot touch themselves and exhibit a strong defence against sexual urges, as can be expressed by fears of masturbation, among other ways. They avoid conversations about the body and sexuality, noticeably avoid games with sexual themes and emphatically remain on the factual level. Countertransference in the examiner gives rise to an especially gender-neutral, fact-based demeanor as the main affect.	At issue are children and adolescents who dress themselves so as to accentuate their gender, are constantly curious and explore their own sex organs and the sexual characteristics of their peers. They also emphasize different gender roles unusually, often in play or play pretend sexual scenes. During latency, they may approach adults in an inappropriately flirtatious and seductive way. During adolescence, they may provocatively display their bodies, especially in a sexual way. On the relationship plane, triangular constellations and constant rivalries are noticeable. In the examiner's countertransference, inappropriate sexualization is clearly perceptible.

Age Group 1 (3 to 5 Years)

Children recognize themselves as boys or girls and occupy themselves during the oedipal phase with their own sexuality and the sexuality of their parents. Against the backdrop of an enduring oedipal conflict on the part of the parents, a special dynamic may develop. Children in this age group accept attributions as masculine or feminine, and greatly base their behavior on masculine or feminine role activities. Observable at the end of this development phase is an exaggerated or noticeably absent preoccupation by the child with his or her own sexuality. The basic experience is that relationships always have an oedipal connotation and that relationships without a sexual dimension are not possible. At the end of this phase, rivalries with the same-sex parent over the parental love object are clearly perceptible.

Age Group 2 (6 to 12 Years)

Gender identity is now clear: Boys play only with boys, girls play only with girls and each side teases or denigrates the opposite sex. As noted above, during latency precursors of an internalized oedipal conflict may reveal itself and may already lead to impaired development. In the passive mode, this condition is manifested by the anxious exclusion of all sexual matters. In the active mode, play, behavior and contact with others noticeably focus on sexuality. Behavior towards children of the same age and towards adults exceeds boundaries set on the physical level, and manifests inappropriate curiosity. A typical impression in countertransference is that something in the relationship "is not right," that childlike aspects are missing. In the relationship, triangular constellations make themselves known. The strong emphasis on sexuality is also manifested through daydreaming and masturbation.

Areas of Life	
Family	
The relationships in the *family* appear fact-based or childlike. These children are notable for their overly prevalent latency. Relationships are formed on a very factual basis, erotic-sexual aspects having no place in them. Seductive aspects have a disturbing effect and are ignored or denigrated. Problems and tensions in the *family*, especially those with a sexual background, cannot be perceived.	There exist close ties to the *family*, especially to the parent of the opposite sex, accompanied by the corresponding rivalries with the same-sex parent ("Mum's little man"). Bodily contact is especially offered in the case of adults. Sibling rivalries have a special connotation of being struggles for the loved parent.
Peers	
Relationships with *peers* are notable for their neutrality and objectivity ("unremarkable"), but also for their very childish need for protection. Nor can situations with clearly sexual content be perceived as such, or they arouse anxiety and rejection. An age-inappropriate insistence on gender-neutral and childish toys is notable.	Relationships with *peers* are contradictory and conflictual. The emphasis on gender roles ('Macho' and 'Little Princess') seems inappropriately imposed for the child's age. Play and recreational activities increasingly become impoverished in an age-inappropriate way as exclusively masculine or feminine role aspects come to dominate.

School

In *school*, their strong focus on facts can make these children very popular among teachers. Schoolmates are more irritated by their neutrality towards and defence against sexual humor. The lack of curiosity may also negatively affect school performance.

Relationships in *school* are impaired by the incipient sexualization and rivalry. Learning problems can arise from the distraction due to excessive preoccupation with sexuality and oedipal matters.

Body/Illness

Illnesses can be problematic for these children, since the *body*, which they had been avoiding dealing with, now becomes the centre of attention. They present their *body* only in terms of efficiency and functionality, not perceiving it also as something with which to impress and attract others sexually. They lack an age-appropriate curiosity about sexual matters, the sex lives of adults, and their peers' bodies.

Illness may afford a welcome opportunity to these children, allowing them to deal with their bodies, particularly in sexual aspects, in a more intensified way. Feminine or masculine sexual characteristics play a comparatively large role in the *body concept*.

Age Group 3 (13 to 18 Years)

At this age, preoccupation with the oedipal conflict intensifies, triggered by physical maturity and by the fact that the genitals can now be directly used for satisfying instinctual needs. Central is the excessive sexualization, or defence against it, which stands out in the overall picture of adolescent development and occurs at the expense of development in other areas. Relationships with people of the same sex also exhibit an unreasonable rivalry or the lack of any rivalry. It should be kept in mind that the development of the negative Oedipus complex can lead to a change in sexual orientation.

In the passive mode, the enormous energy expended in keeping sexual aspects out of one's life is particularly noticeable. This can lead to self-chastisement and asceticism in "more harmless" areas of life. The examiner encounters adolescents conspicuous by their harmlessness, innocence, and naiveté. Indications of fending off sexuality exist, however.

In the active mode, these adolescents are marked by a strong emphasis on sexuality in the form of frequent daydreaming and excessive masturbation, constant preoccupation with sexuality and with acting on sexual urges. These adolescents seem to have little free emotional valence for dealing with nonsexual content. The behavior in contact with peers and with adults is seductive and exceeds limits up to the point of being provocatively sexual through parading the body. Countertransference in the examiner gives rise to clearly noticeable eroticization.

Areas of Life	
Family	
Family relationships are idealized and de-eroticized. Family conflicts and rivalries are denied.	There exist close ties to the *family*, especially to the opposite-sex parent, although they may also be completely unaware of these ties and deny them. The opposite-sex parent may be idealized, and the same-sex parent extremely denigrated. The parents' sexual relationships are pursued with great curiosity. Sibling rivalries are often pronounced and have the quality of wanting to outdo rivals.
Peers	
In *friendships and partner relationships*, these adolescents shut out any form of eroticism and sexuality, forming such relationships solely on an objective, neutral level. Any opportunity to meet people of the opposite sex or to meet with same-sex competitors is anxiously avoided. The result is a drastic constriction of social life. Adult partners and close relationships with younger or same-sex friends are sought with the exclusion of erotic-sexual elements (sibling-like relationships).	Inconsistent, sexualizing behavior (attracting/repelling) makes relationships with *peers* (friendship and partnerships) conflictual or unsatisfactory. The relationships are constellated so that the adolescents intrude into existing relationships, but avoid enduring couple relationships in particular. Chosen partners often resemble the primary objects, but these partners prove disappointing given their contrast with the primary objects. Recreational activities are specifically sought that will allow competition and sexualization, while the person's own potency is also put on display symbolically (possessions, clothing, cars). The desire to beat out rivals is also manifested in denigrations of their *physicality*, among other ways.
School/Vocation	
Relationships at *school* and at *work* resemble the family relationships with inconspicuous, partly good relationships.	Relationships at *school/training/work* are also problematic because of intense sexualization and competitive behavior that

The priority is to avoid rivalries of sexual origin, which will "disrupt work." Striking is an exaggerated emphasis on factuality, even in areas of school and work that do not admit erotic-sexual aspects (during breaks, at parties).

is barely warded off. Open conflicts and hostility may occur, such as jealousy of fellow students or colleagues and the sexualization of relationships with superiors.

Body/Illness

Dealing with *illness* can be experienced as threatening, medical care is endured with anxiety and *physical* examinations are strongly avoided. These adolescents are afraid to masturbate or to have heterosexual contact. An inappropriately large fear of sexually transmitted *diseases* (AIDS) may arise.

Illnesses and the associated invalid role afford these adolescents an opportunity to deal with their own *bodies*. In the physician–patient relationship they are associated with eroticization and competition. The patients can be experienced either as seductive or threatening; generally one of these two dimensions will dominate. The *body* is presented provocatively and especially sexually; excessive masturbation is possible.

Oedipal Conflict – Active Mode

Case Vignette: Daniel, Age 9 Years

Daniel, 9 years at the time of presentation, is the first-born child and has two younger sisters. His parents are very worried about his "repeated thefts." In his mother's words: "Bags of toys from his cousin, stuffed animals, favorite things ('personal trophies'), but also money (up to 500 Euros)." Even during kindergarten he stole things every now and then, such as the mother's jewellery. Daniel is the first child from the couple's relationship, which is still quite young and decidedly ambivalent. His mother weaned him at the age of three months and had to put him in day-care, otherwise she would have lost her job; she weeps as she relates this fact. Until the age of two he cried whenever his mother left the room. To date all children still sleep in the parents' bed.

In the initial interview, the patient approaches the therapist in an almost comradely way, seems precocious, looks small and compact, but quite masculine, wiry, and muscular; his head is almost shaven, though. The father, too, is completely bald. The patient talks his head off about his current projects in the building area at the day centre. He's building a city, and he's the boss. Although he is impressive with his ambitious and imaginative plans, the therapist feels kept in check.

The therapist also notices the following during the preliminary interview: When Daniel talks about how he plays with the other children, his account sounds lively and imaginative. The therapist internally responds with a highly suspenseful feeling that she can interpret only later, however: Daniel does not mention playing with the other boys, but the most important thing is that he can be the boss, and, to this end, he needs to have the others around, hanging on his every word.

The Family as Animals (FAT) drawing is quite remarkable. Dominating everything is the father elephant on the left on the picture, standing on his front legs as in a handstand, his tail high up in the air, his giant head at the centre of the picture leaning forward with huge teeth, a pointed and blackened tusk and large, equally blackened eyes. Head to head is the mummy dog that is much smaller, however, with a blackened throat and blackened between the front legs, looking back at the children. Daniel already becomes agitated while drawing, as he adds in eight hamsters (himself, his sisters and his cousins), 17 birds (uncles and aunts), five dogs (grandpa, grandma), all small-sized. He can hardly talk about the drawing as he becomes so agitated that using the punching bag is the only thing that helps. The further course of therapy confirms the "inner beware sign." (Caution: The relationship level is wrong, he presents himself as a macho to the therapist, tries to seduce her, get her to admire his manliness.) During the play with puppets that are more or less randomly distributed between the two, a battle soon takes place very close to the therapist's abdomen. Daniel is doubtlessly trying by all tricks and means to make the struggle end in his favor and in the complete annihilation of the puppets the therapist is vainly trying to protect. The therapist's countertransference gives rise to the feeling of the two being tightly bound together in an erotically tinged, sadistic struggle.

The patient's mother is an achievement-oriented, delicate creature who can accept being touched. The father stresses his objectivity. The therapist perceives the father's way of speaking (ironic and sarcastic) both about himself and about his children as brutal. The mother complains about her husband's knife collection and that he is always leaving weapons magazines lying about. The therapist does not like to picture a relationship between the parents. Feeling very uncomfortable, the therapist has the sense of standing in the middle of their bedroom and having to witness the conception and birth of the children.

Only during the further course of therapy does the therapist confirm her suspicions related to the obtrusive fantasies she had about the father's sadistic streaks at her initial contact with the parents. For example, after the son had fought with his little sisters over a desired seat between the parents, the father punished him (quite coolly and in a business-like manner) by carrying him together with his chair into the backyard and tipping him into the snow. The father counters his son's oedipal hatred with a chummy offer: Ever since the son was little, he was allowed to accompany the father to music pubs, and got to drink cola and coffee – also in order to calm him down directly in the midst of the conflict.

A moment occurs quite at the beginning of therapy when the therapist is overcome by a very tender feeling, namely when Daniel returns with his parents from the Oktoberfest dressed in *Lederhose* and a traditional costume jacket. Since his father had not shaved Daniel's head in a while, the boy's blond hair was now quite adorable. So for the first, and so far only time, he looked like a normal little boy.

8.7 Identity Conflict

The identity of children and young people encompasses the totality of internal images they have of themselves, and comprises numerous, differentiated, and even contradictory, positive as well as negative, aspects of self. In the course of development, experiences lead to the integration of newly acquired images of the self into the pre-existing identity system. This continual process of integration is differentiated from others and stabilized through supportive and mirroring measures, resulting finally in a sense of coherence and continuity of identity over time. As development progresses, contradictory internal images can co-exist and be tolerated.

We speak of an identity conflict only if contradictory representations of the self produce a life-determining confusion, disorientation, and fear of self-dissonance. In case of an identity conflict, the search for and assurance of identity will govern experience and behavior. There exists a chronic struggle to establish a coherent identity, accompanied by the fear that one's own identity could be jeopardized by inconsistencies to the point of self-dissonance.

The formation of an identity conflict presupposes an at least moderately integrated structural level and differentiated self-representations. Identity diffusion must be distinguished from identity conflict.

Transgenerational migration issues can compel the formation of an identity conflict in children and adolescents. It should be noted, however, that an immigrant background may also contain greater potential for identity development through a culturally determined plurality of forms of identity. As with children and adolescents without an immigrant background, the available resources play a crucial role: If the defence mechanisms are functional and flexible in conflict cases, no enduring conflict will be able to form.

Clinical Anchor-Point Descriptions	
Passive Mode	**Active Mode**
The regressive defence against the fear of self-dissonance prevents an identity-defining exploration on the part of the children or adolescents. Nor do they show any desire for testing identity-promoting ego functions such as language, motor skills, and imagination. They also avoid identity-promoting object relations, with either adults or peers. In interviews, these children and adolescents appear disinterested, indifferent, and adaptive. Their self-perception is dominated by insecurity and disorientation. They superficially adopt assigned roles (identities) without really embodying them and using them for defining identity. The prominent affects are anxiety, confusion, and disorientation. Countertransference gives rise to feelings of helplessness and compassion, but also strain.	A counterphobic defence against the fear of self-dissonance leads to uncritical and constantly changing identifications ("chameleon"). Children and adolescents in the active mode try to use identity-promoting ego functions to arrive at a coherent self-image. They try to fill the lack of a coherent internal self-image with extraneous images and roles with which they can identify (changing "idols"). They use their own bodies and presentations of their bodies as a way to express their (pseudo-)identity, which, however, can appear peculiar because of the quick change in roles ("today one way, tomorrow another"). During the interview these children and adolescents appear driven and restless. Their self-perception is marked by restlessness and changing identification. The lead affects are anxiety warded off counterphobically, restlessness, and the feeling of being driven. Countertransference gives rise to concern and compassion, as well as to alienation and the urge to assign the child or adolescent a specific identity.

Age Group 1 (3 to 5 Years)

The child develops the ability to differentiate between self and objects and to use the space between the self and the objects. At the age of three, the child uses and understands the words "I," "you," "mine," and "yours."

During this phase of development, constant reassurances from the parents as to the stability and coherence of the child's own image of her-/himself often occur and are necessary. At the end of this phase, the first internalized conflicts will already exist.

Areas of Life	
Family	
The child is uncertain about his/her self within the *family*, and often finds that his/her endeavors in mirroring and coherence do not meet with reliably recurring reactions by the parents.	Within the *family* these children begin to replace the actual family situation by a fictitious, idealized one ("Dad is a king"), which leads to interactional conflicts. The real parents may feel rejected by the children's efforts to acquire identity in fantasized roles. The child's adaptation to the parents' notions ("Princess") and ideologies lead to no interactional conflicts.
Peers	
These children have difficulty forming active relationships with their *peers*. They have difficulties in recognizing themselves in comparisons with others, and avoid contact with domineering children assured of their identities. They show no desire for trying out identity-promoting ego functions. They remain inactive both verbally and in their motor behavior.	Among their *peers* these children eagerly grab every opportunity to play a role, but often appear to strain themselves and lose sight of their own concerns. They constantly take on new roles while playing, without having a favorite role or character. This arbitrariness can irritate other children.
Kindergarten	
In *kindergarten* conflicts come to the surface. The child stands out through his/her adaptive behavior and rarely takes the initiative. He/she stays at the edge of the group, appearing indifferent, at times perplexed, and confused in socially complex situations, but, on the other hand, willingly accepts assigned roles. The child finds little pleasure in his/her own games and is insecure and unimaginative.	In *kindergarten* these children stand out because of their attachment to adults and dominant peers in their search for identity and because of their attempts to exhibit the qualities desired by the latter. Since this constitutes their own search for identity, these children prove "disloyal" in relationships, following the person who offers them the stronger identification. This imitation is often disconcerting, since they seem to act inappropriately to the reality and to their situation.
Body/Illness	
During *illness*, they use statements and assessments from the treating physicians to stabilize their identity. *Illnesses* may reinforce role insecurity and make them clueless, or alternatively allow them to assume a "secure," regressive role ("I can't").	*Illness* represents for these children a regressive limitation of their options for action. On the other hand, assuming the designated role of invalid can promote identity formation.

Conflict

Age Group 2 (6 to 12 Years)

Comprehensive disruptions in the child's relationship with him-/herself now become more defined. There exists a basic insecurity in the social context that is enormously broadened by starting school. In most cases, this insecurity will not lead to regression to familial structures, because of the desire for identification on the one hand; on the other hand, the child experiences that familial structures do not ensure identity either or even greatly oppose the surrounding social identities (conscious/unconscious dissonances as with second or third generation immigrants).

Areas of Life	
Family	
These children often do not like to be at home because of the absence of clear-cut identities in the *family*, or they withdraw to home in order avoid role conflicts in other contexts. There exist no or only conflicting and highly problematic offers of roles from either parent, so that the children do not know with whom they are supposed to identify. Identification of children with extra-familial structures and persons are often denigrated by the *family* and not encouraged.	At this age, the children recognize the identity disorders in the *family realm*. Often they construct a fictitious and idealized family history or myth ("family legend"). Lying behind this construction is the conscious or unconscious desire to break away from the familial identity systems, experienced as meaningless or confusing, which have not afforded them any secure sense of identity. The children direct themselves outwards, find substitute families, and pursue close friendships with peers who are secure in their roles.
Peers	
In relationships, *friends* are avoided who, because of their clear-cut and constant qualities, remind the children of their own lack of identity. This discrepancy is difficult to endure. *Peers* are sought who are also socially marginal for similar or other reasons. The children turn to adults with the desire for an affirmation of themselves, and in these relationships seem rather colorless compared with other children.	In their relationships with *peers,* these children are popular playmates, as they enthusiastically accept offers to play and do things together. Given a sufficient ability for empathy, continual creative cooperation may develop from this basis. The children may remain at the level of enthusiastic but occasional contacts, however, which do not lead to permanent relationships. The children seek and maintain membership in groups providing identity (Scouts or Guides, sport clubs).

School

In *school*, the children have particular difficulties with subjects touching on identity dissonances. They also have difficulty in taking a stand and voicing their opinion in a discussion. They have greater success in areas of school less related to identity dissonance. In severe cases, the children do not succeed in identifying with the role of student at all, and they endure the situation adaptively with apparent compliance.

These children give *school* an inordinate role in shaping their identity. They regard *school* as an opportunity to develop a satisfying sense of self through learning and performance. They enthusiastically take up the possibilities of ideological development and opinion formation through subjects like Literature, History, Social Studies, Civics, and Religion. Permanent or alternating substantive ties to these areas may also arise, depending on how long the subject is useful for promoting identity.

Body/Illness

Identity-constituting *physical* activities (such as being a good climber) are not sought, and, while offers to participate are accepted, the activities are not further pursued. *Illness* reinforces the lack of a sense of identity (lack of physical stability and coherence). Distance from the social environment becomes greater and isolation is reinforced. Even as patients the children appear indifferent and distant from their own condition.

Physical activities are enthusiastically sought and conducted, but only as long as they have an identity-creating effect. The result may be rapidly changing sports activities, for example, without any particular activity being coherently pursued in depth. The *body* is dressed appropriately for the currently preferred identity or role. An *illness* is difficult to endure for some children of this age, as illness is associated with a restriction on identity-promoting activities, so that a fixed role ("invalid") must be assumed. On the other hand, some children will actively take up the role of invalid and shape that role in forming an identity.

Age Group 3 (13 to 18 Years)

In this phase, the main internal task lies in developing a stable sense of self, with earlier identifications being challenged and new aspects of identity incorporated, including those pertaining to bodily changes. Pubertal development intensifies conflicts, which in the case of adolescents either intensifies social isolation, with a perplexity as to who one is or wants to be, or the person enters into rapidly changing roles and relationships in order to compensate for his/her own lack of identity. Disappointed, the adolescent will drop these roles and relationships if the lack of identity remains noticeable.

Areas of Life

Family

These adolescents also withdraw within their *families* and develop self-related anxieties. They act shy and insecure, do not understand themselves, and feel they are not understood by others. Within the *family*, there exist unclear or conflicting identities, with no attractive opportunities for identification.

Due to the separation from *parental objects*, fantasies about fictitious and idealized family stories and their own identity can greatly increase. These adolescents fantasize about themselves in different roles and develop a strong interest in biographies. They substitute utopias for concrete life-historical perspectives. In some cases, there is also the conscious desire to play a different role than the one from their *families of origin* in future life.

Peers

These adolescents have a limited ability to explore new life and relationship situations, and they are painfully aware of this limitation ("I don't know who I am"). They avoid relationships with *friends* and *partners*, who could provide identity and support through their evident and admired qualities. The discrepancy between their own lack of identity and the role security of their *peers* is difficult to endure. Age-appropriate sexual relationships tend to be avoided and are frightening, since the insecure self threatens to merge with others or to dissolve.

In their relationships with *peers*, the adolescents show themselves to be unpretentious and easy to handle. They are constantly on the lookout for further possibilities of identification and tend more to dissipate than concentrate their energy. In favorable cases, however, stable relationships develop with *friends* and *partners,* whose qualities can provide identity and support. There is a danger of identifying with groups that promise a strong identity (goths, emos). These adolescents are susceptible to ideologies, which they may change rapidly, however. A strong emphasis on asceticism as an identity-creating form of existence may alternatively prevail.

School/Vocation

In *school relationships* and *performance situations*, such as early working life, questions of the perspective on life and career choices enter the foreground and cannot be answered by the adolescents. They are aware of their helplessness, loss of orientation, and the inability to develop their own perspectives for the future that would be felt as satisfactory, and become worried ("I don't know what

The adolescents accord *school* and the *work world* an inappropriate role in shaping identity (overly dedicated, "always on duty"). These adolescents take every possibility for learning and performing and every proffered social role as an opportunity for stabilizing their own sense of identity. In doing so, they pursue values and ideas as over-valued principles, and appear as fanatical reformers,

I want to do"). They cannot perceive their own self in its continuity over time.

discoverers, or inventors. They gladly take part in student exchange programmes, for example, searching for themselves in foreign lands.

Body/Illness

Externally and internally, no identification with a corresponding peer group occurs. They clothe their *bodies* not according to age or gender roles, but in a neutral way. Owing to their insecurity, *illness* does not afford these adolescents an adequate invalid role that they can accept. They act indifferently towards their own illness, are passive-indolent or use their illness as a regressive form of escape.

They often change their styling and their particular identity does not gain substance and depth, so that these adolescents often seem disguised. They enter into sexual relationships – including those deviating from the norm – in the hope of gaining an identity and finding affirmation. In *illness*, these adolescents tend actively to take up and shape their role as invalids. They use this role for the purpose of finding themselves and presenting themselves, possibly turning the condition into a chronic one.

Identity Conflict – Passive Mode

Case Vignette: Samira, Age 5 Years

The nearly five-year-old Samira comes to the initial interview with her mother and young-looking maternal grandfather. "A father with his two daughters" immediately comes to the therapist's mind.

The mother reports that Samira speaks only with her parents and grandparents, and occasionally utters one-word sentences to a kindergarten friend. She does not speak a single word with other members of her Turkish family. Samira has been a quiet child who sleeps well and has always eaten very little. At the age of one and a half, she was already talking a lot – at home now with her parents and grandparents, she "talks her head off." Outside her family surroundings the daughter is very anxious, her mother reports, and only takes food from her mother. In kindergarten, Samira would rather die of thirst than take a drink of water, being very strong-willed. Samira makes no eye contact with the therapist and cannot be moved to look into the play room or to take crayons in hand; she appears altogether insecure and passive.

Her family comes from Turkey. Her likeable, corpulent mother (with a degree in law) reports in perfect German that Samira was "a grandparents' child." She has a sisterly relationship with the mother's own younger sister (age 14 years), who lives with them. Everyone lives in the same house, as a large family. The other members of the family having rejected the name "D." (Kurdish and not gender-specific) chosen by the mother for her child, Samira is now called by her middle name. Ever since she could talk, Samira has repeatedly changed her name, however; at present she calls herself "Caterpillar." At home only Turkish is spoken and Turkish traditions followed. The mother specifically chose a German Catholic kindergarten for Samira, however. On entering kindergarten at the age of three, Samira spoke only Turkish; no great value was placed on German. Two of the mother's siblings (brother and sister) suffered from heart defects and following years of treatment and many hospital stays, died at the ages of 14 and 12 years, respectively. The now 14-year old aunt was named after her deceased sister. Samira was also originally diagnosed with a heart defect, which she has outgrown, however. The mother expresses several times her idea that Samira has perhaps lived once before. The mother became pregnant because the grandmother longed for a grandson. Samira was raised from the outset and for the most part by the grandmother; she also often sleeps with the grandparents.

Countertransference gives rise to a feeling of confusion and perplexity in the therapist, who senses a desire to become "Turkish" and who experiences herself as being both dangerous and invasive. The family conveys two messages: Having come to Germany as Gastarbeiter (literally translated as "guest worker"), the grandparents remain internally closely tied to their home country and intensively maintain Turkish traditions, which they also pass on to Samira. Samira's father seems not to be fully integrated here and is also tied to Turkey. On the other hand, the mother has become Germanized and wants Samira to grow up "inconspicuously as a German child." Samira has difficulty with orientation and identification; possibly this intelligent and alert child could have managed if she had not been trapped in the unconscious task of replacing the mother's dead siblings for the grandmother and perhaps for the mother herself. It may be that she is primarily supposed to replace the dead uncle, as the dead aunt has already been replaced by the now 14-year-old aunt. That this is the case is suggested by the confusion over her name from early on and by the gender-neutral first name chosen by her mother. The generational confusion is exacerbated by the sisterly relationship between the aunt and Samira. Samira's parents do not identify with their parental role, but live like other children in the extended family, so that the original family seems restored. Samira's mutistic behavior became conspicuous two years ago, namely at the vulnerable time when her aunt reached the age of the deceased uncle and the deceased aunt. Samira has to suppress her progressive impulses, as she experiences them as a threat to or betrayal of her family, and has a fear of impending misfortune, such as death, which had also befallen the aunt and the uncle. After about 30 sessions, during which communication was exclusively nonverbal, Samira begins exchanging her first words with the therapist. In the therapist's attempt to learn some Turkish words, she herself enters the role of "not being able to speak," feels insecure and even "alien." Who is speaking which language becomes blurred during the sessions. The therapist becomes worried that she is manipulating Samira into becoming a German child. In the course of treatment, Samira becomes able to detach herself from the different delegations. The treatment focusses on Samira's no longer seeing progressive impulses as a threat to or betrayal of her family and on her coming to experience that no misfortune will occur as she further develops, defines herself, and finds her own identity. Her parents, and especially her mother, had to be encouraged more clearly to assume the role of parents towards their daughter and clearly to convey the generational boundaries. At the examination for beginning school, Samira did not stand out as odd, she answered all questions fluently in German and was concurrently able to affirm her Turkish identity.

8.8 Information for the Diagnostic Assessment

As already described, temporally enduring intrapsychic conflicts contain conflicting perspectives of experience and action that the person cannot successfully integrate. This is also the reason why these conflicts are considered to be dysfunctional and not, say, conducive to development.

It is important in conducting the assessment that the examiner be clear about *everyday conflicts* not being the issue, since they are generally conducive to development and normative. Indeed, everyday conflicts between parents and children promote the development of autonomy and separation, especially during adolescence (Seiffge-Krenke, 1999).

Also important is that intrapsychic conflicts be distinguished from *severe forms of stress in life* that can affect children and adolescents. These sorts of stress include critical events in life such as the parents' separation, severe illness within the family, relocation, and migration (Perrez, 2004), but also traumas like maltreatment, abuse, and neglect (Egle et al., 2015). As is well known, children and adolescents seeking psychotherapeutic help have a high propensity for such severe burdens in life. Our classification scheme in Appendix B.6 distinguishes between current, severe stress in life, i.e., stress occurring within the six months preceding the interview, and stress occurring before this period. Current and severe stress in life can depress the structure, but possibly also even exacerbate conflicts, while the preceding, severe stress will more likely altogether lower the structural level.

In arriving at the diagnosis, the examiner should pay particular attention to the most important conflict (finding a focus of the conflict), which can provide information for proceeding with or planning the treatment. If, possibly due to structural deficits, no conflict has become clearly defined, but a conflict theme is noticeable, this fact may also be entered in the diagnostic documentation (see Appendix B.6).

Conflict

9. Third Axis: Structure

Mental structure is operationalized and assessed on the basis of children's and adolescents' observable behavior, on the basis of what they tell us about how they behave in play situations (symbolization), and on the basis of externally provided histories. Mental structure comprises individual structural abilities, summarized according to three dimensions in the previous versions of the OPD-CA (Arbeitskreis OPD-KJ, 2003, 2007) (see Table 1). The Assessment Sheet for Structure can be found in Appendix B.7.

Our experiences in training suggested a further differentiation of the structural dimensions in the OPD-CA-2, as shown in Table 2.

The OPD-CA-2 describes an additional dimension as compared to the OPD-CA (Arbeitskreis OPD-KJ, 2003, 2007). *Affect tolerance* has been added to the *Control* dimension, while *conflict resolution* (defence mechanisms) has been removed, being generally incorporated in the assessment of the structural level.

The dimension of self and object perception has been renamed *Identity*; the structural capabilities of *coherence* and *belonging* have been added. The ability to empathize has been moved to the *interpersonality* dimension (formerly communication skills).

The *interpersonality* dimension in the OPD-CA-2 now includes *fantasies* as the key element of internal communication. The aspects of *initiating emotional contact* and *reciprocity* have remained, while new additions include responsiveness to the affects of others (*affective experience*) and the *capacity to separate*.

The *attachment* dimension, represented in the old operationalization of mental structure merely by the capacity for internalized communication, comprises the aspects of *access to attachment representations*, *secure internal base*, the *capacity to be alone*, and the *use of attachment relationships*.

The assessment of the structure should always be resource-oriented and extend beyond the symptom, given the context-dependence of dysfunctional or functional modes of reaction. The assessment of the readiness to act should refer to the preceding six months and is related to the biographical context, in addition to the assessment of situational behavior within and outside the examined situation.

The four structural assessment dimensions are thus described in terms of certain abilities and assessed according to anchor-point descriptions for each level of integration. On the basis of these age-typical examples, which can serve as clinical illustrations, adjustments to an age-independent "structural scale" can be assessed and assigned to a structural level. The no longer primarily quantitative, but rather qualitative, criteria for assessing the structural level are the child's or adolescent's relation to reality, his/her contact with the external world, his/her accessibility during, e.g., impulsive outbreaks, the use of defence mechanisms (flexibility, functionality, variability, continuity), the predictability of his/her behavior, the emphatic possibility of understanding what the child or adolescent is doing, his/her premeditated nature and consciousness, his/her ability to recall, e.g., conflictual situations, his/her capacity for reflection, and his/her level of suffering.

Besides the four values of integration, namely 1 = *good integration,* 2 = *limited integration,* 3 = *low integration,* and 4 = *disintegration,* three intermediate values are possible (1.5; 2.5; 3.5).

In cases of doubt, (for example, when divergent structural levels become evident in the examination), assignment to a structural level is determined by including anamnestic data on the extent of the child's or adolescent's impairment under everyday conditions. The predominant source for the assessment (symbolization in play, interaction, history) can be stated in the assessment sheet (see Appendix B.7).

The following describes the individual structural abilities of the four dimensions *control, identity, interpersonality,* and *attachment* for each age group and operationalizes these capacities in terms of the four structural levels. For each structural ability, relative to the age of the child or adolescent, you will therefore find a description of what type of behavior and experience of that child or adolescent is to be expected on the individual structural levels (1 to 4). For the intermediate values you will not find any operationalizations; they are to be included if the child or the young person cannot be clearly assigned to the better or worse structure level or the child or adolescent oscillates between two structural levels.

In the following, you will find anchor-point descriptions for the respective structural abilities of the dimensions *control, identity, interpersonality,* and *attachment* according to the age group (1 to 3). You can document your assessments on the assessment sheets contained at the end of this book (see Appendix B and Appendix C).

9.1 Control

Clinical Anchor-Point Descriptions	
Control Dimension – Age Group 1 (3 to 5 Years)	
Structural Ability: *Impulse Control*	
Good integration	The child can express his/her own feelings and his/her need for regulation. With parental aid, the child can endure a delay of gratification. In behavior and expression, the child reacts in a neither over-regulated nor under-regulated way. He/she can break away from his/her fantasy play, if the demands of reality requires so and if the child is urged to do so. The child can more or less calmly endure a familiar situation of age-appropriate duration as the situation requires, often with the aid of an adult.
Limited integration	The child can register feelings to a limited extent within their emotional valence (good vs. bad) or describe them with appropriate, feeling-related actions ("I cry ..."). The child is only able to express his/her need for regulation unclearly, however. The child can endure delay of gratification only with assistance and only for a short period. Over-regulation or under-regulation may occur in the child's behavior, which remains externally controllable, however. The child has difficulty in detaching him-/herself from pretend play, and his/her aggressive affects seem partly aimless. The child can only calmly endure a familiar situation of age-appropriate duration with difficulty and as the situation requires.
Low integration	The child cannot consistently name or describe the emotional valence of his/her feelings and can express his/her need for control either unintelligibly or not at all. The child can hardly endure the delay of gratification, even if distracted. Over-regulation or under-regulation in behavior constantly occurs, and can be controlled only with difficulty. The child can break away from pretend play only with considerable effort, after intensive urging, and with

	prestructured transitions; aggressive affects then seem aimless and undirected. The child cannot calmly endure even familiar situations of age-appropriate duration, as befitting these situations.
Disintegration	The child cannot name or describe feelings or his/her need for regulation. He or she cannot endure the delay of gratification, even if distracted. Over-regulation or under-regulation occur regularly, without appearing to be controllable. The child can hardly break away from pretend play, even with considerable effort, after intensive urging, and with pre-structured transitions. Aggressive affects surface aimlessly, without direction, and very vehemently. The child cannot even begin to enter familiar situations of age-appropriate duration.

Structural Ability: *Affect Tolerance*

Good integration	The child can endure negative affects of fear, anger, and grief in appropriate intensities. The child can express different sides of his/her feelings in play and can make transitions. While the child endures the ambivalence and does not oscillate back and forth in his/her emotional state, he/she still does not remain rigidly fixed in a single mood.
Limited integration	The child can endure negative affects only with difficulty and such affects linked to the situation very quickly turn into nonplayful actions. The child tends to deny the existence of ambivalent feelings, or rapid changes in feelings occur. The child manages better with outside assistance, which he/she accepts only from certain, very well-known people, however.
Low integration	The child can hardly endure negative affects, which regularly and abruptly come to the surface, especially in unfamiliar situations. The child cannot articulate affects nor express them through play, but primarily acts them out in order to rid him-/herself of them. Different feelings then appear merely juxtaposed and continually alternate without transitions.
Disintegration	Negative affects cannot be endured and surface abruptly and usually without an object in undirected behavior. They appear in an undifferentiated manner as intense excitement or as mental freezing. Expression seems wholly inappropriate, bizarre, or out of place.

Structural Ability: *Controlling Instances*	
Good integration	The child can distinguish between what is permitted and what is forbidden. Rules are adhered to, at least in the presence of authority figures, but, alone or among other children, the child may occasionally transgress rules, with these transgressions being retrospectively acknowledged, however. The child generally endeavors to comply with norms and rules. Noncompliance leads to unpleasant feelings and often to attempts to make amends.
Limited integration	The child knows his/her parents' norms and rules and also generally endeavors to comply with them. The child is primarily geared to satisfying his/her needs, however. The child suspends rules conflicting with his/her own desires, without developing a bad conscience. Rules and norms are often transgressed even in the presence of authority figures. Noncompliance then rarely leads to attempts to make amends.
Low integration	The child seems to have little understanding of rules and prohibitions, and can merely follow rules in the given situation and in the short term, when expressly instructed to do so, but this compliance does not last. The child becomes extremely upset if external demands conflict with his/her own wants. Even if his or her behavior harms other people, the child does not feel bad, appearing not to have any sense of guilt.
Disintegration	The child acts solely according to his or her own standards and can hardly be controlled through external demands. The child reacts indiscriminately and unpredictably, without recourse to internal or external controlling instances.
Structural Ability: *Self-Worth Regulation*	
Good integration	After having been criticized or experiencing failure, the child finds his/her own way to feel comfortable again. While the child reacts to criticism and slights by feeling unwell, he/she also endeavors to make a good impression again. While occasionally the child requires his/her parents' temporary aid in restoring his balance, he/she succeeds in doing so regularly and dependably.
Limited integration	The child reacts to criticism or slights with withdrawal or aggression, while repeatedly depending on external affirmation. The child's sense of self-worth is clearly unstable and susceptible to interference, and capriciously affects his/her behavior. The child rarely endeavors to restore a positive impression following criticism. Instead, he/she tends to hide or intensively defend him-/herself for reasons of shame.

Low integration	Even in the absence of criticism and slights, the child reacts to experiences of failure with withdrawal or aggression. Even regular external affirmation has an effect, if at all positive, only very briefly. Self-worth is at a continually low level. Criticism and slights often lead to belittling or insulting others. Feelings of shame cannot be endured.
Disintegration	The child is incapable of self-regulation and can be controlled only with difficulty even externally. The child's experiences changeable states is irrespective of praise or criticism, possibly in conjunction with behavior and experiences that are babyish and regressive or out of touch with the real world and delusional. Occasionally incomprehensible freezing-up may also occur.

Control Dimension – Age Group 2 (6 to 12 Years)

Structural Ability: Impulse Control

Good integration	The child can control and verbally communicate feelings, in particular in stressful conflicts. The conflicts are tied to persons or objects. With the aid of his/her parents, the child can distance him-/herself from these conflicts and defer gratification (the child has a tolerance of frustration). The child reacts in neither an over-regulated nor an under-regulated way. The child can disengage from playful, aggressive activity (childish scuffling) if the general situation requires doing so. Aggressive affects do not continue aimlessly and devoid of purpose. The child can endure a familiar situation (e.g., a class period) from beginning to end more or less calmly and as befitting the situation. The child can handle delayed gratification.
Limited integration	In stressful situations, the child cannot fall back on controlling and regulating abilities which are otherwise at his/her disposal; intensive outside support is then necessary. Impulsive behavior (unrest, disruptions, talking out of turn) or over-regulated modes of behavior may also arise in situations familiar to the child (e.g., school lessons). Delay of gratification is often hard to endure.
Low integration	In unstructured or threatening situations the child "loses it," having no impulse control and reacts with behavior destructive to him-/herself and to others. Alternatively, the child may exhibit extreme over-regulation to prevent eruptions of impulses. Extremely over-regulated or under-regulated behavior may also regularly occur in situations familiar to the child, such as school lessons. The child cannot endure

	delay of gratification. Behavior is geared to the immediate satisfaction of desires.
Disintegration	The child is not able to control his/her impulses in any context (kindergarten, school, peer group, family), and repeatedly shows, also in familiar situations, a lack of impulse control that is mostly not understandable from the outside and that is difficult for the child to reflect on afterwards.
Structural Ability: *Affect Tolerance*	
Good integration	The child can perceive and endure negative affects of fear, anger, and grief. The child can express different aspects of his/her feelings and achieves a balance, with smooth transitions between both sides of his/her ambivalence. While the child is labile in his/her emotional state, he/she does not remain frozen in a single mood.
Limited integration	Negative affects tied to the given situation are uncontrollable for the child and occasionally break forth in actions. The child has difficulty enduring ambivalent feelings and tends to deny their existence, or rapid changes in feelings occur. Structuring by other persons is partly possible, or it is averted.
Low integration	Negative affects break through spontaneously and uncontrollably, often in unstructured situations. Affects cannot be articulated by the child and are primarily acted out (body, behavior). Feelings are haphazardly juxtaposed and continually alternate with one another.
Disintegration	Negative affects erupt unexpectedly and possibly unrelated to anything, the child becoming agitated or freezing up. They seem inappropriate, bizarre, or out of place.
Structural Ability: *Controlling Instances*	
Good integration	The child knows what is allowed and what is forbidden. It is important for the child to follow the norms and rules provided by his/her parents. If the child fails to do so, perhaps because he/she allows him-/herself to be led astray by his/her peers, he/she feels bad. The child sees through the harmful consequences of his/her own actions for others, even if often retrospectively. The child can admit his/her mistakes.
Limited integration	The child lets him-/herself be governed by his/her desires and needs, especially when confronted with difficult and stressful situations. Parents are at best partially perceived in their supportive role. The child knows his/her parents' norms and rules and also generally endeavors to comply

	with them. On the other hand, the child disobeys rules that greatly conflict with his/her own desires, without developing a bad conscience. The child lays the blame for some of his/her mistakes on other people, in order to evade negative consequences.
Low integration	Confronted with demands and stress, the child does not have recourse to any controlling instances. The child becomes extremely upset and often feels badly treated. The parents' norms and rules have no priority for the child, who primarily acts according to his/her own (need-oriented) standards, that may be also outside the normal standards. Even when his/her behavior harms others, the child feels no remorse, but always places the blame on others or on the outside world.
Disintegration	The child cannot distinguish between a rigid controlling instance which is externally determined and his/her own ideas, or he/she rigidly follows external commands.

Structural Ability: *Self-Worth Regulation*

Good integration	After having been critisized or experiencing failure, the child finds his/her own way to feel comfortable again. The child can tolerate, without undergoing a significant crisis, that someone from his/her social surroundings does not share his/her positive self-concept. The child can restore his/her equilibrium with the aid of his/her parents. or through other activities.
Limited integration	The child depends on external positive affirmation. The child reacts violently to criticism and slights – with withdrawal, aggression, or cockiness. His/her self-worth is easily disrupted, which can negatively affect his/her coping with everyday life (school performance, contact behavior).
Low integration	Self-worth is constantly questioned; coherence is lacking. Criticism and slights often lead to belittling others or the child him-/herself. In doing so, the child often projects his/her own state onto others.
Disintegration	The child is incapable of self-regulation. Irrespective of praise or criticism, the child often changes states that may be accompanied by experiences and behavior that are babyish, regressive, cocky, removed from reality, or delusional in character, or the child may end up in incomprehensibly rigid states.

Control Dimension – Age Group 3 (13 to 18 Years)	
Structural Ability: *Impulse Control*	
Good integration	The adolescent can make use of his/her impulses, for instance in connection with aggression, regulate his/her relationships with him-/herself and with others. Through this regulation, the adolescent can avoid over-regulation (e.g., rigid behavior) and, in particular, under-regulation (e.g., loss of impulse control). The adolescent can endure delay of gratification. Aggressive or sexual impulses, and the longing for material goods often have the character of needing immediate satisfaction, but can often be deferred owing to values or moral judgments.
Limited integration	Depending on the situation, the adolescent reacts with loss of impulse control or over-regulation. The exorbitant superego is either highly critical or selectively shut off. Following loss of impulse control, the superego can regulate itself again, once the adolescent is able to consider the situation objectively. His/her emotional flexibility is limited.
Low integration	The adolescent enters into exceptional states in which he/she can no longer control his/her impulses and reacts with self-destructive modes of behavior or destructive modes directed towards others. Sexualization in compensation for the lack of relationships, inadequate control of the longing for material goods linked to addictive behavior, and perverse problem solving are observed. The capacity for deferment and sublimation is limited, resulting in states with a pronounced loss of control in delinquent behavior or in the abuse of alcohol and drugs.
Disintegration	Trivial matters can lead to violent loss of impulse control or to uncontrollable and destructive hatred, accompanied by a loss of reality or freezing or dissociation.
Structural Ability: *Affect Tolerance*	
Good integration	The adolescent can master negative affects through defense mechanisms (criticism, sarcasm, rationalization). He/she can tolerate ambivalence, i.e., recognise ambivalence within him-/herself and consciously experience, communicate, and balance this ambivalence. Intense, ambivalent affects may also be experienced and expressed.
Limited integration	Affects, especially negative affects, are for the most part controllable, but may erupt in stressful situations. Defense mechanisms like reaction formation, isolation, and denial

	occur in part. Distancing from affects is possible to a limited extent; it is often successful through external structuring. The adolescent finds it difficult to tolerate intense, negative affects, and prefers dealing with them through over-regulation.
Low integration	Affects, especially negative affects, erupt spontaneously, uncontrollably and violently. Splitting tendencies become evident. Negative affects can flood the adolescent and become so unendurable as to trigger impulsive behavior. The other person is perceived only in his/her positive or negative aspects. Under structured conditions affects cannot be articulated and are unavailable.
Disintegration	Incommensurate to the situation, affects erupt and can trigger a highly agitated state, so that the adolescent responds reactively with counter-measures or rigidly fends them off. The affects are not related to the external conditions and thus seem rather inappropriate and out of place.
Structural Ability: *Controlling Instances*	
Good integration	The adolescent can readily understand that his/her desires conflict with other people and, in cases of conflict, seeks compromises (see also the assessment of empathy in the sense of perceiving the needs of others). The complexity of some moral issues is perceived within a socially constructed framework, general norms are increasingly examined by the individual, and personally understandable decisions are made under certain circumstances.
Limited integration	The adolescent is partly able to adopt different points of views, but lacks the ability in stressful moments and situations of conflict to fall back on these perspectives. He/she then loses sight of the other person. The satisfaction of egoistic needs has priority.
Low integration	Through the disregard for his/her interests, the adolescent's loses the ability to control his/her behavior and becomes caught up in states that are no longer appropriate to the original situation. He/she is generally able to check reality, however.
Disintegration	Eruptions of physical urges can occur up to the point of psychotic excitation, possibly irrespective of the external situation. The adolescent has an inadequate understanding of the initiation of his/her own actions.

Structural Ability: *Self-Worth Regulation*	
Good integration	The adolescent can maintain positive self-esteem in the face of conflictual limitations. The adolescent finds ways to regain his/her positive self-esteem when experiencing criticism.
Limited integration	In stressful situations, the adolescent falls back on configurations of an aggrandized self or reacts with withdrawal. This condition is manifested by sensitivity, self-aggrandizement, self-deprecation, or self-punishment and withdrawal. These modes of reaction occur in stressful situations and can be qualified. While the adolescent's self-esteem is not continually lowered, it is dependent on the affirmation of others.
Low integration	The adolescent constantly questions his/her sense of self-worth and his/her sense of self, with a lack of coherence. He/she oscillates between self-deprecation and the deprecation of others. He/she shows sensitivity to slights, has unrealistic ideas of grandeur, exhibits shame, disgust with him-/herself, debasement, and irritability, breaks off relationships, and is incapable of accepting his/her own limits.
Disintegration	The adolescent has no sense of self. A rigid or fragmentary state exists, as is expressed in considerable distortions of his/her own self-judgement (grandiosity or chronically low self-esteem), or distorted perceptions of reality.

9.2 Identity

Clinical Anchor-Point Descriptions	
Identity Dimension – Age Group 1 (3 to 5 Years)	
Structural Ability: *Coherence*	
Good integration	The child can persistently perceive him-/herself as a whole person in different situations and emotional states. The child also experiences different feelings and needs in specific situations as belonging to him-/herself and is able to express this fact symbolically (through play, language, etc.).
Limited integration	The child can perceive him-/herself as a whole person in different situations and emotional states. This condition is susceptible to stress and not always stable, however. The child frequently experiences different feelings and needs in specific situations, but not always as belonging to him-/herself, so that the capacity for symbolic expression (play,

	language) may be limited. Clinically, this is manifested by contradictory or ambivalent behavior and by easily being susceptible to influence. Support from others has a positive effect, however.
Low integration	The child is hardly recognisable as his/her own person, he/she is highly suggestible and exhibits few character traits of his/her own, as is shown by his/her easily influenceable behavior. There is little differentiation between him-/herself and others. Intrinsic motivation is hardly discernible and a symbolic representation of his/her own person seems hardly possible. The child appears barely independent.
Disintegration	There exists no stable, enduring self-image. The child appears as a wholly different person depending on the situation. He/she has no internal image of who he/she really is.
Structural Ability: *Self-Experience*	
Good integration	The child can describe his/her own person in terms of external variables (appearance, clothing, sexual characteristics), but they are also starting to describe skills (e.g., in sports). Ideas about his/her own person are partly governed by desires. The child is sure about being a boy or a girl. The child can describe him-/herself in terms of positive as well as negative qualities. The child experiences him-/herself as effective in action and takes pleasure in his/her activity. Feelings of guilt and of shame are discernible.
Limited integration	The child can attribute characteristics and abilities to him-/herself, but dependent on the situational aspects. The child experiences shame and guilt as well as pride, while appearing to be very dependent on external influences. The child appears affirmed or offended very quickly and in an exaggerated way. In the child's playful representation of and coping with experiential states in an "as if" mode, rather rigid patterns of behavior are discernible that become more relaxed with the participation and support of an adult.
Low integration	The child succeeds in describing him-/herself only in terms of external characteristics and preferred activities (e.g., playing football) and exhibits greatly limited continuity. Others have difficulty forming a coherent picture of the child's emotional state and self-esteem. Self-limits appear blurred, and no sense of self-effectiveness can be discerned. Negative emotional states are projected externally and can, if at all, be recalled as one's own only after the fact and with assistance. "As if" situations unsettle the child instead of being experienced as fun.

Disintegration	Self-description is not possible or understandable; the child lacks even a rudimentary image of his/her own person. Feelings and expressions of emotions often appear inappropriate in a negative way and detached from the situation. The child appears not to experience self-limits or self-effectiveness.

Structural Ability: *Self–Object Differentiation*

Good integration	The child experiences him-/herself as distinct from other people and can recognize and tolerate discrepancies emerging between his/her own and other people's interests and desires. The child can also recognize that his/her feelings differ from others' in the same situation. The child has an understanding of relations of ownership ("mine" and "yours"). This capability need not be consistently stable and may especially be impaired regarding the child's closest attachment figure. In play and in conversation, the child can perceive his/her own role and that of the examiner, and also act out other roles.
Limited integration	The child has difficulty in ascribing the initiation of actions, intentions, and impulses to him-/herself or to others. Discrepancies emerging between his/her own and others' interests and desires are hardly tolerated and partially denied. The child's understanding of relations of ownership ("mine" and "yours") seems limited and the boundaries appear fluid during play. The child's ability to differentiate improves significantly through the directive and clarifying interventions of trusted others, however.
Low integration	The child cannot recognize his/her initiation of actions, intentions, and impulses, and ascribes it all to the outside world. The child does not discern discrepancies between his/her own and others' interests and desires, and his/her perception of others is governed by his/her own interests and is often lost through projections and polarizations. The child has no understanding of ownership relations ("mine" and "yours"), and even the boundaries during play become blurred. The child often seems beside him-/herself, but he/she does retain contact with the external world, which considerably limits his/her development of autonomy.
Disintegration	There exists a serious disorder, with emotional outbursts, loss of reality, and confusion over the initiation of impulses, thoughts, and needs. The child has no recollection of these states, and does not relate them to experience in its continuity. The reasons for such outbursts are difficult to grasp. The child cannot develop and preserve any level of autonomy appropriate for his/her age.

Structural Ability: *Object Perception*	
Good integration	The child is able to view the examiner as an individual person. The other person is not only an object satisfying needs, but is also differentiated. The child can recognize that objects are not purely good or purely evil, and that he/she can turn to someone after verifying their trustworthiness. The child noticeably endeavors constantly to test objects. Instead of a patterned, stereotypical attitude towards objects, the child maintains a differentiated attitude, depending on the object.
Limited integration	Under stress (physical discomfort, disappointment, or slights) the child has a limited perception of the other person's role and function. The child shows little interest in developing a picture of the other through testing, but appears simply to accept what is immediately visible. Interactive play seems a bit rigid; the child has difficulty taking up the other person's ideas for play.
Low integration	Gratification of needs clearly has priority, with the child not distinguishing between familiar persons and strangers. Play is stereotyped, with no interest in including others or taking up the other person's ideas. The child repeatedly exhibits states (irritations in self-worth regulation, bad moods) in which his/her comprehension of whole objects fails. Other people, even familiar persons, are then experienced as threatening and bad.
Disintegration	Comprehension of whole objects is not possible. The child's view of others is guided only by the success ("good") and failure ("bad") of the gratification of his/her needs. Contact with other people is oppressive, or there is no apparent interest in others. It doesn't seem to make a difference about who the other person is.
Structural Ability: *Belonging*	
Good integration	The child feels he/she belongs to the *peer group* with whom he/she spends time outside of the family (kindergarten, day nursery, day care family, etc.), irrespective of gender. The child can respond to offers of interaction and join in play (e.g., role-playing games), and need not always "dictate" what is to be done. The child is regularly invited to birthday parties, and others accept his/her return invitations. Towards the end of this age range (transition to primary school), the child is already able to distinguish clearly between good friends and casual acquaintances.

	The child has a sense of belonging to the *ethnic* group in which he/she is growing up, and accepts its child rearing practices, its language, culture, and rituals, its nonverbal forms of communication and its specific patterns of interaction (facial expressions, gestures). The child may also approve and enjoy rituals of the new culture (such as eating habits, birthday parties, and Christmas carols), without falling into conflict. Towards the end of this age range (transition to primary school), the child can increasingly reconcile the two systems of reference.
Limited integration	The child often feels uncomfortable in the *peer group* with whom he/she spends time outside of the family (kindergarten, day nursery, day care family, etc.), regardless of gender. Offers of interaction are repeatedly rejected or the child only joins in play (as in role-playing games) if he/she can "dictate" what is to be done. The child is often not invited to birthday celebrations, and other children do not always accept his/her invitations in return. Towards the end of this age range (transition to primary school), the child cannot reliably distinguish between good friends and casual acquaintances. The child has only a limited sense of belonging to the *ethnic* group in which he/she is growing up, or he/she feels he/she belongs exclusively to this group. The child's sense of belonging is fragile and prone to disruption. In his/her experience, the child seems to switch back and forth between groups without being able to establish a connection. The change between the two cultures (bi-cultural identity) is problematic or managed only with difficulty.
Low integration	The child is not well integrated in the peer group with whom he/she spends time outside of the family (kindergarten, day nursery, day care family, etc.), regardless of gender. Only few offers of interaction come from other children; what offers there are, are either declined or dominated by the child. The child is only rarely invited to birthday parties, and other children seldom accept return invitations. Towards the end of this age range (transition to primary school) the child has had little opportunity to experience friendships. Ethnic belongingness: the child does not cope with the cultural differences successfully or does so only inadequately; one of the two cultures is rejected and devalued, the other over idealized. Recognition of the values of the other culture or religion is hardly achieved, even with outside support.

Structure

Disintegration	The child is not integrated in the *peer group* with whom he/she spends time outside of the family (kindergarten, day nursery, day care family, etc.), and relationships do not succeed, regardless of gender. There are no offers of interaction as the child is known to immediately spoil the play by strongly dominating the situation. The child is not invited to birthday parties or to games, and children do not accept his/her return invitations. Towards the end of this age range (transition to primary school), the child has no friends and is socially isolated. *Ethnic belongingness:* Complete rejection of the child's original culture or the culture in which the child is living. No acknowledgement of external reality regarding norms, rules, or regulations. Culture or religion is used as an excuse to ignore prescribed standards.

Identity Dimension – Age Group 2 (6 to 12 Years)	
Structural Ability: *Coherence*	
Good integration	The child can persistently perceive him-/herself as a whole person in different situations and emotional states. The child also experiences various feelings and needs in specific situations as belonging to him-/herself and is able to express this in a symbolical way (through play, language, etc.). The child has a stable internal image of him-/herself and others, and consequently clearly distinguishes him-/herself from others without feeling lonely.
Limited integration	The child is not consistently perceivable as his/her own person in difficult situations or crises. The child's internal (mental) representation of him-/herself and others is only partially stable and is lost under stress, as is clinically manifested in contradictory or ambivalent behavior and in susceptibility to influence. However, the child can recognize and remedy this deficit with aid from others or in noncritical situations.
Low integration	The child is hardly recognizable as his/her own person, is highly suggestible, and exhibits few personality traits of his/her own. He/she clinically manifests this deficit by chameleon-like behavior with little differentiation between him-/herself and others. The child shows little willingness to exert him-/herself cognitively or motivationally, and his/her behavior is accompanied by superficial and diffuse mental representations of him-/herself and of others.

Disintegration	The child's mental representation of him-/herself and of others hardly exists or is totally absent (identity diffusion). The child has a painful sense of incoherence, clinically manifested by, for example, his/her playing a role in order to fulfil the supposed expectations and desires of others in his/her environment, with no internal image existing as to who he/she really is.

Structural Ability: *Self-Perception*

Good integration	In the child's description of him-/herself, internal, more detailed attributions (skills, qualities) play a greater role, leading to a more accurate idea about him-/herself, which the child is also able to articulate verbally. The child perceives and discernibly examines how he/she appears and is perceived by others. The child is secure in his/her individuality. He/she can distinguish between feelings and the expressions of feelings. The child can also experience and describe different emotional states as belonging to him-/herself. The child can behave "as if" (especially discernible in play) and can talk about it. Thus, humour and lies are possible.
Limited integration	The child attributes to him-/herself qualities and abilities in a more differentiated form, but these attributions are liable to disturbances depending on the (conflictual) situation and theme. The child reacts to compliments with an unrealistic sense of importance, and, on the other hand, is very touchy in his/her sense of self and deprecates him-/herself. The child's sense of self-assuredness can be restored through affirmation and appreciative support. Negatively tinged emotional states like anxiety, grief, or anger tend to be blocked, but can afterwards be integrated through external support. In the child's playful handling of experiential states in an "as if" mode, rather rigid patterns of behavior are discernible; his/her ability to play improves if an adult participates.
Low integration	The child shows no continuity in his/her self-attributions of qualities and abilities, which tend to vary according to his/her states of self. He/she projects negative emotional states onto the outside world and can, if at all, recall them as belonging to him-/herself only afterwards and with assistance. Handling "as if" situations unsettles the child. Humour and other self-distancing processes are clearly impeded.
Disintegration	The child's description of him-/herself cannot be followed and yields no coherent picture of his/her own individuality. Feelings and their expressions do not seem authentic.

Structure

Structural Ability: *Self–Object Differentiation*	
Good integration	In play and in conversation, the child can perceive his/her own role and that of the examiner. The child shapes his/her social roles in the deliberate imitation of and reliance on social role models. The child can see that there exist other interests and motivations, and can attune them both to adults and to peers. The child is increasingly able to discern conflicts of interest and then to negotiate. The child can flexibly move back and forth between the level of the "as if" (in play and in conversation) and that of relationship.
Limited integration	The self–object differentiation becomes blurred if the child does not view the actual presence of and attention from others as a given or cannot him-/herself establish this fact. In play, the child shows a strong tendency to dominate and a striving for superiority, with rigidity in the ascription and development of roles. Coordination with the interests and motivations of others often fails, but is possible with the support of adults.
Low integration	The child repeatedly exhibits states in which self–object differentiation becomes blurred and the perception of other people is governed by his/her own interests and gets lost due to projections and polarizations. Reactions seem inappropriate given the occasion and are not age-appropriate. While the child often seems beside him-/herself, he/she retains contact with the outside world. While the child can recall such states, he/she has no emotional connection to them, which significantly hinders the development of autonomy.
Disintegration	Frequent losses of narcissistic balance with confusion over who is initiating actions and impulses. The child seems markedly limited in his/her development and preservation of autonomy. The child is unable to perceive and to handle conflicts of interest and motivation.
Structural Ability: *Object Perception*	
Good integration	The child is consistently able to recognize others in his/her function and as representing a particular social role. There exists a willingness to deal with the viewpoints of others. Towards adults and peers there is a gradation of intimacy (strangers – acquaintances – friends).
Limited integration	The child's perception of others in their functions and roles is limited given the situation (relative to conflict and issue), but can be restored through support. In interactions with

	peers, the child manifests a limited ability to deal with others' points of view, making the ability to form relationships fragile and prone to disruption. Recognition of the graduation of intimacy succeeds with support.
Low integration	The comprehension of whole objects repeatedly breaks down. The experience and recognition of the other in various functional and role-related aspects shows no consistency, and can change abruptly. Hostile projections then prevail. The reasons for such outbursts are difficult to comprehend. The sense of connectedness, even to persons close to the child, can abruptly cease.
Disintegration	The experience of objects is governed by the child's own needs, and a comprehensive perception of other people in their different aspects is not available. The child seems to be in contact with objects in an arbitrary and chaotic manner. Extreme closeness or distancing can be observed.

Structural Ability: *Belonging*

Good integration	The child feels he/she belongs to the *peer group* with whom he/she spends time outside of the family (school, after-school care, sports club), but in an increasingly gender-dependent way (same sex). The child can respond to offers of interaction, join in play, and usually keep to the rules of the game, or at least understand them well, and does not always have to "dictate" things. The child is invited regularly to birthday parties or games, and the other children accept his/her return invitations. Towards the end of this age range (transition to secondary school), the child has steadfast friends who are not easily replaceable and with whom he/she exchanges confidentialities. The child has a sense of belonging to the *ethnic* group in which he/she is growing up, and accepts its child-rearing practices, its language, its culture, its nonverbal forms of communication, and its specific patterns of interaction (facial expressions, gestures). The child also has a secure sense of belonging to the community or nation in which he/she lives. Shifting between the two identities (bi-cultural identity) is possible without major problems.
Limited integration	The child has only a partial sense of belonging to the *peer group* with whom he/she spends time outside of the family (school, after-school care, sports club). Relationships with the same gender in particular often do not succeed. The child can respond to offers of interaction only to a limited extent, as he/she often does not keep the rules of play, does

Structure

	not reliably understand them, or always wants to "dictate" things. The child is often not invited to birthday parties or to games, and other children often do not accept his/her return invitations. Towards the end of this age range (transition to secondary school), the child has few or frequently changing friends who are easily replaceable and with whom a confidential relationship rarely exists. *Ethnic belongingness:* The child has only a limited sense of belonging to the ethnic group in which he/she is growing up, or feels he/she belongs exclusively to that group; the practices of upbringing as well as the language, culture, non-verbal communication, and specific patterns of interaction (facial expressions, gestures) are not or only partly known and are rejected or over-idealised. Moreover, the child has no secure sense of belonging to the community or nation in which he/she lives. The shift between the two identities (bi-cultural identity) is problematic or managed only with difficulty. External symbols can have an identity-establishing function (headscarf, dietary rules, etc.), which may be flexibly handled depending on the situation.
Low integration	The child is not well integrated in the *peer group* with whom he/she spends time outside of the family (school, after-school care, sports club), and relationships neither with the same-sex nor the opposite-sex generally succeed. Offers of interaction, if they exist at all, are not recognized or accepted, or they are immediately undermined by a strong domination of the situation. The child is very rarely invited to birthday parties or to games, or invited only at his/her parents' instigation, and the other children often do not accept his/her return invitations. Towards the end of this age range (transition to secondary school), the child has no steadfast friends or constantly changing acquaintances of short duration and who are easily replaced. *Ethnic belongingness:* The shift between the different cultures is not successful or is only inadequate; one of the two cultures is rejected and devalued, the other overly idealized. Recognition of the values of the other culture or religion is hardly possible, even with outside support. External symbols have a strong identity-establishing character (e.g., headscarf, dietary rules, etc.), which may not be handled flexibly in a given situation.
Disintegration	The child is not integrated in the *peer group* with whom he/she spends time outside of the family (school, after-school care, sports club), and relationships neither with the same-sex nor with the opposite-sex succeed. There are no offers

of interaction, the child is never invited to birthday parties or to games, and the other children do not accept his/her return invitations. Towards the end of this age range (transition to secondary school), the child has no friends and is socially isolated.

Ethnic belongingness: Complete rejection of the original culture or the culture in which the child is living. No acknowledgement of external reality regarding norms, rules, or regulations. Culture or religion are used as an excuse to ignore prescribed standards.

Identity Dimension – Age Group 3 (13 to 18 Years)	
Structural Ability: *Coherence*	
Good integration	The adolescent is consistently able to experience him-/herself as a whole person across different emotional states and contexts of life. The adolescent can also integrate conflicting feelings, desires, and ideas, regardless of the situation. The feeling of coherence endures and is context independent; it can be expressed in a well-considered and symbolic way. The adolescent has a stable internal image of him-/herself and of others. The adolescent is accordingly clearly distinct from others without being lonely.
Limited integration	In situations of crisis (disputes with peers, physical changes, first intimate encounters, development of autonomy, etc.), the adolescent has problems consistently perceiving him-/herself as his/her own person. The adolescent's internal (mental) representation of him-/herself and others is only partially stable and gets lost under stress (identity crisis), as is clinically manifested in contradictory or ambivalent behavior and in his/her susceptibility to influence. However, the adolescent can recognize and remedy this deficit with aid from others or in noncritical situations.
Low integration	The adolescent is hardly recognizable as his/her own person, is highly suggestible, and shows few personality characteristics of his/her own in distinction from other persons. This deficit is clinically manifested by chameleon-like behavior, with little differentiation between him-/herself and others, a so-called "as-if personality." The adolescent's mental representation of him-/herself and others is barely integrated or even not at all, as is clinically manifested by superficial and diffuse descriptions of him-/herself and others (identity diffusion) and which leads to a painful sense of incoherence.

Disintegration	The adolescent is persistently unable to describe him-/herself, and there is a deficit in goals, values, and standards, an inability to retain relationships, or an over-identification with groups and their leaders. This is clinically manifested by a high risk of his/her developing problems in school, with peers, in the family, and in any other interpersonal relationship. The adolescent behaves erratically and his/her moods are difficult or impossible to follow.

Structural Ability: *Self-Perception*

Good integration	Self-description succeeds in terms of authentic and differentiable personal qualities (such as body image, gender identity, social status, personal abilities and their limits), and understandable collective values (political opinions, opinions about the environment). The adolescent can distinguish between feelings and the expressions of feelings. He/she can also experience and describe different emotional states as belonging to him-/herself. A sense of identity persists across different emotional states and different stages of development (ego activity, coherence, consistency, distinctness, vitality). The adolescent has a basic idea of his/her self-effectiveness.
Limited integration	Self-description requires confirming feedback from the outside world. The adolescent's narcissistic equilibrium can be jeopardized depending on the situation. Frustration scenarios are definable (neurotic conflicts). Collective values and opinions seem rigid or blurred. Negative emotional states limit feelings of autonomy, resulting in greater withdrawal or an inflated need for affirmation. The adolescent retains his/her sense of identity.
Low integration	Self-description in terms of personal qualities is undifferentiated and fluctuates between exaggeration and self-deprecation. Confirmatory or corrective feedback from the outside has little effect. Self-worth regulation is unstable, with rigid functional patterns. Setbacks in self-perception are triggered for no apparent reason and without relation to the given situation. The adolescent is highly sensitive to slights. Collective values and norms can be abruptly thrown out. His/her sense of identity is incoherent.
Disintegration	Self-description is confused. Self-perception lacks coherence.

Structural Ability: Self–Object Differentiation	
Good integration	The adolescent generally succeeds in ascribing affects, impulses or thoughts either to him-/herself or to others. The adolescent can increasingly delimitate him-/herself from familial frameworks, recognize membership in his/her peer group as being important and accept this membership. Important relationships are preserved and increasingly redefined. Transient polarizations triggered by conflicts can arise. The adolescent can recognise that he/she has other interests and motives relative to other important figures and can check these interests and motives against theirs. The adolescent is increasingly able to recognize conflicts of interest.
Limited integration	Depending on the given subject or situation, the adolescent has a limited ability to ascribe affects, impulses, and thoughts to him-/herself or to others. Delimitation from the familial framework is often unsuccessful, as is manifested in recurring disputes standing in the way of solutions and considerably impeding steps towards detachment. The images of the parents remain within a childish, dyadically oriented horizon of expectations. Illness can occur frequently. Membership in the peer group is unstable; feeling at one with others is difficult.
	Depending on the issue and situation, other adolescents' views, their interests and motives cause the adolescent to lose his/her own interests and motives as well as his/her sense of independence. He/she is able to realize this afterwards.
Low integration	The ascription of affects, impulses, and thoughts to him-/herself or to others repeatedly becomes confused, and becomes manifest in polarizations, splitting, projections and projective identifications. Connections to situations cannot be discerned, but a sense of reality does remain. Delimitation from the familial framework is consistently polarizing. The demand for the gratification of infantile needs coexists in unrelated form with a significantly reduced libidinous cathexis of the parents. Confrontation with distortions of reality perception improves the self–object differentiation. The adolescent can recall different self-states, but cannot organize them according to experiences (emotionally). The relationship to the peer group is fragile according to the different self-states.
Disintegration	The self–object differentiation is consistently confused and dissociative. Impulsive behavior like suddenly breaking off contact (freezing reactions) are incomprehensible and

	cannot be recalled. The adolescent can no longer distinguish what is to be ascribed to him-/herself and what to others.
Structural Ability: *Object Perception*	
Good integration	The adolescent is consistently able to perceive the other as a whole person in his/her different aspects and roles. The adolescent recognizes the other's independence. There is a willingness to deal with the other's point of view. He/she feels connected to other people. The pressure of conflicts gives rise to minor projective distortions. Towards adults and peers there exists a gradation of closeness (adult/friend/acquaintance/stranger). In his/her descriptions, the adolescent is able to bring to life persons close to him/her. The adolescent can empathize with and understand the other's experiential world as an independent perspective. Internalization of objects is stable, absences can be endured, and relatedness is preserved.
Limited integration	The adolescent fluctuates in his/her ability to perceive the other as a whole person representing a particular role. The willingness to deal with the perspectives of others is limited, especially if conflict themes or specific transference triggers are present in the given situation. These situations usually involve three people. The adolescent can make people close to him/her come alive in his/her descriptions, even if they are a bit one-sided. The adolescent is receptive to corrective comments. Object constancy is fragile, the adolescent feels easily rejected and slighted, experiences him-/herself as depending on others or overcomes the fear of dependence counter-phobically.
Low integration	The adolescent's perception of others is determined by his/her own needs, which, in turn, are governed by dual (early childhood) relationship needs. This perception is distorted by projections and projective identifications, which overlay the ability to recognize others in their various aspects, i.e., as whole persons, and in their autonomy. The adolescent describes persons close to him/her in an unrealistically one-sided way, according to his/her own needs. He/she has few bonds with other people. A gradation of closeness (friend/acquaintance/stranger) is not accompanied by any understandable and realistic assessment. The adolescent is hardly open to corrections. Contact with the outside world is retained, however. Adults are recognized (generational boundaries) only after clear-cut intervention by an adult other. Confrontation with the distorted object perception is accepted, but not placed in a remembrable relationship with experienced ego states.

Disintegration	The description of the other is empty and incomprehensible, also threatening and disconcerting, wholly dominated by the adolescent's own neediness, sometimes rigidly one-sided (good vs. evil), and sometimes blurred. A confrontation with distorted object perception is ineffectual. The sense of reality is seriously disturbed both in terms of quality and quantity.
Structural Ability: *Belonging*	
Good integration	The adolescent feels he/she belongs to the *peer group* with whom he/she spends time with outside the family (school, sports club, recreation), and increasingly so regardless of gender, with same-sex friendships having an identity-establishing role (friends as "aid workers," Seiffge-Krenke & Seiffge, 2005). Norms and rules of the peer group are known and upheld, but can also be individually shaped (dress code, rituals, morals). Regular get-togethers are the rule; peers take the place of parents, providing support and protection. Towards the end of this age range, the first steady romantic relationships often develop. The adolescent has a sense of belonging to the *ethnic* group in which he/she is growing up in, and accepts its child-rearing practices, its language, culture, its nonverbal forms of communication, and its specific patterns of interaction (facial expressions, gestures). however, the adolescent also has a secure sense of belonging to the community or nation in which he/she lives. These adolescents can recognize and endure different value systems, bring them into harmony with one another, and confidently move back and forth between them. They can easily shift between the two identities (bi-cultural identity).
Limited integration	The adolescent has only a partial sense of belonging to the *peer group* with whom he/she spends time outside the family (school, sports club, recreation), irrespective of gender. Same-sex friendships serving to establish identity (friends as "aid workers," Seiffge-Krenke & Seiffge, 2005) are often absent, but are missed. Although norms and rules of the peer group are known and respected, they cannot be individually shaped (dress code, rituals, morals), which leads to the search for subcultures (Gothic, Punks, Emos, etc.) or to peer group pressure. Regular get-togethers outside the adolescent's own subculture are rare. Adolescents also engage in romantic relationships only within their own subculture. The adolescent has only a limited sense of belonging to the *ethnic* group in which he/she is growing up, or feels he/she

Structure

	exclusively belongs to that group, he/she either rejects its practices of upbringing, language, and culture, or over-idealizes them, respectively. His/her sense of belonging to the community or nation in which he/she lives is unstable. The shift between the two identities (bi-cultural identity) is problematic or managed only with difficulty. Religion and/or tradition become exceedingly important, external symbols can have an identity-forming character (e.g., headscarf, dietary rules), which the adolescent may be able to handle flexibly depending on the situation.
Low integration	The adolescent has no sense of belonging to any *peer group* with which he/she spends time outside the family (school, sports club, recreation), irrespective of gender; even same-sex friendships with an identity-forming function (friends as "aid workers," Seiffge-Krenke & Seiffge, 2005) are completely absent, although greatly missed. As get-togethers hardly ever occur, the precondition for breaking away from his/her parents is not met (no "developmental aid" from peers for coping with developmental tasks). While he/she does long for romantic relationships, he/she declines them for fear of being rejected. *Ethnic belongingness:* The adolescent does not succeed in shifting between the two cultural identities– one of the two cultures is rejected and devalued, the other over-idealized. Recognition of the values of the other culture or religion is hardly ever achieved, even with outside support. External symbols have a strong identity-forming character (e.g., headscarf, dietary rules, rules of attire), which are not flexibly manageable in a given situation. Ideological leaders are sought and acknowledged in an identity-forming way.
Disintegration	The adolescent has no sense of belonging to any *peer group* (irrespective of gender) and consequently totally withdraws socially. Friendships with adolescents of the same or the opposite-sex are lacking. No get-togethers occur, so that the "developmental aid" from peers for mastering developmental tasks is wholly absent. Romantic relationships are devalued and rejected. *Ethnic belongingness:* Complete rejection of the culture of origin or the culture in which the adolescent is living. No acknowledgement of external reality regarding norms, rules, or regulations. Culture or religion is used as an excuse to ignore prescribed standards. Radical groups have an identity-forming function and are not questioned.

9.3 Interpersonality

Clinical Anchor-Point Descriptions	
Interpersonality Dimension – Age Group 1 (3 to 5 Years)	
Structural Ability: *Fantasies*	
Good integration	The child can report on his/her mental world, he/she can name his/her thoughts, feelings, and fantasies and clearly indicates the existence of an inner private space. This is an important regulator in experiencing emotional states; fantasies can replace actions or contribute to creative, functional solutions. Depending on the age these fantasies may be limited in stressful situations or appear rigid, an imaginative space is always present, however.
Limited integration	The child's fantasizing activity is significantly limited. While a private space for thoughts is present, it appears thoroughly rigid and inflexible, and, to a large extent, is permeable to the outside. The child sometimes gives the impression of bubbling over. He/she can keep little to him-/herself and puts many things immediately into practice. Outside support can help stabilize this interface, however.
Low integration	Even in protected and supportive situations the child hardly manages to relate to his/her inner world. He/she appears mainly to live in reaction to concrete situations and not to have any mental space of experience. Experiencing is immediately directed outwards without the possibility of carrying out actions mentally. Fantasies can then appear excessive, limitless, and threatening, or lifelessly tied to what is concrete. Discharge through impulsive action is possible, however.
Disintegration	Fragments of fantasies cannot be perceived as separate from reality; they have a concrete character, are threatening for the child, press towards immediate discharge, and lead to destructive, bizarre, and incomprehensible behavior.
Structural Ability: *Initiating Emotional Contact*	
Good integration	The desire for contact with other people is expressed, but varies depending on the person. The child's need is understandable and his/her relatedness to the other person is noticeable. That other person is not easily replaceable. In different situations, contact with some people is clearly preferred and actively sought, in part, although others would do just as well (as playmates, solace-givers, attachment figures, etc.).

Structure

Limited integration	Contact is either sought very intensely or clearly avoided. However, the search for intimacy seems rather nonspecific as to persons, and the child's need is not always clearly expressed. Little distinction is made between preferred persons for a particular need, but rather they are chosen according to familiarity. If access to the other person is somehow hindered, the child will seldom actively strive towards contact.
Low integration	Contact is sought in a very unspecific way, with apparently little relation to the object. That person is chosen as a counterpart who seems most accessible, and not the person who could best satisfy the child's need. It is often very difficult to understand the child's message. The child seems altogether hardly selective in making contact and seems significantly unsure about him-/herself.
Disintegration	The child makes contact with others by intensely drawing attention to him-/herself and not through directive communicative signals. The child appears to have less the need for contact than an intensive desire to dissolve and disappear.

Structural Ability: *Reciprocity*

Good integration	In contact with peers, but also with adults (as in the examination situation), a lively and mutual give-and-take occurs. The child is noticeably pleased with playful exchanges, accepts suggestions, and contributes ideas of his/her own.
Limited integration	The child can either take up suggestions by others or contribute his/her own ideas, but has difficulty in coordinating these two aspects for the sake of a lively exchange. Yet with support he/she succeeds in doing this, and he/she can develop a sense of togetherness, but generally more so with adults than with peers. Under stress, limitations may arise even in this case, however.
Low integration	Lively and mutual exchanges practically never occur, regardless of whether adults or peers are concerned. Extreme forms of behavior hindering communication quickly arise, as do polarizations and projections, rendering lively and mutual exchanges impossible, even in play, since no common frame of reference seems to exist.
Disintegration	Extreme forms of behavior hindering communication quickly arise, accompanied by vehement affects. There exists neither a common frame of reference nor a shared reality. The child is no longer susceptible to influence from the outside.

Structural Ability: *Affective Experience*	
Good integration	The child can admit and understand his/her own emotional experience, without interrupting his/her present activity or communication with significant other persons. Affects are experienced as pleasant or unpleasant, as well as, in principle, controllable and not disruptive. The child is generally able to perceive and name or describe his/her own affects.
Limited integration	Different feelings can be perceived and named only with little differentiation, namely between good and bad. The child has little confidence in the persistent controllability of bad states in particular, which often leads him/her to initiate contact with a familiar person. Affects tend more to be recognized from expressive features than experienced in a differentiated form.
Low integration	The child has little connection with his/her inner experiences; feelings tend to be perceived in a poorly differentiated form as internal tensions; practically incomprehensible emotional eruptions repeatedly occur to give way to a discharge of tensions. The range of qualities of feeling is quite reduced, and there is only very limited confidence in their controllability.
Disintegration	Feelings are perceived as undifferentiated states of tension and appear threatening, alien, and empty. Violent impulses or hostile distancing regularly occur. Behavior is no longer predictable or understandable. Confrontation leads to further escalations. The child seems beside him-/herself.
Structural Ability: *Empathy*	
Good integration	In play situations the child can express object-directed affects like caring, gratitude, disappointment, and concern. The child can display intentions to put things right and console. He/she can understand the other's emotions or needs and let them guide his/her behavior.
Limited integration	The child rarely expresses pro-social impulses on his/her own, but only with adult support. Even if he/she understands the other's needs, he/she has difficulty letting them guide his/her behavior.
Low integration	Besides moderate integration, the child repeatedly reveals him-/herself to be in a state (affective flooding, anxiety, ill humour) where there is no room for object-directed affects or altruistic impulses. The interest in connecting with others is inconstant.

Structure

Disintegration	The child shows him-/herself incapable of feeling empathy for others, registering their needs, and connecting with others through pro-social impulses. The child appears consistently reliant on the support and control from adults.

Structural Ability: *Capacity to Separate*	
Good integration	The child reacts to separation with considerable demonstrations of aversion. The resentment expressed depends on the other person in question, however, and on the availability of alternative offers. Generally the child appears more to trust in the temporariness of the separation than to suppose the opposite.
Limited integration	The child avoids goodbyes and separations with a tendency to cling to the object and to express his/her displeasure intensely. This tendency depends on the person, however, and becomes more intense the closer the person is to the child. In other cases, the child acts as if the separation had little emotional significance.
Low integration	Separations lead to violent expressions of discontent on the part of the child and also to his/her actively running after the person who has left. In the event of failure, stagnation occurs and the child seems to regard the separation not as temporary but as permanent, and to struggle against this loss.
Disintegration	Either separations are simply accepted with no visible emotional response, as if they were totally insignificant, or violent, undirected signals of extremely high urgency occur. The child then seems either frozen or frantically combative.

***Interpersonality* Dimension – Age Group 2 (6 to 12 Years)**	
Structural Ability: *Fantasies*	
Good integration	Fantasies increasingly enrich the child's experiences and can be observed both in play and in coping with the world. At the beginning of this age range the child cannot yet always reliably distinguish between fantasy and reality; his/her sense of reality can become secure with the aid of a third party, however.
Limited integration	The child's activity in fantasy is limited, being revealed in play and in his/her coping with reality. A certain lack of fantasy is observable; the child cannot use fantasies to make a more flexible and playful interaction possible.

Low integration	Even with support and in a protected environment, the child hardly manages to establish a connection with his/her own fantasy world and to make use of that world in play. Threatening content that cannot be reliably distinguished from reality repeatedly overwhelms the child.
Disintegration	As with Age Group 3, certain fragments of fantasies cannot be distinguished from reality; they have a concrete character and lead to destructive and bizarre and no longer really comprehensible actions.

Structural Ability: *Initiating Emotional Contact*

Good integration	The desire for intimacy with other people is expressed understandably and varies according to the person in question. To a small extent, the child gives the impression of an existential, emotional dependence on the attachment figure. If need be, the child clearly prefers and sometimes actively seeks contact with the primary attachment figures.
Limited integration	The child either seeks contact very intensely or clearly avoids it. The impression arises of either a very clinging or a very independent child. The child's search for intimacy seems unspecific as to persons, as does the reason for taking up contact. His/her medium of expression is often not primarily language, but motor skills and physicality.
Low integration	Intimacy is sought in a very unspecific way, with apparently little relation to the object. The child chooses that person as an attachment figure who seems most accessible. Contact is made through nonverbal channels and the active search for intimacy. The child hardly avails him-/herself of his/her pre-existing linguistic competence when it would be appropriate to do so.
Disintegration	Contact is made rather through intensely attracting attention and not through directed communicative signals. Language practically no longer serves as a medium of expression. Neediness is expressed in a way not at all appropriate for this age group, and is practically incomprehensible.

Structural Ability: *Reciprocity*

Good integration	Contact with adults and with peers is characterized by a lively give-and-take, manifested in play but also in exchanges on the greatest variety of subjects. In the peer group, age-related subjects lead to an enriching, mutual dialog. Give-and-take with opening, acceptance, and counteroffer is possible at all times.

Structure

Limited integration	The child needs outside support to develop a sense of togetherness. Reciprocal contact in the dyad can be built up and maintained with assistance, however. Still, stress may result in limitations. The capacity for a sense of togetherness still exists in principle.
Low integration	A sense of togetherness rarely occurs; extreme forms of behavior hindering communication, distorted perceptions and mistrust quickly arise and prevent lively and mutual experiencing.
Disintegration	A lively, mutual sense of togetherness is not possible, even with support and in a protected space. Interruptions and terminations of reciprocity occur abruptly. An opening or offer to reciprocity cannot be accepted.

Structural Ability: *Affective Experience*

Good integration	The child's own affects can (at the beginning of this age range, possibly still with support) be perceived in the interpersonal context and experienced as separate from others' affects. Communication with the other person is not interrupted, or can (again at the beginning of this age range) be maintained with external support.
Limited integration	The child can perceive individual feelings on a global level. A differentiated perception of his/her own emotions is possible for the child only to a limited extent. Affective experience and affective expression are sometimes reduced to bodily reactions accompanying the affect, for example.
Low integration	The child has an inadequate perception of and capacity for verbalizing affective states. Negative affects generally predominate, with emotional outbursts that are difficult to understand and to empathize with.
Disintegration	The child cannot consciously perceive his/her own affects as such. They appear threatening, alien, and empty, and can be expressed only through violent impulses. Affective stimuli trigger fierce autonomous-vegetative reactions.

Structural Ability: Empathy

Good integration	The child is able to form a picture of others' needs and moods and can also express this in play and in conversation. The child perceives what feelings he/she triggers in others and can act accordingly. The child distinguishes between a momentary expression of feeling and a persisting, basic emotional attitude on the part of the other person.

Limited integration	The ability to perceive the other person's needs and moods is fragile in the case of conflict. The child's own neediness and experience of frustration lead to a loss of emphatic abilities. To expressions of negative feelings, the child reacts, feeling offended, and generalizes the other person's attitude toward him/her.
Low integration	The child repeatedly exhibits states lacking pro-social affects due to loss of a holistic perception of the other person. The interest in connecting with others and maintaining that connection is low.
Disintegration	The ability to empathize with others is low; the child's handling of relationships seems to lack a need or interest.

Structural Ability: *Capacity to Separate*

Good integration	The child reacts to separation with considerable demonstrations of aversion. The expressed aversion depends on the other person in question, however, and on the availability of alternative offers. The primary medium of expression is language, and the child succeeds in making him-/herself understood through this channel. There is a basic confidence in being understood.
Limited integration	Despite positive experiences, the child avoids farewells and separations and tends to cling to the object, even though he/she temporarily manages well. Sometimes the child appears unaffected by the separation. Expressions of displeasure are intense, but not very clear and conveyed verbally only to a small extent. The child copes well with being alone over a certain period of time, however.
Low integration	Separations lead to expressions of discontent by the child and to his/her actively running after the person who has left. Often transitional objects are needed in order to endure the separation. If this is also not successful, stagnation and resignation are to be observed. In other cases, these expressions of resentment are lacking, but the child can make constructive use of being alone only to a limited extent.
Disintegration	Separations are either simply accepted with no visible emotional response, as if they were totally insignificant, or violent, barely directed signals of extremely high urgency occur. Despite the child's linguistic competence, these signals are not conveyed verbally. The child appears either frozen or frantically combative.

Structure

Interpersonality Dimension – Age Group 3 (13 to 18 Years)	
Structural Ability: *Fantasies*	
Good integration	Fantasies can be reported and have a stimulating and enriching effect. They are an important regulator in experiencing emotional states and can either replace action or contribute to creative, functional solutions. In intrapsychic conflicts, these fantasies are contained and limited (mobilizing or rigid) and subject to defence.
Limited integration	The adolescent's activity in fantasy is limited. These limitations appear to be either clearly dependent on the context and related to the topic or they are, to a certain degree, rigid and lifeless. Fantasizing that can no longer be controlled can partially influence action.
Low integration	Even in protected and supportive situations the adolescent can hardly relate to a vibrant imaginative life. Fantasies can appear excessive and limitlessly threatening or lifelessly tied to what is concrete. Discharge through impulsive action is possible.
Disintegration	Fragments of fantasies cannot be perceived as separate from reality; they are concrete in character and lead to destructive, bizarre, and incomprehensible actions.
Structural Ability: *Emotional Contact*	
Good integration	The adolescent is consistently able to make appropriate emotional contact with peers and adults, depending on the respective context. Temporary neurotic aspects can be corrected. The adolescent can express desires and needs understandably even in difficult social situations. The adolescent endeavors to safeguard relationships and to maintain contact with persons important to him/her.
Limited integration	Making emotional contact often appears limited and is possible only towards certain persons in certain contexts. Contact appears sometimes rigid, unstable, vacillating, and inflexible. Under stress contact, behavior tends to diminish, and contact may be broken off. The emotional significance of the other person is clearly exaggerated and the adolescent gives the impression of emotional object dependence, with frequent searching for intimacy. Occasionally there is also the impression of exaggerated independence. In addition, contact behavior seems directed towards very few people.

Low integration	Emotional contact is hardly possible for the adolescent; breaking off of contact and misunderstandings are frequent. Regulation of distance and intimacy is very limited and reactions appear wholly inappropriate. Emotional significance is clearly tied to the actual presence of the object. Contact is constantly being made with whoever is available. Little preference for particular persons is discernible, often resulting in frequently changing and merely short-term relationships.
Disintegration	Making emotional contact is not possible. The adolescent's behavior is unpredictable and incomprehensible. Emotions are either rigid or impulsive. A form of making contact understandable from the outside does not occur. The person loses him-/herself either in symbiosis or in striving for autonomy. There is no way to let others become emotionally significant and to enter into interactions with them, without surrendering oneself. The two messages sent are: "I want nothing to do with you." Or: "I'm completely at your disposal, so that you can save me."

Structural Ability: *Reciprocity*

Good integration	Contact with adults and with peers is characterized by lively interactions, which makes even exchanges on more difficult subjects possible. Mutual understanding and the sense of togetherness are possible. Temporary neurotic aspects can be corrected.
Limited integration	For developing a sense of togetherness, the adolescent needs external support, but he/she can develop and maintain reciprocal contact in the dyad with assistance. Even then, stress may result in limitations, although the capacity for a sense of togetherness remains in principle.
Low integration	A sense of togetherness rarely occurs. Extreme forms of behavior hindering communication and polarizations and projections preventing lively and mutual exchanges quickly arise.
Disintegration	No sense of togetherness can be established. The attempt to frame a "common work" is prevented by distortions of reality and vehement affects. The adolescent is no longer susceptible to external influence.

Structural Ability: *Affective Experience*

Good integration	The adolescent can admit and understand his/her own, emotional life in a differentiated way. The adolescent does not break off communication with significant others. Inter-

	nal dialogs are experienced as enriching. Differentiated perception of his/her own emotions is possible for the adolescent.
Limited integration	The adolescent cannot easily differentiate between emotional states and often does not have a good understanding of his/her own emotions. Usually he/she can describe being in this condition, however. A certain level of suffering exists.
Low integration	The adolescent has hardly any connection with his/her inner experiences. He/she has no differentiated perception of his/her feelings, and hardly comprehensible emotional eruptions repeatedly occur. The range of qualities of feeling is quite reduced and negative feelings predominate.
Disintegration	The adolescent's own emotions appear threatening, alien, and empty, and can be expressed only by violent impulses or distrustful and hostile distancing. Behavior is no longer predictable or understandable. Confrontation leads to further escalation.

Structural Ability: *Empathy*

Good integration	With his/her own mental experiences, the adolescent is consistently able to empathize with the other person's inner world and thereby understand the other's attitudes, motives, and actions. The adolescent is able to relate his/her own perspectives to other people's.
Limited integration	The capacity for empathy is limited in stressful situations. The adolescent then does not perceive what feelings he/she triggers in the other person, and takes the others's momentary expression of feeling to be a persistent basic emotional state. Forms of treatment typical for the adolescent's age and tolerated by his/her peer group (coolness, taunting, insults, "dissing") are used inappropriately (too much/too little). He/she can be approached in this regard, and shows a degree of suffering.
Low integration	The adolescent is dominated by his/her own states, confusing his/her own feelings with those of others. He/she experiences the perception of a person with feelings of his/her own as threatening. Other people's emotional states corresponding with the adolescent's are registered with great sensitivity, without appropriate action on the adolescent's part. The adolescent's own affective states are often reflected in states of tension.

Disintegration	Motives, attitudes, and needs can no longer be assigned to the object or to the self in terms of their origin. The adolescent is accordingly unable to take the appropriate approach to the other person. Recognition of other interests and situations of conflict is no longer possible.
Structural Ability: *Capacity to Separate*	
Good integration	The adolescent reacts to separation with appropriate sadness. This includes being able to regulate oneself after an appropriate period of time, and not just to endure the separation. The adolescent also succeeds in withdrawing affective cathexes from objects if they appear to be or actually are lost.
Limited integration	The adolescent avoids farewells and separations with a tendency to cling to the object. Losses are ignored and only with a great effort does affective cathexis gradually diminish.
Low integration	There is no internal representation of separation or loss. Any experience in this regard is denied. Should actual loss occur, pathological reactions of mourning will often occur in the form of depression and helplessness.
Disintegration	Separations are simply accepted without visible emotional reaction, as if they were totally insignificant, or the mere idea of separation already triggers extreme emotional responses that appear uncontrollable.

9.4 Attachment

Clinical Anchor-Point Descriptions	
Attachment Dimension – Age Group 1 (3 to 5 Years)	
Structural Ability: *Access to Representations of Attachment*	
Good integration	The child can clearly express his disapproval of the absence of the attachment figure and the desire for intimacy and security. At the same time, the child does not fall into a state of impotence and helplessness, but tries, appropriate for his/her age, to fall back on self-regulatory skills. The extent of his/her success in doing so is not of importance here.
Limited integration	With attachment activation, the child expresses tension and concern in either an increased or decreased manner. The child has little recourse to self-regulatory skills, but tries to bridge the time gap by making an increased effort or by simply waiting and enduring.

Low integration	With attachment activation, the child shows quick and intense stress reactions; there is no clear expression of a need for intimacy, and no internal images of an attachment figure seem available. Physical presence can bring the attachment stress back under control again, however. Prevalent is a clear expression of fear of a permanent loss of the attachment figure.
Disintegration	Each activation of attachment leads directly to very intense, partly panicky reactions of anxiety. The child feels threatened when alone, but also the physical presence of the attachment figure can bring relief only in a makeshift way. Intrapsychically no functioning strategy seems to be available.

Structural Ability: *Secure Internal Base*

Good integration	In situations where he/she is alone, the child has ways to calm him-/herself down and console him-/herself until external regulatory aids become available again. The attachment system may then certainly remain activated, especially in the case of small children, but states of helplessness or despair will not arise. The child can strike a balance by him-/herself between attachment and exploration.
Limited integration	In situations where he/she is alone, the child has only limited ways to calm him-/herself. Tension is always high and external regulatory aids are actively sought, but with little precision or requested without vigour. States of helplessness or desperation are hardly expressed, depending on the child's exact age. The child cannot strike a balance between attachment and exploration. Activation of attachment remains dominant until external aid becomes available.
Low integration	The child is practically unable to calm him-/herself down. The child can bridge short periods of time through distractions or transitional objects, but cannot activate any internal images which would help to satisfy attachment needs. The child either quickly and fiercely combats being alone or he/she endures this condition as well as he/she can until external regulatory opportunities become tangible.
Disintegration	Being alone is impossible during attachment activation. Even the threat of being alone triggers reactions of panic. Considerable confusion and increasing agitation predominate. Being alone then induces almost immediately feelings of despair, helplessness, and impotence.

Structural Ability: *Capacity to Be Alone*	
Good integration	The child can symbolize different characters as well as relationships, even in their absence. The child can then vary these symbols according to the situation – as in play, for example – and bring them into relationship with one another.
Limited integration	While characters are distinctly differentiated from one another, flexibly entering into a relationship occurs only to a limited extent and only for functional reasons. The ability to symbolize is then considerably susceptible to changes in basic conditions.
Low integration	Even types of characters are hardly differentiated and are not clearly distinguished from one another in representations. The corresponding images are also hardly positive. The situation does not seem to have any influence, it appears "always the same."
Disintegration	No complete internal images exist. Accordingly, the ability to symbolize is also limited, since the child regularly reacts with despair, as can be observed in the various situations involving attachment stress.
Structural Ability: *Use of Attachment Relationships*	
Good integration	The child manages to make use of the people available, and to calm and to console him-/herself and to resume exploring with the aid of the attachment figure. The child then clearly discerns which person is offering regulatory assistance. The regulation of the attachment system appears as a communicative act involving a specific other.
Limited integration	The interactive regulation of the attachment system appears inflexible and cumbersome. It seems more like a negotiation than communication. Regulation becomes difficult because the child cannot clearly express his/her needs and because the other person does not seem to understand the child's signals. This interactive adaptation will vary in character depending on the other person in the interaction, however.
Low integration	Irrespective of the partner in interaction, the child seems to have great difficulty in self-regulation. The interactive patterns of communication appear rigid and partly independent of the other person's reactions. While the child can calm down a bit and take a step towards exploration, attachment stress then quickly resurges with an active demand for intimacy.

Structure

| Disintegration | The attachment system seems to calm down more from exhaustion than from regulation. The child seems torn between the despair of being alone and the feeling of being threatened by intimacy. The child can then hardly differentiate between different interaction partners. He/she even tends to be more successful with strangers than with attachment figures. |

Attachment Dimension – Age Group 2 (6 to 12 Years)

Structural Ability: Access to Representations of Attachment

Good integration	The school child has internalized objects and relationship patterns. In activating attachment, the child employs his / her verbal possibilities to articulate his/her neediness. Images of attachment figures are complete and differentiable parts. There is a noticeable difference in significance between persons relevant to attachment and other people.
Limited integration	There exist internalized parts that can be distinguished from one another. These parts are not differentiated very much, however, and the stability of the internal images diminishes as the absence of the real object persists. While a difference in significance between persons relevant to attachment and other people is noticeable, it too diminishes over time.
Low integration	The school child has few and predominantly negative internal images at his/her disposition. The internalized relationship patterns appear to have little flexibility and are reduced to functional aspects of basic care. Emotional aspects are primarily anxiety, neglect, or persecution. The internal objects can be used for stabilization, but only at certain times and in certain situations.
Disintegration	Activation of attachment seems very threatening, as only partial objects are available. They pertain to persecution, threat, and anxiety. In attachment-relevant situations they do not even seem to suffice for short-term stabilization, so that the child strives only for the physical presence of a person. Intrapsychically, no resources seem available for regulating the attachment stress.

Structural Ability: Secure Internal Base

| Good integration | Given the activation of attachment, the school child has ways to calm down and to console him-/herself and to deactivate attachment stress even without external regulatory aids. In this respect, the child does not always have to |

	succeed without external assistance, but at least most of the time. Even after a longer period of time, no states of helplessness or despair will arise in solitary situations, however.
Limited integration	With the activation of attachment, the child has only limited ways to calm him-/herself. Usually this deactivation will persist only for a limited period of time, after which external regulatory aids will be needed again to deactivate the attachment system. However, no state of helplessness or despair is experienced.
Low integration	The capacity to be alone and calm down is significantly limited once attachment stress arises. Shorter periods of time can be bridged through distraction or with transitional objects. No internal images can be activated that could give a sense of intimacy and security, however. Help from attachment figures is then necessary, and the child subsequently manages to calm down.
Disintegration	Being alone is nearly impossible during activation of attachment. Deactivation can be brought about solely by others. The internal images themselves appear threatening and produce anxiety. Considerable confusion and increasing agitation prevail that can be brought under control only with difficulty, even with assistance.

Structural Ability: *Capacity to Be Alone*

Good integration	The child has various and differentiated representations of persons and relationship patterns with which he/she can reduce attachment-related stress. The situational context is then clearly included. The child manages to talk about this stress on the meta-level after the event.
Limited integration	While internal images of attachment figures and relationship patterns exist, the situational context seems to have little influence on which of these images are to be used for regulation. The ability to reflect upon this is existent, though limited.
Low integration	The child seems to have only one internal image to deactivate attachment stress. The same strategy is always used, which may sometimes succeed, but usually does not produce the desired result. The situational context seems to have little effect on how the child attempts to regulate him-/herself.
Disintegration	There exist no complete internal images. Upon acitivation of attachment the possibilities of regulation are therefore severely restricted, as the child regularly reacts with helplessness and despair, which can be observed in the widest variety of situations in which attachment stress occurs.

Structural Ability: *Use of Attachment Relationships*	
Good integration	The child manages to make use of the people available and, with their aid, to calm and console him-/herself if need be, and to turn back towards the outside world. Language then becomes the preferred medium. Physical contact remains important in the case of the primary attachment figures, however. The child clearly discerns which person is offering regulatory assistance.
Limited integration	While the interactive regulation of the attachment system succeeds, this regulation seems inflexible and cumbersome. The child cannot always clearly express his/her needs, nor can the other person sufficiently understand the child's signals, which leads to misunderstandings. There is a difficulty in finding a common "language."
Low integration	Irrespective of the partner in interaction, the child seems to have great difficulty in self-regulation when it is required. The child's expression seems rigid and unresponsive to the other person's reactions. Sometimes expression is wholly suppressed. While calm does return, the attachment stress will now and then resurge. The child will then only be able to make limited use of his/her available communicative resources.
Disintegration	The attachment system seems to settle down more because of exhaustion. The child seems torn and cannot make use of interactive offers and the availability of people in order to calm him-/herself. He/she then hardly distinguishes between different interaction partners, and even tends to become calmer in the presence of persons who are not primary attachment figures.

Attachment Dimension – Age Group 3 (13 to 18 Years)	
Structural Ability: *Access to Representations of Attachment*	
Good integration	The adolescent has internal images of significant persons, who are also invested with positive emotions. The attention and affection from these people are noticeably important, and the adolescent fears and worries about losing this affection.
Limited integration	Generally images of significant persons are present, but only momentarily, and the adolescent has only a limited ability to maintain these images in difficult situations. The adolescent's anxiety is primarily related to object loss and not so much to the loss of affection.

Low integration	In the absence of other person(s), internal images exist only in the form of neglectful, persecutory, or harmful objects. Without the physical presence of the object, the adolescent cannot sketch any positive picture. His/her anxiety refers in particular to the threat of being harmed by the object.
Disintegration	There are no internal representations of real objects. The internal images are destructive, frightening, or threatening. The child even has difficulty investing the object with positive emotion when present. There exists a distinct fear of merging with the object and losing identity.

Structural Ability: *Secure Internal Base*

Good integration	If need be, the adolescent can calm down if he/she is alone and activate and make use of his/her internal images of important relationships. This strategy need not be successful in the long term, and, in the event of high attachment stress, it may also serve only to bridge the time until external regulatory opportunities become available again.
Limited integration	The adolescent has difficulty calming down by him-/herself, as he/she is increasingly driven by his/her internal images and flees into some distracting activity without really being able to deal with the trigger and his/her inner state.
Low integration	The adolescent is practically unable to calm down by him-/herself or care for him-/herself. No internal images can be activated which would help to do so, and the adolescent manages to distract him-/herself only to a limited extent. The adolescent endures being alone as well as he/she can until external regulatory possibilities become tangible.
Disintegration	When attachment is activated, only partial objects are available. The adolescent manages neither to distract him-/herself nor simply to endure this state. Confusion and increasing agitation predominate. Being alone induces feelings of despair, helplessness, and impotence. Even if external regulatory opportunities exist, the adolescent finds it difficult to make use of them.

Structural Ability: *Capacity to Be Alone*

Good integration	The internal images of significant others are differentiated and diverse. The images appear demarcated from one another and self-subsistent, and can also be partially interrelated. In this way the adolescent can deactivate the attachment system and turn back towards the outside world.

Structure

Limited integration	While the internal images are present, there is little differentiation. In part, they are not clearly demarcated from one another, and they can hardly be placed into relationship with one another. Activation of attachment is successful only to a limited extent, and appears more as a makeshift solution.
Low integration	Positive internal images are virtually nonexistent. There exist no clearly definable internal parts, and they also exhibit little differentiation within themselves. Representations of relationships are functionalized and limited to a dyadic contact. Attachment stress can be mostly endured, but not deactivated by the adolescent's themself.
Disintegration	No internal images exist which could be activated. If anything, internal objects are threatening and persecutory. Attachment stress is so threatening that the adolescent immediately seeks contact with the outside world once he/she is alone. This is also the primary and sole goal that is pursued.

Structural Ability: *Use of Attachment Relationships*	
Good integration	If necessary, the adolescent can actively seek the help of others and avail him-/herself of this aid. He/she can understandably express a need for intimacy. This expressiveness seems to vary according to the other person and the situation. On the other hand, he/she will also be able to provide adequate assistance to others, if required.
Limited integration	The adolescent has difficulty in accepting help, on the one hand, because he/she can express this need for help only when there are clear indications that he/she feels overwhelmed; and, on the other hand, because he/she does not regard many offers of help as useful. Conversely, he/she has a tendency to offer too much help to others.
Low integration	The adolescent is hardly able to accept aid or to express his/her need for support, and this deficit is accompanied by distrust, deprecation, and aggressive rejection. Furthermore, he/she cannot imagine possibly being of help to others.
Disintegration	To the adolescent, others cannot be of any help. He/she does not express the need for help, and in needy situations he/she often fully ignores object boundaries. In the event of contact and intimacy, the adolescent tends to strive towards symbiosis.

9.5 Identity Diffusion as a Structural Problem and the Identity Conflict as an Intrapsychic Conflict

Identity diffusion is characterized by the inability to integrate a harmonious, stable and coherent concept of oneself and significant other persons (Clarkin, Yeomans, & Kernberg, 1999). Clinically, this condition is manifested by an unreflected, chaotic, and inconsistent description of oneself and others, without this inconsistency itself being recognized.

In contrast to identity diffusion (Foelsch et al., 2010), which presents a structural problem, an identity conflict presupposes a more integrated structural level, as the formation of an intrapsychic conflict is modulated by the integration level of the mental structure. Mentzos (2005) differentiates in the individual stages of development primary conflicts that can lead to crises in the identity development of children and adolescents, and which, if overcome, lead to new self-image aspects. Failure to integrate these new self-image aspects into an existing self-image leads to conflicting and confused self-images in the sense of an exceedingly intense adoption of changing identifications or to disorientation and helplessness. Our concept of identity conflict incorporates this idea and thereby makes an assessment possible.

Structure

10. Fourth Axis: Prerequisites for Treatment

In contrast to the *interpersonal relations, conflict* and *structure* axes, the definitions and operationalizations of the individual items and dimensions of the *prerequisites for treatment* axis require less theoretical embedding based on psychodynamic constructs. An exception is the gain from illness item, based on the psychoanalytic theory of neurosis with the corresponding assumptions about unconscious motives in the development of neurotic symptoms.

  Given a brief description of the theoretical context, each item is thus individually defined and operationalized with anchor-point descriptions according to the age groups of the OPD-CA. The Assessment Sheet for Prerequisites for Treatment can be found in Appendix B.8.

10.1 Subjective Dimensions

Subjective Impairment Through Somatic and Mental Complaints/ Problems

Theoretical Background
The subjective experience of physical discomfort and/or mental problems plays a central role in the patient's willingness to undergo therapy, in his/her ability and will to change, and in the course taken by his/her illness. If subjective experience does not accord with the degree of impairment as externally assessed, discrepancies will occur between the two dimensions that must be taken into account in the diagnostic assessment. The subjectively experienced impairment is also influenced by the patient's coping with the illness, which is sex- and age-dependent in children and adolescents (Hampel & Petermann, 2005). Among children, the subjective experience of a functional im-

pairment may differ greatly from the assessment from an adult's perspective. Consequently, besides the examiner's objective assessment of the severity of the psychosocial impairment according to Axis VI of MAS/ICD-10 diagnostics, the subjectively experienced degree of the impairment from the child's or adolescent's perspective is ascertained separately.

Operationalization

The subjective impairment from somatic and/or psychical complaints or problems is a situational criterion that is subjective in character. The criterion captures the particular degree of subjective impairment from physical complaints and/or problems as experienced by the particular child or adolescent. It is not to be equated with a professional (medical, psychological) assessment of the severity of an illness or impairment of the psychosocial adaptation level, as occurs along the MAS Axis VI, for example, or as operationalized in the International Classification of Functioning, Disability, and Health (ICF) of the World Health Organization. The degree of subjective impairment is captured irrespective of these professional assessments of severity given the particular impairment as experienced from somatic complaints and psychical problems.

If the degree of subjective impairment cannot be inferred from the patient's spontaneous utterances, a direct question must be asked. A negative response to the question about subjective impairment (see Appendix A: Interview Guide) would have to be considered equivalent to the assessment: *absent*. As of Age Group 2 (6 to 12 years), the degree of the impairment is assessed with the aid of graphic symbols. According to current findings on the health-related quality of life, children from an age of eight years are able to provide appropriate information about all aspects of their health (Rebok et al., 2001). The rating incorporates only the information provided by the child or adolescent. In the case of complex disorder patterns, the question pertains always to the complaints and problems constituting the reason for presentation at the diagnostic assessment and the interview. If the degree of impairment is not verbally expressed, the assessment should refer to other clear-cut signals of subjective impairment. In case of doubt, the lower level of impairment is to be assumed. The subjective degree of impairment cannot be equated with the separately assessed level of suffering. Even if these two items are often pronounced to an equal degree, they need not be so. In particular, in the case of a high *gain from illness*, an expressed high degree of subjective impairment (along with, for example, persistent school absenteeism due to a school phobia) may be accompanied by a noticeably low level of suffering. In this case, clear information is provided on the patient's failure to manage his/her life in an age-appropriate way because of his/her illness. The child or adolescent seems to have nicely accommodated him-/herself to this degree of psychosocial impairment, however, with the result of little suffering. For assessing *subjective impairment* as opposed to the level of suffering, selective questioning in the interview should allow elaboration of the failure to manage his/her life in an age-appropriate way due to his/her problems or symptoms, or his/her failure to handle age-related developmental tasks, from the child's or adolescent's perspective. The key diagnostic question could be: "How would your life be different if you didn't have this problem?" (e.g., "have more friends," "return to school," etc.). On the basis of the child's or adolescent's replies, the examiner can then ask about *subjective level of suffering* (see below, e.g., "How bad is it for you that …"). In sum, *subjective impairment* can be distinguished from *level of suffering* in that the former comprises more the cognitive orientation towards the degree of illness-related limitations, while the latter corresponds more to the emotional stress from these limitations. Finally, the degree of subjective impairment from somatic symptoms and/or mental problems is coded on the assessment sheet according to the scale: 0 = *absent*, 1 = *low degree*, 2 = *moderate degree*, and 3 = *severe or high degree*.

Subjective Illness Theory

Theoretical Background

Subjective theories about certain physical or mental states crucially influence both coping with illness and the motivation for therapy, and form an integral part of these processes (e.g., Resch & Schulte-Markwort, 2008; Schulte-Markwort, 1996; Wiehe, 2006). In children and adolescents, subjective conceptions and implicit theories about the origins of illnesses can diverge from the therapist's view during the diagnostic assessment and treatment even more than those of adults. If a child fantasizes that his/her illness is punishment for undesirable or "evil" behavior, for example, the therapist's understanding of the symptom will not reach the child as long as this unspoken conception is not discussed and dispersed. For example, an antisocial adolescent may not acquiesce to treatment as long as he/she cognitively and emotionally retains the conception that the problem lies with his/her surroundings and not with him-/herself.

Following Faltermaier, Kühnlein, and Burda-Viering (1998), we may describe subjective conceptions of illness as follows:

> Lay people have thoughts about how illnesses arise, how their health is affected and how health can be preserved. While these thoughts may vary in complexity, they do not necessarily adhere to the pattern of scientific theories; we must rather assume that lay theories follow a different logic of development and have a different empirical basis. However, it is obvious that people's beliefs about the conditions of health and the causes of illness very much influence their actions regarding health and whether they act at all and in what direction." (p. 312; translated by T. Talbot)

Studies on conceptions of illness in mentally ill children and adolescents indicate that subjective hypotheses about illness may trigger or sustain anxieties and fears that can exacerbate a pre-existing psychiatric illness in the patient (Schulte-Markwort, 1996).

Operationalization

A subjective theory about illness is defined as the subjective assumption or fantasy on the part of a child or adolescent regarding the origin of his/her physical and/or mental illness (Faltermaier et al., 1998). The hypothesis is verbally documented in order to acquire illustrative original material.

To be distinguished from the subjective illness theory is the *insight into biopsychosocial interrelations* (see below): The former concerns the initial "raw state" of the etiological model of the child or adolescent, i.e., the patient's theory about the origin of his/her own illness or about the issue leading to the presentation, as expressed in the diagnostic interview when simply asked. This hypothesis is assessed only qualitatively and employed for diagnostic hypothesis formation. *Not* (yet) assessed is the ability for introspection and self-reflection, which plays a significant role only in the assessment of the *insight into biopsychosocial interrelations* (see below). In children and adolescents without prior experience of psychotherapy, we generally expect that introspective and self-reflective processes leading to verbalizable insight into biopsychosocial interrelations pertaining to the child's or adolescent's own illness or problem must first develop through the dialog of the psychodynamic interview (see below). The following are typical examples of subjective theories about illness for the respective age groups.

Examples

Age Group 1 (3 to 5 Years)
"Sometimes I get so mad, it just happens."
"I get scared when Mum and Dad go away – I have to be careful that they don't leave."
"… since that bad thing [the patient had observed a bad accident] happened."

Age Group 2 (6 to 12 Years)
"I can be really mean … My Mum once beat me really hard. Maybe I take after her."
"I get mad so fast because I'm quick to feel wronged."
"It's my body's fault. I have to throw up, and I get dizzy. I want to go to school, but I can't."

Age Group 3 (13 to 18 Years)
"I'm sick because I feel responsible for everything."
"My break-up with my girlfriend is why I couldn't cope."
"It makes me so sick that my mother is doing so badly. I can't help her."

Level of Suffering

Theoretical Background

The severity of psychosocial impairment from an illness (according to Axis VI of the MAS) as externally ascertained, i.e., by health professionals, the level of suffering from psychological/somatic symptoms (see above) and the *level of suffering* of the child or adolescent need not be equally pronounced. Discrepancies between the above categories are always particularly revealing from a psychodynamic perspective. For this reason, the OPD-CA-2 captures these categories in a differentiated way. In particular, children sometimes experience the smallest physical injuries with considerable suffering, whereas they may patiently endure severe chronic neglect or even chronic physical illness for years without letting on that they are suffering. *Level of suffering* has great significance for many aspects of the treatment, however. The assessment of a child's or adolescent's level of suffering must take into account the psychosocial, familial, and interactional pressure to which the patient may have to adapt. *Level of suffering* is an essential precondition for the *motivation for change* and for the *specific motivation for therapy* (see below), but is in no way to be equated with either. In particular, given a high *gain from illness* (see below), which may also include a subjective gain from suffering, the *motivation for change*, for example, may be low despite a high level of suffering.

Operationalization

Level of suffering refers to the expressed, subjectively felt degree of suffering from a psychical and/or somatic illness or from a mental state. Consequently only situational information provided by the child or adolescent on the extent of their suffering should be coded. For example, if the patient expressly denies suffering when asked, his/her level of suffering is coded as "absent," even in the case of pronounced depressive facial expressions.

If the *level of suffering* cannot be reliably assessed from the patient's spontaneous utterances, he/she must be questioned directly. In this case, the patient should be asked about his/her *level of suffering*, if possible, in direct connection with *subjective impairment* (for sample questions, see above and Appendix A: Interview Guide). A negative reply to the question about suffering (see Appendix A) is to be equated with the severity level "absent." Should no spontaneous reply occur to the questions, the child or adolescent in question should be offered the four levels of "not at all," "a little," "quite a lot," and "a lot" in the dialog.

In the case of younger children, the four smileys displayed in the assessment sheet can be used as an aid. The rating is determined solely on the basis of the information provided by the child or adolescent. In the presence of combined disorder patterns, the questioning always concerns the illness constituting the reason for the patient's presentation at the interview. The assessment of the level of suffering not explicitly expressed requires a high degree of clarity pertaining to otherwise communicated conscious suffering. In case of doubt, the lower level must always be assumed.

Motivation for Change

In contrast to adults, children and adolescents are often presented for psychotherapeutic diagnostic assessment and treatment planning because of external factors (school, kindergarten) or through mediation by their parents. Often these patients say there's nothing they want to change, but wish instead that something would change in their family or school, for example. Children and adolescents also often wish that changes would occur without therapy or external influences.

With this item, the child's or adolescent's desire for change should be expressly assessed. On the other hand, the family's desire for change is coded in *family resources* (see below).

To be set apart is the *specific motivation for psychotherapy* (see below), involving the child's unequivocally expressed desire to overcome a set of symptoms with therapeutic assistance. The motivation for change, in contrast, indicates possible solutions that can also be sought externally, irrespective of a desire for therapy. Also to be set apart is the *level of suffering* (see above), i.e., the subjective feeling of suffering irrespective of possible changes.

Operationalization

The child or adolescent is dissatisfied and expresses verbally or non-verbally the need for change. If the desire for change is not verbally expressed, it must be evident from the patient's behavior, if this characteristic is to be coded. The motivation for change is the more pronounced the more the child or adolescent is prepared to recognize his or her own possibilities of change and does not only expect change to come from the outside. This includes taking responsibility for his/her own actions. The desire to change may be connected with the desire for specific therapy (*specific motivation for therapy*, see below), but need not be.

The *motivation for change* is to be coded as "low" if change is desired only in one partial aspect of the disorder pattern and/or its psychosocial effects. If changes are desired in several partial aspects, the motivation for change is moderate. A high motivation for change at the age of six years or more will require the clearly expressed willingness to change things not only externally but in the child or adolescent him-/herself.

Examples

Age Group 1 (3 to 5 Years)	
Absent	Change and discontent are not addressed in play or in conversation.
Low	These children are only a little dissatisfied with their current situation and desire change, especially on the part of others.
Moderate	These children express a desire to change their current situation, or bring this up in play.
High	These children express a desire to change their current situation, or bring this up in play.
Age Group 2 (6 to 12 Years)	
Absent	The child shows no interest in change. These children are passive and do not answer questions or do so only tersely.
Low	In the interview, these children behave for the most part passively regarding their discontent with their symptoms and the desire for change, and answer questions tersely, expressing only a slight desire for change.
Moderate	These children bring up their dissatisfaction over their symptoms and verbally express the wish to change when asked or in the play situation, although rather as an aside. They assume rudimentary responsibility for their problems.
High	These children independently articulate both their dissatisfaction over their symptoms as well as a strong desire for change.
Age Group 3 (13 to 18 Years)	
Absent	These adolescents are fully content with their present situation. If problems exist at all, then it's the fault of others.
Low	These adolescents express little desire for change in their current situation. Change is for the most part expected from their surroundings.
Moderate	These adolescents express the desire for change in several aspects. They admit to being dissatisfied, and assume partial responsibility for their problems.
High	These adolescents are very dissatisfied, make suggestions of their own for change or have already done so within their families. They then accept responsibility for themselves and partly for the issues.

10.2 Resources

Theoretical Background

Psychosocial and individual resources must be appropriately considered in all child and adolescent psychiatric and psychodynamic diagnostics and therapy. Research on resilient children and children at risk over the last 30 years has left the concept uncontested, and salutogenic concepts have been more greatly integrated in routine diagnostics, not least because of the shift towards family therapy. Recent longitudinal studies (Werner, 2013), but also the large-scale international epidemiological studies, indicate the existence of protective factors against the occurrence of mental disorders, even among multiply stressed children. As part of the child's power of mental resistance or resilience, the situational flexibility of affective and cognitive response patterns appears to increase the likelihood of long-term mental health. The resistance to stressful events and relationships interacts with the general cognitive level (see MAS Axis III), physical development and performance (see MAS Axis IV), and the abnormal psychosocial conditions (see MAS Axis V) in a complex, interdependent interplay.

Definition

The concept of resources in the OPD-CA-2 comprises all protective factors, albeit with a clear emphasis on interactions. Here we refer not to abilities measurable in isolation (like intelligence), but to psychosocial skills as demonstrated in dyads or groups. To be assessed is the extent to which a child and his/her family can utilize the resources available to them in the real life in order to overcome problems. Section 14.2 on *resources* in the OPD-CA-2 also contains factually existing conditions co-determining the life situation, the psychodynamics and the psychotherapeutic and prognostic situation of a child and his/her family. This includes, for example, coping with socio-economic risks such as poverty, a socially isolated residential area, and inadequate access to schools and health care systems. External anamnestic data must be reliably integrated in these contexts, and the interview will usually require explicit questioning in order to clarify matters as much as possible.

The categories of this section are closely related in content and operation to the MAS Axes III to VI as well as to the category of *inter-*

personality (formerly communicative skills) of the *structure* axis of the OPD-CA-2, and should therefore be interpreted for the most part on the basis of knowledge of the mental structure and typical relationship patterns (see the *interpersonal relations axis*).

Relationships With Peers

Theoretical Background

Experiences within the parent–child relationship form the basis of the ability for group integration. This area contains considerable interindividual variability in development between the middle of the 2nd and 6th years of life, depending on the family and social influential situations (kindergarten, extended family, patchwork family, etc.). Nevertheless, the development of play relationships as an area of social learning is also behaviorally innate (Hassenstein, 1986).

During preschool age, the child usually makes his/her initial contacts outside the family (extended family, Prague-Parent-Child-Program (PEKiP, German: Prager-Eltern-Kind-Programm) courses, toddler sports, playgroups, early musical education, etc.), the interactional arrangements and continuity of which indicate the child's mental resources.

In the period between 6 to 12 years, integration into the group of peers is one of the key developmental tasks. Forming lasting and yet flexible contacts outside the family, coping with school demands, and the child's prepubertal struggle with his/her own gender role occur during this period. They are increasingly regulated through peer relationships as well. The patterns of upbringing acquired in the parent–child relationship prove in many situations to be hardly functional or in need of modification, and must be revised for the peer group. Phases of social withdrawal can alternate with phases involving seemingly indiscriminate contact. An alternation between regressive and progressive elements of mental development occurs, with the connection to the family usually not being questioned, as will sometimes occur during adolescence.

During adolescence, integration in different groups of peers becomes the primary psychosocial developmental task, always in interplay with a partially distancing reorientation in the adolescent's relationship with his/her parents. Besides many other factors, the increasing importance of "best" male or female friends and the transient fixation on the first romantic partners govern healthy, youthful social behavior. The peer relationships of clinically abnormal adolescents may considerably differ.

In all age groups, types of behavior typical of the gender and ethnic group must always be carefully investigated and considered in the classification or rating.

Operationalization

The assessment of resources for *relationships with peers* concerns the extent to which, given the social development tasks of the particular age group and irrespective of the relationships with the family and with adults outside the family, friendships with peers are available, are maintained, and can be experienced and used as a source of social and emotional support. The assessment accordingly incorporates, across all age levels, concepts of social support insofar as they basically pertain to contact with peers. Of particular importance are participation in social networks among peers, such as kindergarten, sports clubs, school study groups, informal groups, church groups, virtual networks, etc., the subjective perception of support, i.e., the experienced emotional solidarity and loyalty in friendships, and the clear and critically questionable naming of male or female friends.

The assessment should also include considerations of how the children cope with their externalenvironment, with virtual environments playing an increasing role, depending on the individual constellation. The real availability of peers (possibly hampered by an isolated residential location, physical illness, age stratification of the residential environment, etc.) should also be considered, as should the child's individual ability (even given limited opportunities) to maintain real social contacts.

Examples

Age Group 1 (3 to 5 Years)	
Absent	This applies only to extremely salient cases of children growing up in extremely isolated conditions or impaired by considerable neuropsychiatric or organic disorders.
Low	Peers have only a low subjective and objective importance for the child's social behavior. While the child does take part in occasional group activities, he/she shows little initiative and does not differentiate between peers. For play, the child

	tends to seek younger children, but also especially adults. For children in this category, spontaneous invitations to birthday parties or recreational activities are extremely rare. Included in this category are children who, due to actual external life circumstances (chronic hospitalization, extremely isolated residential area, socially over-protective family system, etc.), can hardly make contact with their peers. While the child can mention contacts for playing when asked, play relationships with particular peers seem largely interchangeable and hardly an independent source for positive emotional experiences.
Moderate	These children regularly take part in externally organised or partly self-initiated group activities (play groups, parent–child sports, spontaneous games in the street), and obtain generally positive experiences of social acceptance from them. They tend to withdraw in reaction to irritations such as separations, temporal inconstancy of activities, and little support by adults, and are only partially able to maintain stability of internal representations of peers over longer periods of time. After a two-week interval, memories of play experiences have greatly faded and can be reactivated only through outside intervention (photos, accounts). While the child can express the independent subjective value of play relationships in a rudimentary way as a source of positive social and emotional experiences, this sense is not fully developed.
High	These children have stable relationships with peers outside the family. Especially noteworthy is kindergarten, but also informal play groups, sports activities, musical groups, and more distant relatives. These relationships, of course, depend significantly on the emotional and practical support in life from the primary attachment figures or possibly other adults. These children are able to maintain contact with their peers by themselves and to compensate for separations of longer than four weeks through intrapsychic object constancy. Parental influence needs especially to be regarded. The child's subjective experience has priority in the assessment. The child describes his/her relationships in play in a way indicating their role as a stable source of positive emotional and social experience.
Age Group 2 (6 to 12 Years)	
Absent	These are the most severely disturbed children, who de facto are unable to establish or maintain relationships with their peers. Only extreme cases of children growing up in thoroughly isolated conditions or affected by considerable neu-

	ropsychiatric or organic disorders (see again MAS Axis IV: organic disorders) fall in this category).
Low	These children maintain sporadic and superficial relationships with their peers. They cannot name relevant classmates or playmates, do not have their names ready at hand or simply refer to the entire group as "my friends." Especially regarding this question, external information should be obtained from parents, teachers, and siblings. This group also includes children with peer relationships solely initiated by adults. These children are very seldom invited to birthday parties, and tend more to have contact with smaller children or older people. On the one hand, the child may respond affirmatively in the interview when asked about friends in the socially desirable sense. On the other hand, the child's answer when asked about particular friendships and the corresponding experiences is rather vague, diffuse, or generalizing.
Moderate	Children in this group regularly have peer contacts, generally experienced as positive, and are based, at least in part, on the children's own initiative. Relatively stable relationships with peers develop which in their subjective significance lie well below relationships with the primary attachment figures and provide the child with only partial support in psychosocial crises. In the interview, these children are largely able to differentiate between peers as independent personalities and in a rudimentary way name shared activities or experiences with friends that they have especially appreciated.
High	These children are distinctly sociable and engage in regular exchanges with peers. Their relationships with other children form an essential part of their life, the subjective importance of which can certainly match that of parents and family. Intense involvement in sports, musical, or religious activities may be included here, with the child's initiative and activity significantly exceeding the levels already commonly encountered in this age group. Also to be coded here are cases in which the child's position in the peer group has been crucial for his/her mental and social survival, given the failure of other socialization factors (anti-social cliques and gang membership, mutual "upbringing" between neglected children). In psychosocial crisis situations, these children experience important support within the group. When asked, these children can name, in addition to specific activities they enjoy sharing with peers, values which for them make up a good friendship and which underscore the importance of friendship as an independent source of social support.

Age Group 3 (13 to 18 Years)	
Absent	These are the most severely disturbed adolescents, who de facto are unable to establish or maintain relationships with their peers. Only extreme cases of adolescents growing up in very isolated conditions affected by considerable neuropsychiatric or organic disorders fall in this category.
Low	This category comprises adolescents having very little contact with peers and hardly ever taking part in group activities typical for their age (sports, recreation, "hanging out," chatting online, virtual internet games, etc.). Here adolescents are coded who can report on a single apparently viable friendship. Beyond this friendship they have hardly had any positively experienced group contact. Therefore they seem locked in an exclusively dyadic relationship pattern. Clinical example: "Only my best friend understands me – no one else."
Moderate	The peer group functions as an important frame of reference for this developmental stage and forms the background for social activities. Contact with the family and with primary attachment figures is of equal importance.
High	In this age group, relationships with peer groups make up a central part of life, in the interest of which areas of life previously more important are now revaluated as subjectively less significant. To be rated high in the coding are such adolescents whose activities take place almost exclusively with their peers, whether at the expense of other relationships or as an enriching supplement to generally stable relationships with primary attachment figures or family members. In psychosocial stress situations, friends are the key contacts and supports, or are significantly involved in resolving a general issue.

Family Resources

Theoretical Background

Dysfunctional familial structures have high importance as a risk factor in the development of mental disorders in children and adolescents. Functional and sustainable family relationships accordingly play an important protective and salutogenic role. In the assessment of the *family resources,* the salutogenic view of the family system is crucial. As there exists no unambiguous theoretical frame of reference for family-related resources, nor is this to be expected in the foreseeable future, the OPD-CA-2 lists individual factors. Altogether, they provide information on the skills and abilities of families for coping adequately with children's and adolescents' problems.

The following familial resources are regarded as particularly important within the OPD-CA-2:

- Intense relationships with primary attachment figures
- Helpful relationships with other family members
- Constructive culture of exchanges between the parents
- Mandatory family rules
- Predictability of parental behavior
- Stable bond with a parent, even if the other parent may often be aggressive or deprecating
- Stable relationship with siblings

In addition to these areas, observations of the following are also incorporated:

- Open communication among family members
- Mental flexibility of family members
- Emotional ties between family members
- Exchanges between the family and the outside world

Also considered is how open-minded and interested family members are in reaction to verbal interventions (e.g., clarifications, confrontations, interpretations).

Examples

Age Group 1 (3 to 5 Years)	
Absent	Neither a primary nor surrogate family exists. The child grows up in an institutional environment from birth. No experience of familial structures (street children, Kasper Hauser Syndrome). There are no fantasies about parents, not even idealizations. This is an extreme category, seldom to be assigned in coding.

Low	Parents (single or both) or familial surrogate parents are available only to a limited extent, are inconsistent and un-clear in their treatment of the child, and not available to the child with much reliability. The bond between the child and relevant family members is fragile or at least highly ambiv-alent and can be activated as a support in crisis situations only in exceptional cases. Communication between the adult members of the family or siblings is partly problem-atic, incoherent, and characterized by misunderstandings and projections (see MAS Axis V, distorted intrafamilial communication). Nonetheless, the child is partially able to integrate individual relationship episodes or positive mem-ories of parental figures in basically positive representations, and develop simple idealizations. With the appropriate sup-port, the parents have a rudimentary ability to reflect on and change their relationship with their child.
Moderate	Many of the factors mentioned in the definition can be found in these families. Communication is in principle open-ended and geared to the child's interests. Contact with parental figures is supportive and central. Other family members are integrated in the child's inner world. In the interview, the parents can describe and discuss problems and the respective approaches to a solution in an emotion-ally adequate way. They respond to suggestions and trial in-terpretations.
High	These families tackle emotional as well as cognitive prob-lems and sources of irritation regarding their child in a very open way. They can perceive ambivalent feelings towards the toddler, verbalize them and creatively use them for fur-ther development. At the same time, the parents are aware of the importance and value of their relationship as a cou-ple as well as the transgenerational boundaries. They use exchanges with their own families of origin as well as with any siblings of the child in order to arrive at a sophisticated view of the symptomatic child. The parents recognize and appreciate their child's age-related possibilities and limita-tions and adjust their demands to an age-appropriate level. The child him-/herself is able to perceive and possibly de-scribe his/her father and mother in a detailed way and to recognize the differences between them without being over-come by anxious impulses. In projective tests, the child ex-presses internal images of the family that simultaneously depict coherence and distinguish between the individuals. The child can also discern and express ambivalent impulses towards his/her parents.

Age Group 2 (6 to 12 Years)	
Absent	Neither a primary nor a surrogate family exists. The child grows up in an institutional environment from birth. No experience of familial structures (street children, etc.). There are no positive fantasies about parents, not even idealizations. This is a rarely coded category for cases of extreme developmental disorders.
Low	Parents (single or both) or familial surrogate parents are available only to a limited extent, are inconsistent in their treatment of the child, and are hardly emotionally available to the child. The bond between the child and relevant family members is fragile or at least ambivalent and can rarely be activated as a support in crisis situations. Communication between the adult members of the family or siblings is partly problematic, incoherent, and characterised by misunderstandings and projections (see MAS Axis V, distorted intrafamilial communication). Nonetheless, the child is able to integrate repeated, pleasant relationship episodes or positive memories of his/her parental figures in a generally positive representational world, and develop clear idealisations.
Moderate	Many of the factors mentioned in the definition can be found in these families. Communication is in principle open-ended and geared to the child's developing interests. Contact with parental figures is supportive and central. Other family members are integrated in the child's inner world. In the interview, the parents can describe and discuss in a sophisticated and emotionally adequate way the particular development of the family, problems, and appropriate approaches to solutions. They respond creatively to suggestions and trial interpretations.
High	The family as a whole is aware of the issues and presents a united attitude towards the outside world and the diagnostician, with individual idiosyncrasies being respected. The child is supported appropriately to his/her age and in his/her steps towards individuation. New peer relationships are integrated in the familial framework in a positive way and this integration is supported by the parents. Sibling relationships are sincere, respectful, and provide support for the individual child in times of crisis.

Age Group 3 (13 to 18 Years)	
Absent	Neither a primary nor a surrogate family exists. The adolescent grows up in an institutional environment from birth. There is no experience of familial structures (street children, long-term stays in a home, etc.). There are no positive fantasies about parents, not even idealizations. This is a rarely coded category for cases of extreme and chronic developmental disorders.
Low	Parents (single or both) or familial surrogate parents have been and are available only to a limited extent, are inconsistent in their treatment of the adolescent, and are hardly emotionally available to the adolescent. The bond between the adolescent and relevant family members is fragile or at least ambivalent, and in crisis situations can only rarely be activated as a support. Communication among family members is in part problematic, incoherent, and subject to misunderstandings and projections (see MAS Axis V, distorted intrafamilial communication). Nevertheless, the adolescent is now and then able to report recurrent, pleasant relationship episodes or positive memories of the parental figures when asked. The adolescent can partially accept his/her parents with their weaknesses and discern their positive qualities. The parents are partially willing and able to reflect on and change their relationship with their child.
Moderate	Most of the factors mentioned in the definition can be found in these families. Communication is in principle open-ended and at least partially geared to the adolescent's developmental needs. Contact with parental figures is important for the adolescent, and other family members are integrated in the adolescent's inner world. In the interview, the adolescent and his/her parents can describe and discuss in a sophisticated and emotionally adequate way the particular development of the family, problems, and appropriate approaches to solutions. They respond to suggestions and trial interpretations.
High	The overall family is aware of issues and presents a generally united attitude towards the outside world and the diagnostician, with individual idiosyncrasies being respected. The adolescent is supported appropriately to his/her age and in his/her steps towards individuation. New peer relationships are integrated in the family in a positive way and this integration is supported by the parents. Sibling relationships are sincere, respectful, and provide the individual with support in times of crisis.

Intrapsychic Resources

Theoretical Background

In the attempt to operationalize the corresponding strengths and abilities already present in the child or adolescent within a subjective dimension (i.e., in separation from dimensions captured in the MAS, such as intelligence), in psychoanalytic theory we inevitably encounter the agency of the ego, its structure, and its abilities. In the operationalization of intrapsychic resources, intentional components of the ego, i.e., the person's own consciously experienced abilities available to that individual for controlling and shaping external reality or for approaching the object world and acting in relation to it (Rudolf, 1995), were to form essential determinants for the assessment.

On the other hand, the aim was to avoid redundancies in the assessment along the *structure* axis and to find an operationalization that, for the most part, dispenses with metapsychological constructs.

As to the conceptual orientation of the psychoanalytically trained user, we note that the concept of ego strength, but also certain ego functions and ego achievements (in particular external and internal perception, anticipation, self-reflection, the ability for action and functional zest), are theoretically closely related to the intrapsychic resources, or are essential parts of the same thing. We finally chose a theoretically neutral, generally understandable definition corresponding to a resultant, rateable in the interview, of the aforementioned abilities of the ego with regard to internalized confidence. Utilizing the conceptual system of attachment theory (Bowlby, 1998), we could also speak of an internal working model of "confidence in coping with problems". Expressly to be distinguished here, on the other hand, is the concept of internal convictions of control (Lohaus & Schmitt, 1989), designating the subjective independence from the support system.

Operationalization

By intrapsychic resources we mean the specific psychosocial abilities available to children and adolescents for coping with stress, problems, and conflicts, and therefore also for coping with problems in subjective experience responsible for the diagnostic presentation. These consciously experienced abilities significantly determine the degree of expressed confidence in children and adolescents in overcoming the existing disorder or illness with therapeutic assistance. The classification gives particular importance to spontaneous utterances of confidence in overcoming mental illness (example: "I do need help, but I can do it!"). If no confidence in overcoming the disorder is expressed owing to a symptom-related high level of suffering, internal working models for coping with problems in other contexts will have to be considered and must generally be inquired about.

Examples

Age Group 1 (3 to 5 Years) (can generally be assessed only if speech sufficiently developed)	
Absent	A preschool child with symptoms of anxiety does not indicate either in his/her utterances or scenic play the conceivability of these anxieties being overcome, not even with the aid of other people.
Low	A preschool child offers, e.g., in scenic play a solution initiated by the child-protagonist or playfully takes up a corresponding offer from the examiner, but reacts with hesitant withdrawal or avoidance behavior when the examiner draws attention to this problem-solving model as an achievement of the child-protagonist and as possibly applicable to the child's own situation (example: "As we've just seen playing together, a child can do something to make him-/herself feel less afraid").
Moderate	A preschool child reacts with curiosity and interest to the examiner's verbalized suggestion that a solution developed in the scenic play and initiated by the child protagonist could be helpful for coping with his/her own problems.
High	When asked, a pre-schooler verbalizes a strategy available to him/her for reducing anxiety (example: "What do you do when you're alone and you get scared?" – "I put the scariness under my pillow, and then it's gone").
Age Group 2 (6 to 12 Years)	
Absent	A depressive schoolchild appears completely helpless and full of despair, and, on questioning, expresses no confidence or belief in problem resolution.
Low	During the interview, a schoolchild with difficulties in making contact and anxieties can take up verbally or in play the idea of a child being able to resolve issues or of being confident, but reacts hesitantly or with avoidance to a mirror-

	ing intervention that attempts to relate this subject to his/her own situation (example: "Has it ever happened that you found someone who could help you and that you felt better afterwards?").
Moderate	On questioning, a schoolchild with difficulty making contact and with anxieties begins to express an internalized confidence that he/she will feel better soon if someone helps him/her (example: "It would be good if someone were there for me; maybe then things would get better").
High	On questioning, a schoolchild expresses clearly that he/she has an internalized idea of confidence or problem resolution, specifically in reference to either existing issues or to other situations that may well be fictitious (example: "I think I can do this." Or: "If I were as strong as Pippi Longstocking, I would ...").
Age Group 3 (13 to 18 Years)	
Absent	A depressive schoolchild appears completely helpless and full of despair, and, on questioning, expresses no notion of confidence or problem resolution.
Low	An adolescent suffering from compulsions indicates when questioned in the interview that he/she has a rudimentary internal idea of problem resolution, but cannot yet relate this idea either to his/her own abilities or to his/her current situation, so that the feeling of hopelessness predominates even when aid is offered.
Moderate	An adolescent with an eating disorder expresses ambivalence about his/her confidence in finding a way to control his/her eating behavior through therapy, but can name issue-resolving abilities of his/her own in other areas when asked.
High	An adolescent with an anxiety disorder can state significantly subjective experiences of his/her abilities in other problematic situations when asked, and expresses, for the most part, confidence in improving his/her symptoms through therapeutic help.

Extra-Familial Social Support

Theoretical Background

The availability and the possibilities for utilizing a social support system crucially influence the onset and the course of a mental health problem in the child. A network with helpful social support, consisting of tangible social relationships also outside the family system through friends, neighbors, and acquaintances from the occupational or recreational activities of the family, has been often identified in the literature as a protective factor in the healthy development of children from risk groups (Plass & Wiegand-Grefe, 2012; Resnick, Harris, & Blum, 1993; Zolkoski & Bullock, 2012). For example, highly emotionally distressed young or grown-up children of mentally ill parents retrospectively state that they generally did not feel they had sufficient social support during childhood, or that they would have liked to have had greater social support (Sollberger, Byland, & Widmer, 2008). While the majority of children have a certain, mostly small, network of social relationships with relatives or acquaintances at their disposal, they generally avoid using these relationships for coping with everyday problems.

Operationalization

This category concerns the availability and utilization of social support from the child's extra-familial social environment. This social support comprises all socially helpful contacts and relationships with adults outside the nuclear family, irrespective of any professional support and irrespective of support from the child's or adolescent's same-age peer group. The network of extra-familial social support in question thus supplements professional support and support from friendships with peers. This category includes friends and acquaintances of the family, social integration in neighborly affairs as well as social integration in club activities, church activities, music orchestras, or similar social affairs.

The assessment of this availability and the possibilities for using a social support system captures to what extent social relationships are available at all to a family or a child that can be utilized as required. The usability of these available social resources is also assessed. The interview must explicitly inquire into this matter and, in each case, be supplemented by external anamnestic data (usually from the parents).

Examples

Age Group 1 (3 to 5 Years)	
Absent	These families or children have no possibilities of social support available to them because they are not able to develop them or avail themselves of existing opportunities.
Low	This category describes children and families with marginal possibilities of social support. The children grow up with little contact with adult attachment figures beyond their parents (friends, neighbours, colleagues, acquaintances of the parents). The family is largely socially isolated. These children hardly ever speak of people outside the nuclear family, nor can they conceive of such persons being helpful in problematic situations.
Moderate	There exists a theoretical awareness about the possibilities of using a social network of the family. Some contact exists with adult attachment figures outside the family, but this contact is not used extensively. The child takes part in extra-familial activities under external supervision.
High	The parents intensively avail themselves of the social support available for this age group among friends and acquaintances from the family's occupational or recreational circles. The parents maintain much contact and regular exchanges also with, e.g., parents of other children in this age group.
Age Group 2 (6 to 12 Years)	
Absent	Support from a social network plays no role at all with these children. The child has no conception of there being helpful people from the family's environment. There may exist a paranoid-hostile family climate in which the idea of maintaining contact with other people or even availing oneself of help from other people is fraught with anxiety or accompanied by paranoid hostility.
Low	These children are hardly or only marginally capable of availing themselves of extra-familial helpers from the family's social network. While they do find themselves in situations with theoretically helpful people, the children hardly perceive this fact and attribute practically no importance to people outside the family as helpers.
Moderate	While these children are aware of or have contact with extra-familial persons of the family's social network and also possibly maintain relationships with these people, the

	emotional relevance is not very pronounced. The helpful influence of external people is felt as rather low compared with parents or primary attachment figures.
High	Children with a high degree of this characteristic can already have intense trust in extra-familial attachment figures (family friends, neighbors, acquaintances) very early on in life and also avail themselves of their assistance in resolving issues. These children succeed in integrating extra-familial people in their daily life.
Age Group 3 (13 to 18 Years)	
Absent	There exists no possibilities for using social support among children in this age group, or they categorically reject these possibilities.
Low	Potentially helpful social relationships or people are used only marginally. Alternatively, there may exist a high anxiety potential up to the point of paranoid distortions among adolescents strongly tied to their families. Social relationships of the social network are deprecated or ignored and at best ambivalently accepted in unavoidable dramatic emergencies.
Moderate	These adolescents can seek support outside the family, among people of the social network. The extra-familial relationships then have more of a functional than a personal interactional character, and may be configured discontinuously.
High	These adolescents utilize a social network outside the family in a lively and unhindered way. The socially helpful relationships are actively and regularly maintained by these adolescents, and supplement familial structures or constitute a possibly viable compensation for intrafamilial relationship problems.

10.3 Prerequisites for Treatment

Insight Into Biopsychosocial Interrelations

Theoretical Background

The concept of insight is widespread in psychotherapy and serves as an important construct in nearly all therapy approaches. This applies in particular also to analytic psychotherapy (Thomä & Kächele, 1988).

Here, insight is not understood as the "insight into illness," which plays an important role in many areas of medicine, such as the treatment of psychotic patients, forensic-psychiatric assessments, and medical awareness campaigns. *Insight into biopsychosocial interrelations* in our sense also encompasses more than the ability for introspection, which merely involves the general ability for internal perception (Mertens, 1992). Internal perception can initiate self-reflective processes, which, in turn, lead to insights (see Section 5.3 on *Theoretical Conception of the Axes – Structure*). Consequently our construct of insight into biopsychosocial interrelations comprises a continuum encompassing introspection as well as self-reflection.

Whereas Freud (S. Freud, 1914/2000) related insight more to unconscious pathogenic childhood conflicts and their later derivatives and effects, Fenichel (1941) situates insight between the poles of thought and feeling. Insight in this sense pertains only to children's and adolescents' cognitive abilities to discern relationships, as in their understanding present behavior on the basis of earlier events, for example (Fisher & Greenberg, 1977).

Insight and the ability for introspection partly overlap with one another. The OPD-CA-2 represents the ability for introspection along the structure axis under the concept of *self-perception* (see above). Insight primarily incorporates the rational-cognitive aspects of the ability for introspection, while *self-perception* also includes affects and physical sensations.

Operationalization

Insight into biopsychosocial interrelations pertains to the willingness and ability of children and adolescents to discern relationships between external life situations, inner experiences, and their problems or symptoms appropriately for their age. To assess such a self-reflective treatment of biopsychosocial interrelations, it is generally necessary to stimulate and facilitate an appropriately self-reflective approach in the diagnostic dialog with the examiner, by means of specific psychodynamic interventions stimulating introspection and discussing biopsychosocial interrelations (e.g., clarification, confrontation, and interpretation).

For assessing suitable topics of conversation, the interviewer can bring up typical situations triggering the initial occurrence of symptoms or the patient's recognition of benefits from the symptoms of a secondary *gain from illness* (see below). The insight into biopsychosocial interrelations is assessed only on the cognitive-rational level. The patient's ability to perceive his/her own affects is represented along the *structure (affective tolerance)* axis. For coding the insight, it is crucial that the children or adolescents not only confirm relationships or issues brought up by the examiner with a "yes," but also pick up these matters in terms of their content, reproducing them in their own words, and possibly developing them further through reflection. Therapeutic change need not accompany this insight. The insight should be assessed purely on a descriptive level given the child's or adolescent's verbal utterances. From a developmental-psychological perspective, the level of abstraction in the child's rational thought necessary for this operationalization is hardly to be expected before the age of 13, so that this item should be rated only as of age group 3 (13 to 18 years). It must be kept in mind that the rating of the insight depends on the child's level of intelligence, so that an objective assessment of intelligence according to MAS Axis III (at least through a systematic survey of school performance levels) should occur beforehand.

Examples

Age Group 3 (13 to 18 Years)	
Absent	The adolescent recognizes no relationships between constellations of problems and symptoms, even after their presentation by the examiner.
Low	The adolescent can respond to the examiner's suggestions of relationships (confrontations, mirroring, etc.) only in some of their aspects; for example, he/she will recognize the temporal aspect of triggering situations, while denying relationship-dynamic contexts or relationships with other psychosocial conditions.
Moderate	These adolescents do not contribute spontaneous ideas of their own on biopsychosocial relationships. They discuss these relationships if suggested by the examiner, however, even if only hesitantly, and with cognitive comprehension.
High	These adolescents recognize and further develop biopsychosocial relationships spontaneously or through mirroring or confrontations on the examiner's part ("It strikes me that …"). For example, they can recognize their own part in a conflict-ridden detachment-related set of problems from home.

Specific Motivation for Psychotherapy

Theoretical Background

"Specific motivation for psychotherapy" in the OPD-CA-2 refers to the patient's willingness and motivation, as revealed in trial sessions, to engage in a specifically psychodynamic or psychoanalytic mode of working in the psychotherapeutic setting. For rating the specific motivation for psychotherapy, the child's or adolescent's reactions to the following specific characteristics of a psychodynamically-oriented interview are therefore crucial (see **Table 3**).

The differentiation between the items *motivation for change, level of suffering,* and *specific motivation for psychotherapy* aims at obtaining a maximally informative basis for the indication for psychotherapy of a child or adolescent. This includes considerations of the differential indication for different therapeutic approaches. It can be especially enlightening for diagnostic considerations if the motivation for change, level of suffering, and specific motivation for therapy are, contrary to expectations, not equally pronounced. For example, a high level of suffering with a low motivation for change and low specific motivation for therapy can warrant the decision to begin with a clarification phase in the family-therapeutic setting, to shed light on the psychodynamic meaning of this apparent inconsistency in the context of the family system (example: "What is the child doing for the family with his/her symptom?"). Likewise, a high motivation for change with a low specific motivation for therapy can lead to the use of other interventions first (e.g., pedagogical measures), with the motivation for psychotherapy being checked again at a later time.

Table 3. Specific characteristics of psychodynamic interviewing

- The gearing of the interview to the patient's inner experiences.
- The attempt to elaborate on intrapsychic and interpersonal conflicts and their role in existing issues and symptoms.
- The attempt to understand an issue or symptom in its life-historical context.
- The attempt to establish meaningful affect-related connections between apparently irrational behavioral and experiential patterns.
- The attempt to consider an issue or symptom in its interplay with the patient's important relationships (mostly parent–child relationships).

Operationalization

The concept of specific motivation for psychotherapy comprises the specific interest, registered in a psychodynamically oriented initial interview with a child or adolescent (a phase of multiple trial sessions is also possible), in working to ameliorate the reported issues or complaints and symptoms. Here were are referring neither to the motivation for change nor to the general ability for making contact. Nor do we mean a nonspecific positive reaction to the attentiveness and care of the examiner, although these aspects do influence the specific motivation for psychotherapy.

In the assessment of the specific motivation for psychotherapy, the patient's immediate reactions to the dialogical interventions (clarification, confrontation, and interpretation) explained in Section 6.1, *Diagnostic Assessment*, have the greatest value. Ideally, these interventions will be developed in the aforementioned order in the course of the interview. In the initial phase of the interview, empathic listening predominates, with selective questioning in the case of ambiguity, diffuseness of reported feelings, or the omission of apparently important topics and content (clarification). As initial impressions about the typical behavioral patterns of the patient intensify and shape themselves from the participatory observation of the interaction in the course of the interview, they can be mirrored from the dialog (confrontation, example: "It struck me while listening that …"). If an initial, apparently plausible psychodynamic hypothesis about the unconscious dynamics of the described symptoms can be developed in the course of the interview on the basis of the patient's reactions to these clarifications and confrontations, a subsequent phase of the interview can propose this hypothesis to the patient as a provisional interpretation. This is very often not the case, however. If such a dialogically developed provisional interpretation is provided (example: "Can I understand that you mean …"), observation of the further course of the interview as to how the child or adolescent responds to this trial interpretation will be of central importance for the assessment. In addition, it is assessed globally how the child or adolescent reacts to the aforementioned characteristics of a psychodynamic interview. In the final phase of the interview, when the termination as well as possible continuation of the dialog at a later date is discussed, the patient's communication and modes of behavior will also provide valuable information, to be considered in the subsequent rating. In case of doubt, if the assessment cannot be sufficiently grounded in the patient's utterances, the *specific motivation for psychotherapy* can be assessed from the overall impression. But if the patient's communications coming into consideration for this category cannot be reliably differentiated from the *motivation for change* or from the general need for contact, "cannot be rated" must be chosen.

Examples

Age Group 1 (3 to 5 Years)	
Absent	The child completely rejects the examiner's offers of play and contact, or openly displays refusal.
Low	While the child can be reached through age-appropriate offers of contact (play, drawing, etc.), he/she remains largely passive in repetitive play patterns or becomes considerably evasive once the examiner tries to bring up the issue in play symbolically, e.g., in scenic play by offering a mother figure who wants to remove herself.
Moderate	The child rather hesitantly communicates his/her problem symbolically by drawing or in play. When the examiner broaches stressful subjects like danger, anger, anxiety, and separation, or suggests them in play, the child reacts reticently, although signals the desire to continue contact.
High	The child communicates an aspect of his/her problem during contact in play or while drawing, and shows curiosity when the examiner suggests interpretative aids for understanding during play or, while continuing the symbolic game, emphatically supports the child in trying out solutions.
Age Group 2 (6 to 12 Years)	
Absent	The child completely rejects the examiner's offers of play and dialog, or openly displays refusal.
Low	Although reacting with interest to the examiner's offer of dialog or play, the child repeatedly evades the examiner's attempts at understanding (directing the child towards inner experiences, discussing conflicts, relationship context, etc.).

Moderate	The child hesitantly accepts the examiner's endeavors to understand, but clearly shows ambivalence by evading these efforts at other points in the interview (e.g., avoidance behavior, denial, etc.). On the whole, however, the child makes clear that he/she wants to continue the dialog with the examiner.
High	The child reacts with thoughtfulness and interest to the examiner's efforts to understand, and clearly signals a desire to continue the dialog.
Age Group 3 (13 to 18 Years)	
Absent	The adolescent completely rejects the offer of dialog or openly displays refusal.
Low	While the adolescent accepts the examiner's offer of dialog, he/she repeatedly evades the examiner's attempts to understand (directing the child towards inner experiences, discussing conflicts, relationship context, etc.).
Moderate	The adolescent hesitantly accepts the examiner's endeavors to understand, but clearly shows his/her ambivalence by evading these efforts at other points in the interview (e.g., avoidance behavior, denial, etc.). On the whole, however, the adolescent signals that he/she wants to continue the dialog with the examiner.
High	The adolescent is emotionally affected and shows concern and/or thoughtfulness and interest in the examiner's endeavors to understand, and clearly signals the desire to continue the initiated dialog.

Gain From Illness

Theoretical Background

Ever since Freud, the psychoanalytical theory of neurosis has conceptually distinguished between the primary and secondary gain from illness. The "primary gain from illness" refers (along the lines of a dynamic understanding of the symptom as a neurotic compromise between defence and that defended against) to the "success" of the symptom as the attempt at an initially tension-reducing conflict resolution. For example, should repressed separation anxiety result in "school phobia" as a symptom, the primary gain from illness would lie in the avoidance of separation and restored intimacy with the mother, attained by the refusal to go to school. The primary gain from illness is thus causally related to the genesis of the symptom. Freud (1905/1953) emphasized the etiological importance of the primary gain from illness, coining the phrase "flight into illness." Secondary gain from illness, on the other hand, encompasses all other consequences and reactions of the environment following a manifest disorder and subjectively experienced as reinforcement, and that possibly contribute to the patient's retaining his/her symptoms. This particularly includes the increased attentiveness and care resulting from a disorder. Understanding the secondary gain from illness is especially important in cases of psychogenic disorders with predominantly physical symptoms. The somatic-medical attention to the physical symptom can be especially important in these patients' experience for legitimizing their need for help. It should also be considered that certain intrapsychic conflicts, in particular conflicts of *closeness vs. distance* (formerly: *autonomy vs. dependency)* as well as *taking care of oneself vs. being cared for*, can considerably interfere with the gain from illness (see Section 5.2 *Theoretical Conception of the Axes – Conflict*).

In a compilation of various remarks by Freud on the primary and secondary gains from illness, Thomä and Kächele (1985) note his critical stance towards the distinguishability of etiology from the retention of psychogenic symptoms. They conclude that, in particular, the course of stable symptom formations is characterized by such a combination of the primary conditions and secondary motives as to render a distinction nearly impossible (ibid).

In child and adolescent psychiatry and psychotherapy a differentiation between primary and secondary gains from illness also seems rather problematic. A clear distinction between etiology and secondary symptom intensification is often not possible in clinical assessments. For example, the desire for attention is very often integrated in the genesis of complex symptoms. For this reason, the OPD-CA-2 comprehensively rates the gain from illness in its primary and secondary components. This should help raters assess in advance the degree of the expected resistance to treatment or the expected tendency to cling to a symptom. The gain from illness thus, to a certain extent, forms a dynamic counterpoint to the items of *level of suffering, motivation for change,* and *specific motivation for psychotherapy*. From the assessment of the interplay between these items, we can therefore draw conclusions about the assumed ambivalence towards treatment.

Operationalization

The concept of gain from illness comprises all aspects of the patient's subjective experience that have a potentially reinforcing effect on the symptoms. They include, besides (e.g., anxiety-fraught) experiences avoided through the disorder, all reactions by the environment that have a subjectively reinforcing effect, even if they may appear aversive when considered objectively. For example, an aggressively and hyper-actively behaving child can process his/her parents' constantly recurring angry reactions as a form of increased attention, irrespective of the accompanying negative effect. Aspects like "gain in power" in the family are also incorporated here. The gain from illness is generally unconscious. A verbal confirmation is generally not to be expected in the interview. The assessment must therefore rest on the patient's observable behavior or descriptions, allowing indirect but plausible inferences as to the gain from illness.

Examples

All Age Groups (3 to 18 Years)	
Absent	The child's or adolescent's verbal and nonverbal communications give no indications of social or emotional gain from the disorder, diagnosis, or therapy.
Low	While at one to two points in the interview the child's or adolescent's verbal and nonverbal communications discreetly indicate an emotional gain or social advantages from the disorder, diagnosis, or therapy, these are not determinative of the overall impression. • A child signals that he/she feels better because others are worried about him/her, but nothing indicates that this concern is determinative of his/her behavior. • An adolescent smiles during the interview as her mother describes her helplessness over her daughter's anorectic symptoms.
Moderate	The patient's subjective experience as expressed in verbal or nonverbal communications reveals some social advantages or aspects of emotional gain from the disorder, diagnosis, and therapy. These communications occur at more than two points in the interview. The symptom is integrated in the patient's management of relationships. The disorder has resulted in a perceptible "special role" that these children or adolescents play in their families, school, or social surroundings.

High	Several social advantages or aspects of emotional gain become clear from the disorder, diagnosis, and therapy given the patient's verbal and nonverbal communications. The symptom seems to play a significant role in the patient's management of relationships. As a result of the disorder, these children and adolescents play a distinctly "special role" in their families, school, or social surroundings.
	Example: With his/her aggressive behavior at home, a child firmly unites both parents in their anger towards him/her, so that family life practically exclusively centres on the child's behavioral problems. An existing relational conflict between the parents can no longer be settled, but is rather displaced by a permanent parent–child conflict.

Ability to Form Working Alliances

Theoretical Background

The therapeutic working alliance is the psychotherapeutic form of the patient contract. Unlike the case in adult treatment, working alliances in child and adolescent psychotherapy are generally triangular relationships between the parents, the child, and the therapist. However, our concern is mainly with the children's or adolescents' personal prerequisites for entering into a working alliance. Many patients were not able to acquire sufficient experience with reliable "holding objects" (in the broadest sense) in early childhood, affording safety and comfort (Heigl-Evers, Heigl, & Ott, 1993). Consequently the creation as well as preservation of a therapeutic alliance forms an especially important part of the therapist's work. The creation of a working alliance can therefore initially be the primary goal of therapeutic endeavors. The age-specific assessment of the ability to form working alliances brought along by a child or adolescent is also a useful prerequisite of treatment, given the importance of the parents and the therapist's efforts. A prerequisite of the child's ability to form working alliances is his/her willingness to make clear-cut agreements with the therapist and to keep these agreements within the framework of a trusting, sustainable relationship. Such agreements also particularly concern external parameters (punctuality, frequency of sessions, arrangement in the holidays, etc.). Especially in child therapy, the therapist serves as a role model by duly announcing ahead of time any absences or changes.

The parents' share in the realization of the working alliance varies greatly given the therapeutic spectrum – from an out-patient setting with long driving distances to in-patient care. The overall picture in the assessment of the *ability to form working alliances* according to age group and setting should also include the parents' compliance.

In children under the age of six, parental influence is practically the only factor to bear on out-patient treatment. For this reason, the item is assessed only from Age Group 2 (6 to 12 years) on. In adolescents aged 15 years and above, the relevance of the intrinsic ability to form working alliances predominates. Separate documentation in a freely formulated form of the assessment of the attainable working alliance with the parents is recommended, as this documentation is generally important for the interpretation of this category. Note that this category cannot be assessed on the basis of a single initial interview situation. Nevertheless, in order to enable an assessment in terms of a foreseeable ability to form a psychotherapeutic working alliance within a diagnostic phase, the assessment should include at least one other session following the initial interview, in order to rate the patient's motivation and reliability for coming back after an initial session. Note also that the *ability to form working alliances* can only pertain to the given treatment setting. For example, it may happen that certain patients exhibit a high *ability to form working alliances* in the course of in-patient treatment, but after their discharge no longer reliably avail themselves of the provided out-patient setting, which requires greater personal responsibility.

Examples

Age Groups 2 and 3 (6 to 18 Years)	
Absent	Despite supportive surroundings, reminders from parents or guardians, and despite being seen off, the child arrives at the sessions late or not at all. While in pressured situations contact by phone may occur, no committed relationship is established
Low	The children in question are often unpunctual. When confronted about this behavior, they become evasive. Often the prehistory indicates the discontinuation of supportive measures that is not primarily due a lack of cooperation on the part of the parents or because of other limited family or social resources. The therapist begins to feel that no stable

	therapeutic alliance can be attained; instead, the ability to form working alliances seems to be the primary working goal.
Moderate	The establishment of a stable therapeutic setting seems foreseeable. On this basis, deviations can be discussed in a therapeutically fruitful way. During the interview, a basic agreement can develop regarding the primary issue requiring treatment.
High	The patients behave very reliably within the agreed setting and make reliable agreements in due time, so that all parties acquire the sense of a stable mode of initiating relationships. In the relationship, one can discern the patient's willingness to work towards solutions to the jointly defined issue.

Utilization of the Care System

Theoretical Background

The availability and utilization of the care system has a crucial influence on the course of mental disorders. In particular, in the complex care system of a modern welfare state with partly competing and conflicting missions and funding agencies, it is important for a psychodynamic assessment to recognize recurring interactive patterns of patients and their families and to assess these patterns in terms of functionality and importance. Re-enactments of earlier, possibly traumatic or neglected relationships occur especially in patients with a lower level of structural integration, and are important for diagnoses and treatment planning.

Material aspects like social transfer payments and concessions must also be considered here.

Operationalization

The assessment of the *utilization of the care system* captures the extent to which a family or child is aware at all of the offers of aid, the manner in which and since when they avail themselves of this aid, and whether secondary dependencies on aid providers have developed that may impair the child's development of autonomy. Extreme poles can be described in families structured in an anxious to paranoid form who completely ignore offers of help. On the other hand there are very needy families utilizing the services of various helpers and therapists simultaneously. Midway lies a timely, solution- and problem-oriented as well as committed use of offers of help. This category concerns the actual handling of extra-familial care systems offering social support. This practice must be expressly inquired into during the interview (usually with the parents) and in any case supplemented with external anamnestic data. Inner experiences play a subordinate role, but should not be completely neglected.

Examples

Age Group 1 (3 to 5 Years)	
Absent	These families have de facto no awareness of professional offers of assistance, or they strictly and categorically refuse extra-familial assistance. Anxious to paranoid perceptions of the social environment and in particular of institutions prevail. The outside world is strictly separated from the intrafamilial world. The children of these families have de facto no contact with adults outside the family, who are experienced as potentially threatening.
Low	These are families with a marginal knowledge of professional aid facilities. The children grow up having little contact with their peers; the family is largely based on its internal structure, and partly dissociates itself from its surroundings in an anxious to hostile manner. Kindergarten attendance is typically rare or irregular, and contact with attachment figures is precarious or limited to formalities. The children themselves hardly ever mention people outside the family and cannot conceive of them as helpful in problematic situations, except as virtual, superhuman rescuers.
Moderate	There exists a theoretical awareness of professional aid systems in the children's environments. The child takes part in extra-familial activities under external supervision. For the parents, extra-familial counsellors are significantly less important than intrafamilial ones, however, and offers regarding specific behavioral problems are accepted rarely, met with scepticism, or utilized only in the event of clear-cut issues. Typically, reticent ambivalence will prevail.
High	The parents intensively avail themselves of the support offered for this age group, and they have contact with other parents with babies or toddlers, whether in play groups or in kindergarten. The parents regularly seek the advice of kindergarten teachers and other institutions, and participation in parent–teacher conferences goes without saying. Typically, literature and the internet are also used as sources of information on child development.

Age Group 2 (6 to 12 Years)	
Absent	Support from professional aid systems or institutions plays no role for these children. Knowledge about helpers or helpful external institutions does not exist. Typically there will exist a paranoid-hostile family atmosphere in which the idea of accepting aid from outside the family is fraught with anxiety.
Low	These children are rarely capable of accepting assistance from extra-familial helpers. While they find themselves in situations with theoretically helpful adults, they are hardly aware of this opportunity and ascribe practically no constructive power to people outside the family. "Significant others" in the salutogenic sense play only a marginal role in these children's conceptions and reality.
Moderate	While these children are aware of or have contact with extra-familial helpers and may also maintain relationships with them, the emotional relevance is not very pronounced. Helpers are primarily persons acting in some official capacity (trainers, facilitators, specialists, etc.) rather than clearly defined and identified as individuals. In times of crisis, extra-familial persons are only partially helpful and are sought by the children only sporadically or from external urging. The helpful influence of these external people is felt as rather low compared with parents or primary attachment figures.
High	These children intensively trust in extra-familial helpers (kindergarten teacher, home educator, school teacher, etc.) already at an early age and also avail themselves of their assistance in resolving family-related issues. They can easily include persons outside the family in their daily lives, and thus introduce protective external perspectives, if necessary. This may occur, on the one hand, indiscriminately if there is a lack of object constancy (see Structure axis) or continually and sustainably with the development of one or more relationships with constantly relevant external persons.
Age Group 3 (13 to 18 Years)	
Absent	There exists no awareness of aid institutions (e.g., for refugees or adolescents with cognitive impairment), or such institutions are categorically rejected.
Low	The awareness of potentially helpful extra-familial institutions or people is rudimentary and activated only in extreme situations. Alternatively, there exists a high intrafamilial anxiety potential up to paranoid distortion in the case of

	adolescents strongly tied to their families. Offers of help are misconstrued, devalued, or ignored, and, at most, accepted with ambivalence in unavoidable dramatic emergencies.
Moderate	These adolescents are familiar with various ways and strategies for procuring aid outside the family in professional crises. The extra-familial relationships then have more of a functional than a personal interactional character, and are configured discontinuously. Depending on the attachment pattern of the primary family (see the Structure axis), extra-familial persons are viewed with scepticism or anxiety.
High	These adolescents have detailed knowledge about school and institutional assistance outside the family and can avail themselves of this aid unhindered. Contacts are generally positively helpful and are actively maintained by the adolescents, and also regularly sought even in the absence of an acute crisis. These contacts always supplement familial structures or provide a sustainable compensation for intra-familial relationship problems.

Part 3: Clinical Application of the Axes in Diagnostic Assessment and Therapy

11. Interpersonal Relations

11.1 Diagnostics

The *interpersonal relations axis* can be used for describing familial inter-actions, clinical diagnoses of dysfunctional relationship patterns, and as a progression instrument (pre–post measurements) in psychotherapy or quality assurance (Weber, 2012).

Instrument for Describing Familial Interactions

This instrument is suitable for diagnosing familial relationships. For example, the examiner can assess whether and to what extent a child in the course of a session, following an initial desire for contact with his/her father, who is disinterested in the interaction, withdraws or reacts with reproachful and accusatory behavior, and how, in turn, the father reacts to this behavior. In addition, it can be investigated whether there exist certain typical relationship patterns for the individual dyads within the family. Clinically, the OPD-CA instrument is already being used in child custody reports, among other purposes, as it allows a comprehensive description of relationship behavior. In an empirical study, Seifert (2011) investigated the parent–child relationships as predictors of judgments in custody reports in connection with child custody awards.

Clinical Diagnosis of Dysfunctional Relationship Patterns of the Child

In clinical diagnoses, the examiner rates the discernibility of dys-functional relationship patterns in the child on the basis of the child's observable relationship behavior in different dyads (examiner, parents, teachers, friends), either directly experienced or described by third parties, of the reactions of the attachment figures and of the therapist's responses in his/her encounters with the child. Are such relationship aspects indicated which, because of dysfunctional transference patterns, prevent the child from handling relationships in a functional way, and, owing to the strong urge to continue this behavior (repetition compulsion), limit the child in his/her mental development? To illustrate, we refer to a previously described case (Weber, 2012) both here and in our description of the interpersonal relations axis as a outcome instrument (see below):

Peter is a ten year old boy who as a toddler was subject to severe neglect by his parents. Placement in various children's homes proved unsuccessful, as Peter was deemed unmanageable. The degree of his behavioral disorder then led to several months as an in-patient in a child-psychiatric ward, where a reactive attachment disorder was diagnosed.

An OPD-CA-2 assessment was performed, in which a low integration of mental structure as well as a *closeness vs. distance* conflict on the conflict axis were determined. Along the *interpersonal relations* axis the following was found: Peter behaved autonomously to an extreme degree, could not accept any offers of dialog, never told anything personal about himself, showed no positive emotions in relationships, had to retain strong control of contact, and never let himself be guided. Playing with other children was consequently impossible for him. Peter displayed disinterest and strong reticence towards the greatest variety of offers of relationship. When individual fellow patients or clinical staff wanted to establish contact that was too close for him, he could also react with intense aggression. Overall, his relationship behavior was characterized by great rigidity and always had the same form, even in the face of very different attempts to make contact with him by potential interaction partners, which is characteristic of dysfunctional transference processes regarding his present handling of relationships. On the ward, the children largely reacted with disinterest and withdrawal. The ward staff experienced no positive emotions in their relationships with Peter, and often felt an inner anger at his rejection. They felt a strong impulse to withdraw from the relationship altogether, or to comply with him helplessly and reluctantly or to react in a mitigated way with controlling countermeasures.

The OPD-CA-2 circumplex model can represent the dysfunctional relationship patterns between Peter and his interaction partners as exhibited in all areas of the ward and other contexts of life; **Figure 3** illustrates the *subject-directed circle*. We can summarize this relationship pattern as follows:

Peter's behavior in all areas of life is completely autonomous, he shows no friendly-open and happy interest in other people, and reacts to different offers of contact with aggressive withdrawal.

In Peter's case, this relationship pattern was largely due to his dysfunctional transference pattern. With great pressure, he projected his predominantly negative relationship expectations, based on numerous experiences with violence and neglect, onto the ward staff, who in their internal responses were able to feel only a very narrow range of aversive affects (see above).

Outcome Instrument

Unlike the *Strukturierte Analyse Sozialen Beziehungsverhaltens* (SASB; Structured Analysis of Social Relationship Behavior) instrument, which examines the individual speech acts in a micro-analytical approach and was developed as an empirical tool, the *interpersonal relations* axis was developed primarily for clinical use. Besides the aforementioned clinical diagnostics, the axis can also be used during psychotherapy

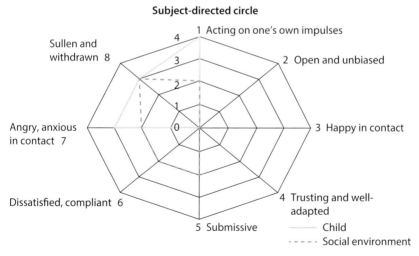

Figure 3. The OPD-CA-2 axis interpersonal relations: Subject-directed circle: Peter and his interaction partners.

to document changes in the individual sessions and also to capture changes in the therapeutic relationships during different stages of therapy. Psychotherapeutic studies have so far rarely used the *interpersonal relations* axis. A single-case study looked at the therapeutic profile of an adolescent in a psychodrama group (Bindernagel, Scherrer, Winzeler, & von Wyl, 2011).

The following diagram (**Figure 4**) illustrates the application of the *interpersonal relations* axis on the basis of an out-patient psychodynamic psychotherapy of Peter, the boy described above. This psychotherapy took place following in-patient treatment.

In this session, Peter exhibits in his relationship with the therapist a broader range of possibilities for interaction compared with his relationship behavior as an in-patient and at the start of out-patient therapy, so that the circumplex model can now incorporate more items of higher levels. Greater flexibility can now be observed along the axis of influence. Peter can thus better subordinate himself, in part with discontent (throwing away an object after limits have been imposed, and yet straightening things up afterwards), in part also accompanied by a joyful emotion in wanting to implement the rules laid down by the ther-

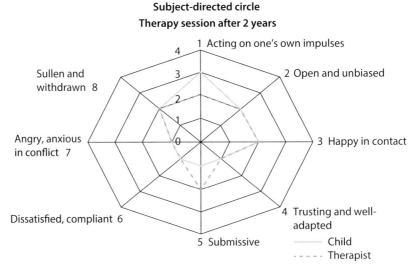

Figure 4. The OPD-CA-2 axis interpersonal relations: Subject-directed circle: Peter and the therapist, two years after discharge.

apist (trusting and well-adapted). For example: After putting back certain toys at the end of the session, he grins as he says he's now straightened up half of the things, so that the therapist has to do the other half – that was the agreement! Also impressive is his independent and decisive manner combined with the expressed desire for a relationship, in contrast to his behavior as an in-patient. For example, after being greeted he runs away, hides behind the door, and wants to be found. He sullenly shuts down to a considerably lesser degree, and appears more open in his remarks and behavior. For example, he spontaneously reports the experiences of his class trip when he injured himself, and shows the therapist his injured toe. Along the affiliation axis there now appear, in addition to vehement aggressive affects (hurling the ball against the window after a small disappointment), several joyful affects in relation to the therapist. For example, his entire face beams when rediscovered after suddenly disappearing at the beginning and end of the session.

The therapist repeatedly has the feeling of a shared experience and of joy in playing. Overall, the therapist develops more positive than negative feelings towards Peter. Troubled and dissatisfied feelings do not persist for long. The therapist feels less under pressure in the relationship, less having to exert himself and feels freer in his interventions, as when he addresses the disappointment of the last session.

Summary of relationship dynamics: Compared with his time as an in-patient and at the beginning of therapy, Peter shows a much broader range of behavioral possibilities. His distinctly independent behavior continues to predominate, although now combined with more joyful emotions. In his internal response, the therapist finds himself quick to accept the child's offers of a relationship, while also generally feeling less irritated and more comfortable in his dialog with the child.

11.2 Application in the In-Patient Treatment Concept

In clinical and multi-professional teams, the *interpersonal relations* axis already provides a tool for developing a common language within the team for describing the interactions of in-patient children and adolescents with one another and with the members of the team. Just as the development of an approach to treatment employing the *interpersonal relations* axis is important in the clinical context, so will such an approach be very helpful for the implementation of measures under juvenile penal law. Often the delinquent development of an adolescent will be closely related to his/her relationship behavior with dysfunctional transference phenomena. Especially pathological relationship patterns expressed along the *interpersonal relations* axis will considerably complicate implementation of these measures, however. If such relationship patterns do not become evident in connection with a measure under juvenile penal law, relationships will often be broken off or shifted, often with a re-enactment character.

The multi-professional team meetings can compile typical dysfunctional relationship patterns of the patient. The currently effective inner mental conflicts and structural deficits, represented along the interpersonal relations axis, express themselves in the patient's relationship towards the treatment team. In the foreground is the question of whether relationships can be experienced as regulating and whether offers of relationships for co-regulation can be accepted or they have to be controlled and combatted.

Perception of the patient's scenic enactment and the function of the in-patient treatment team as a space for resonance and as a container form the central resources for the team in arriving at a better understanding of the patient. All team members are then called upon to take notice of and describe their own relationships and feelings towards the patient as well as to reflect on how this affects the relational structure of the team. On the other hand, this is also about the team members expressing their fantasies about the patient and his/her family and about the motives of his/her actions. In this way, it will thus often become evident how the relationship is handled between subject and object and what basic relationship difficulties exist. Comparing the patient's relationship circles with different people will reveal the variability or constancy of the patient's handling of relationships.

Individual vague expressions of feeling become relevant findings through the team members analysis of the examiner's internal response axis of the OPD-CA-2. Firstly, this processing and reduction to what is observable, and, then, to place this in relationship to the patient, allows the exchange of feelings and fantasies to become a process of reflection about the patient and a more accurate perception and understanding of him/her. A psychodynamically oriented overall therapeutic concept can tie the measures of treatment to a common point of reference, namely the unconscious significance of the relationship. The shared reflection on the dynamics of the child's relationship patterns and the inner response by the treatment team allows the coordination of interventions, reflection on projections and splitting processes, and the individual orientation of the treatment plan. Team meetings can make clear what changes in the relationship formation by the members of the treatment team are necessary. Ideally, psychodynamic understanding can be combined with structurally supportive measures and developed in co-operative contexts.

The effectiveness of past relationship experiences, feelings, and needs that have inscribed themselves into the psyche are recorded. Depending on the child's ability to reflect on and regulate his/her internal activities and his/her social relationships, a shared attitude will come to be incorporated in the treatment plan. The offer of a relationship and the therapeutic interventions can be geared to the child's mental structure. Participation in the child's experience in the relationship allows the maturation of his/her deficiently developed inner mental structure and to describe and evaluate changes in how he/she handles relationships at regular intervals. Treatment focuses, on the one hand, on the patient's ability to form relationships, which can also be described on the affiliation level, and, on the other hand, on the development of self-regulation competence, which can also be seen on the level of interdependence.

The continual perception of and exchanges on the understanding of the significance of the relationship and the contexts of this understanding in escalating interactions also provide an orientation aid in dealing with the child. The regulation of closeness and distance, accommodation, and the drawing of boundaries succeeds in a more sociable form. The child's active dialog is also translated into a shared language and keeps him/her from falling into a dysfunctional relationship dynamic.

In summary, we can say that the *interpersonal relations* axis provides a useful tool for compiling what is observed and one's own experiences of the interactions on the ward between the child and the members of the team. This allows a reflexive understanding of the unconscious configuration of relationship and offers a relationship, resulting from this understanding, and interventions in multiprofessional treatment.

12. Conflict

In this chapter, we present some basic aspects in the assessment of the conflict axis, such as the differentiation between types of stressors and the fact that we need to consider the actual age group, even if the patients seem considerably "younger" to us. This is important because an intrapsychic conflict by definition impairs development. We then describe the diagnostic procedure, i.e., we consider what materials are used in forming a conflict hypothesis and in testing that hypothesis in subsequent diagnostic interviews. The question of why training is important and meaningful is also relevant in this regard. In the following, we explain the advantages of comprehensive OPD-CA-2 diagnostics, in which the conflict axis has its place, and its relation to the *structure* and *prerequisites for treatment* axes. Finally, we explain working with the conflict axis with a case vignette, in which the close relationship between the conflict and structure axes is made clear (see also Seiff-ge-Krenke et al., 2014).

12.1 Conflict Classification: Some General Remarks

As already discussed in Chapter *5: Theoretical Conception of the Axes – 5.2 Conflict*, at issue here is the assessment of a persistent intrapsychic and development-impairing conflict with which the child or adolescent is coping in an active or passive mode. This conflict can reveal itself in different areas of development (family, peers and friends, kindergarten and school, and body and illness). We assume the existence of associations with the structure axis insofar as no conflict is discernible in the case of a poorly integrated, i.e., a rather deficient, structure.

A relatively well integrated structure is a precondition for conflict formation. In the case of a moderately integrated structure, external conflict themes tend to be more apparent than genuine intrapsychic conflicts, which are characterized by a clash between desire and defence.

Following extensive discussion, the OPD-CA-2 Task Force has decided to differentiate between Age Group 1 (3 to 5 years, i.e., toddlers and pre-schoolers), Age Group 2 (6 to 12 years, i.e., middle childhood), and Age Group 3 (13 years and older), based on Piaget (1952). The classification always refers to the actual age, not the developmental age, as experience shows that many children and adolescents with neurotic disorders seem considerably younger. We assume that forerunners of conflicts will exist as well as, potentially, a transgenerational transmission of conflicts. Attention should therefore be given to the existence of similar conflictual themes in the parents.

In applying the classification, it is important to be clear on the following: The *closeness vs. distance conflict* should only be diagnosed if attachment is disturbed at an elementary level. In active mode, this conflict is manifested as the fear of closeness and as an exaggerated emotional independence and as the fear of separation and search for close relationships in the passive mode. This conflict should not be diagnosed if flexible attachments to others are possible, e.g., outside the home to other people. In the conflict of *submission vs. control*, control of self and others governs relationships. In the active mode, constant rebellion against obligations, and compliance and submission in the passive mode will be found. In the conflict of *taking care of oneself vs. being cared for*, the issue of care governs relationships. In the active mode, we find self-sufficiency and self-sacrifice for others, while in the passive mode clinging, and parasitic behavior prevails. The conflict of *self-worth* primarily concerns the regulation of self-worth. In the active mode, we find self-aggrandisement, and in the passive mode significant losses in self-esteem. A *guilt conflict* arises when children and adolescents try to secure their relationships with their parents at all costs, and develop inappropriate levels of guilt because of strong ties of loyalty. In the active mode, we find deprecations, with the children and adolescents appearing as amoral and unconscionable. In passive mode, they seemed to be burdened with heavy guilt, and they show excessive fidelity to their parents. The *oedipal conflict* primarily concerns erotic-sexual desires and the defence against them. Sexuality and triadic relationships are emphasized in the active mode, while children and adolescents in the passive mode tend to be more business-like and sexually unattrac-tive and ambiguous. In the *identity conflict*, finding and securing an identity determines interactions. In the active mode, we find an un-critical adoption of alternating identifications, and disorientation and helplessness in the passive mode.

12.2 An Important Differentiation: Severe Stress in Life, Everyday Conflicts Versus Intrapsychic Conflicts

The patients who come to us experience multiple types of stress. For example, in the last few months before the initial diagnostic interview or the beginning of treatment, severe stress in life (such as separation or severe illness of the parents) may have occurred that will adversely affect the child or adolescent. Usually one finds in children and ado-lescents in out-patient or in-patient psychotherapy numerous forms of severe stress in life, but also severe trauma such as abuse, mistreatment, etc. In fact, the living conditions of children and adolescents have greatly changed in recent years; we find more single parents, higher unemployment, more poverty, and more children and adolescents with an immigrant background (Seiffge-Krenke, 2006). In recent years, the number of children and adolescents who are traumatized and have ex-perienced severe stress such as abuse, mistreatment and neglect (Egle et al., 2015) in health practices and clinics has increased. Of course, we must be wary of an inflated use of the term "traumatized." These severe forms of stress in life must be stated in the diagnostic documentation (Appendix C), with a distinction being made between severe stress in life taking place within the last six months before the diagnostic inter-view and severe stress in life going further back in time. In particular, severe stress occurring shortly before the diagnostic interview, such as the sudden death of family members, may adversely affect the patient's structural level and therefore complicate the assessment of conflicts.

It is important to note that everyday stress is not assessed along the conflict axis. Such stress occurs often and only at moderate levels, and is relatively easily managed by children and adolescents (such as poor grades, arguments with parents, etc.). This stress also includes typical everyday confrontations between parents and children over homework, cleaning up, going out, and the like. Such everyday stress initially has no pathological significance and is regarded as normative. It may even – especially during adolescence – serve development, as greater autonomy will be negotiated with the parents.

In working with the conflict axis, it is important to clearly distinguish intrapsychic conflicts from these other two types of stress. While everyday stress may be noted, but is somewhat different from intrapsychic conflicts according to the OPD-CA-2, the occurrence of severe stress in life (such as critical life events and traumas) should be assessed separately. This separate assessment is necessary because the presence of such severe stress will lower the structural level, as already noted, but may also intensify the intrapsychic conflict or impair the patient's ability to cope with this conflict.

12.3 Conflict Diagnostics for Initial Interviews: Notes on Diagnostic Procedure and Typical "Errors"

Conflict diagnoses conducted in the initial interviews must clarify several important questions, beginning with: On the basis of what materials shall I diagnose such an internalized conflict? Which is the most important conflict? This focus is important for the further planning of treatment.

First, we consider determining the *focus of the conflict*: What conflict theme governs experience and behavior, whereby the unconscious dynamics of the conflict can be perceived via the internal resonance of the therapist and his or her scenic understanding. Even a child's or adolescent's fairy-tales or favorite stories or films can provide important information. Second, it must be asked which conflict has hindered the child's or adolescent's development the most. Thus, *dysfunctionality* will be looked at more closely here. We then rank the conflicts, with the most important one at the top. Since other issues will often become clearer in the course of treatment, it makes sense to glean what other conflicts hindering development are indicated from the ranking list.

In considering the material to be used as supportive evidence for conflict diagnosis, we must keep in mind that the conflict hypothesis rests on the integration of diagnostic materials from four different sources:

1. The interview with children and adolescents and their parents.
2. Observations during play as well as results from (projective) testing methods.
3. Individual development and family history by questioning the parents and, to some extent, the child.
4. The presentation of a scene.

Scenic understanding in particular plays a large role in OPD-CA-2 diagnoses. In order to get information on how the potential conflict may develop in a concrete interaction, it is important to begin trial sessions with an unstructured initial interview with the child or adolescent, for example, according to the Interview Guidelines (see Appendix A) or, as described in Diederichs-Paeschke et al. (2011). We also recommend interviewing children and parents separately, with the father's participation being indispensable. After forming hypotheses about conflict and structure from these initial sessions, the next sessions can be devoted to more detailed questions that possibly provide information on which of the conflicts is more important (at the moment). This approach is especially useful with children and adolescents with co-morbid disorders, where developmental impairment may be the case in multiple areas, which only becomes evident gradually during treatment. The final session should specifically inquire about the prerequisites of treatment, i.e., it is recommended to proceed according to a "funneling principle." Depending on the setting, it may be useful to inquire about the motivation for treatment and the explanations for a disorder ("Why do you think you're here?," "What do you think should change?") also at the beginning of the interview.

Interview questions relating to typical conflicts inquire about clashing motives or endeavors typical of a conflict. We then form a conflict hypothesis and at the end may make a provisional interpretation or offer for discussion whether the issue may indeed be this conflict. We would thus look for which conflict hypothesis the most material is available and would then try to address the specific conflict hypothesis in the next session. The classification should also consider the age group, i.e., classify according to the chronological age in the Manual. The mode must then also be considered more precisely: Does the child or adolescent proceed actively or passively in coping with this conflict, and in which areas does he/she do so? Are many areas affected or only a few? Active coping could indicate resources.

The existence of multiple conflicts could indicate comorbidity and possibly structural deficits as well. A transgenerational perspective should also be considered, e.g., whether the conflicts originate from the parents. Finally, as already noted, we must register whether severe stress has occurred in the recent half year leading up to the initial interview (and what sorts of stress existed before this time). Indeed, as already mentioned, we assume that very severe stress such as critical life events or even trauma affect the child's or adolescent's coping capability and intensify defence, so that not only influences along the structure axis but also influences on handling conflicts will be evident.

The following flow chart can be useful when working with the conflict axis (see **Figure 5**).

Some typical diagnostic "errors" were repeatedly observed during training. For example, we found that the former diagnosis of *depend-*

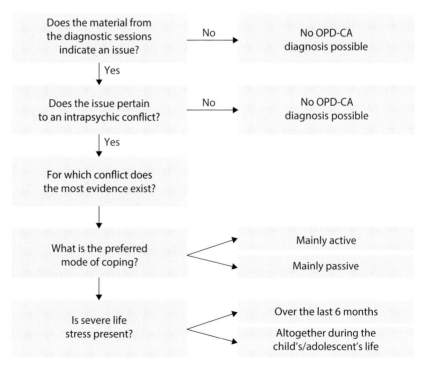

Figure 5. Flow chart for assessing the conflict axis.

ency vs. autonomy conflicts occurred relatively often because the previous formulation of this conflict (Arbeitskreis OPD-KJ, 2007) suggested that autonomy was the issue. We have now reformulated this conflict as *closeness vs. distance* and operationalized the conflict more clearly as an extremely elementary issue, noting that this conflict should be diagnosed only if no attachments exist, including alternatives given the discontinuation of parental attachments, and noting that the behavior of children and adolescents oscillates between the extremes of "fear of being too close" and "fear of being too distant". Moreover, the growing number of children and adolescents from families with separated or divorced parents led to the frequent diagnosis of a (formerly designated) *loyalty conflict* (Arbeitskreis OPD-KJ, 2007). This conflict is not necessarily and not exclusively tied to such a separation issue. We have consequently reformulated this conflict as *guilt conflict*. Finally, it must be borne in mind that nearly all patients have comparatively low self-esteem and that a *self-worth conflict* should be considered only if extremely pronounced. De facto we find the diagnosis of self-worth conflicts to occur relatively often, however. In the past, problems have also occurred in diagnosing the *identity conflict*; it should be diagnosed only when an issue clearly impedes development and not in cases of normal identity issues among children and adolescents.

12.4 Why Is Training Important?

The *conflict* axis is the most psychodynamic axis in the OPD-CA-2. The complex structure – the inclusion of three areas, three age groups, seven types of issues, and two coping modalities – already underscores the necessity of intensive training for effectively applying this axis. Of course, the intervals between the training courses should not be too long, so that gains from the training remain high.

So what does the training accomplish? For the OPD-CA-2, there are three training courses: a basic course and two advanced courses, in which classification according to all axes is practised and certified, for a total of 35 hours. In this regard, we have conducted a study (Seiffge-Krenke et al., 2011) of the possible influential factors, such as the examiner's gender, age, and experience, as well as of the influential factors on the part of the patient (gender, age, and diagnosis), but also of the features of the training course (duration, number of patients and continuous or discontinuous participation in the training). Finally, we addressed the question of whether any individual axes are particularly difficult to apply. A sample of trained students who had completed a total of 35 hours of OPD-CA training showed good agreement between the raters applying the conflict and the structure axis (Seiffge-Krenke et al., 2011). The intraclass correlation as a measure of interrater reliability was ICC = 0.76 over both axes, with agreement between the raters within the conflict axis (ICC = 0.79) being greater than within the structure axis (ICC = 0.58). The age and gender of the raters had no influence on the assessments along the conflict and structure axes. Important, however, is not to let too much time pass between the individual training courses, so that what is newly learned can be consolidated and firmly anchored. It is therefore useful, for example, to apply the OPD-CA-2 regularly in groups with colleagues or quality circles. Having a common language has proven especially important in this regard.

12.5 The Report to the Referrer Based on the Conflict Axis

The hitherto now practice of employing the OPD-CA in the preparation of reports for **referrers** is still in need of improvement. Short keywords are not helpful and can lead to the need for clarification from the referrer. It should therefore be explained in more detail why, say, one is of the opinion that a certain intrapsychic conflict is present. Here the conflict axis can be helpful by providing orientation according to the specified conflict themes and how these are processed.

The report to the referrer contains information on numerous points, such as the current situation that led to seeking a therapist, details on the patient's present mental and physical developmental state, his/her family situation, and the diagnosis of the clinically significant disorder. In addition, the psychodynamics should be presented, i.e., considerations as to what in the patient's life history and family situation contributed to his/her symptomatology. Finally, information must also be provided on the goal of treatment, a treatment plan must be prepared, and the possible prognosis with the proposed treatment stated.

Information for the report to the referrer can above all be incorporated into the *psychiatric findings,* i.e., "What is now?," for example, in relation to the current structure and the relative dominance of a particular conflictual theme in the child's or adolescent's present life. But the OPD-CA-2 can also be fruitfully used with regard to *psychodynamics*: "Where does the problem actually come from?" and "How did these conflicts and structural deficits come about?," namely by clarifying to what extent the child's or adolescent's life and past relationships have been governed by issues to be regarded as early precursors of the actual conflict, to what extent a transgenerational transmission of dysfunctional conflict themes is observable, and what dominant coping mode is constraining the child's or adolescent's life. In addition, regarding *treatment plan and therapeutic aims*, we can explain what goals the child, adolescent, or parents have, i.e., the conflictual focus where a supportive and structuring approach is called for, and where an explorative approach is more the issue. Finally, regarding *prognosis,* some prognostic considerations may be stated, given the fulfilment of prerequisites of treatment as compiled in the OPD-CA-2.

12.6 The Conflict Axis: An Aid for the Indication and Planning of Treatment

Structural prognostic characteristics are important for the therapist to be able to make a differential indication for certain forms of psychotherapy (e.g., psychodynamic vs. analytic psychotherapy). These relate to important aspects of the structure and conflict axes in the OPD-CA-2, and pertain to the psychodynamics (i.e., a central, underlying intrapsychic conflict) and to structural aspects (i.e., affect tolerance, impulse control, the ability for self- and object differentiation, and the ability to make emotional contact). This information can be used for a differential indication for treatment and for supporting treatment planning, namely by indicating whether a more regression-based or a more ego-supportive approach is necessary (Seiffge-Krenke, Mayer et al., 2013c). Moreover, it can be decided on the basis of this information, for example, whether identity diffusion as a structural deficit or an identity conflict implying a relatively good structural level is present (Seiffge-Krenke, 2012b).

At present, the conflict axis is often used by experienced therapists for treatment strategy and planning. It may then be useful to determine diagnostically specific structural deficits (Seiffge-Krenke, Fliedl et al., 2013a). Another area of application is child and adolescent psychiatry. Here experience shows that OPD-CA diagnostics helps the therapist confine his/her efforts by focussing on a conflict that can be worked on, for example, as in the framework of narrowly time-limited in-patient therapy. A comprehensive assessment of structure, conflict, and prerequisites of treatment also has the advantage of providing information about the patient's motivation for treatment and possible available resources, which is especially important with these patients (Seiffge-Krenke, Fliedl, & Katzenschläger, 2013b).

12.7 Working With the Conflict Axis in Ongoing Treatment: Shift in the Focus of Conflict

As explained, the conflict axis can be used in the probatory sessions for obtaining essential information for the report to the referrer, which can also support us in treatment planning by determining a focus of conflict, for example. To conclude, shifts in the conflict focus in ongoing treatment are illustrated, i.e., concrete work with the conflict axis in psychodynamic treatment (Welter & Seiffge-Krenke, 2006), with the case study of Julia, who began psychodynamic therapy at the age of 13 years. She has received 70 hours of individual therapy; 17 hours were set aside for working with her parents. We begin with the probatory sessions, and then discuss the further course of the therapy.

Julia was diagnosed with an eating disorder in the midst of current psychosocial stress from bullying experiences; a lesser degree of dissociative disorder was the secondary diagnosis (enactment, parent participation). *Submission vs. control* was diagnosed as the conflict, while an *oedipal conflict* was only hinted at. On the structural level *good to moderate integration* was found; deficits were revealed especially in object perception, self- and object differentiation and in coping with negative affects (*affect tolerance)*. Julia was conspicuously unremarkable in contact. Concerning the *prerequisites of treatment*, the primary question was who actually wanted the therapy, as the parents seemed very much committed to the idea and spent long nights in bed discussing the problems in their daughter's friendships and romantic relationships. Noteworthy too was that the entire family – both parents but especially Julia herself – remained focus on aggression from external attackers.

In the course of therapy, Julia contributed a mass of material to the sessions and discussed very many relationships with peers, which greatly confused the therapist. During one session Julia mentioned altogether 45 different names, but all the names from her clique of friends seemed interchangeable and not to bear any emotional significance. Countertransference gave rise to feelings of great paralysis and fatigue; it was difficult to keep the patient focussed on a particular relationship. She exhibited little self-reflection on her contribution to the conflicts and was externally oriented. Topics of discussion were often triangular situations and sexual matters in terms of attraction and repulsion. The therapist experienced the countertransference as having voyeuristic elements. Concerning crisis situations, it was clear that Julia would withdraw with diverse physical symptoms such as hyperventilation and fainting when things became too difficult.

The second half of treatment revealed a shift in the focus of conflict. It became more and more clear that the issue of *submission vs. control* had shifted to the *oedipal conflict*. At the same time, her relationships became more coherent and longer lasting. The patient had little awareness of her participation in conflicts with her circle of friends, with whom she generally interacted by turning two girlfriends against one another or by splitting up an adolescent couple. Julia was not at all able to explain why X or Y had become so angry with her. We also found strong involvement by the parents, who often discuss all night long the dangers and consequences of their daughter's sexuality.

By the end of treatment Julia had attained a certain degree of stability in her relationships. Julia now had a boyfriend and was rarely experiencing any more conflicts in school or with girlfriends. Earlier physical symptoms were largely gone. Up to the end, the parents refused to discuss their contribution to the sexual conflict and detachment; they rather insisted that their relationships were harmonious. The intrapsychic conflict continued to indicate, as before, *submission* and *control*, but also clear was the oedipal conflict, i.e., the strong relationship between Julia and her father. At the end of the 70 hours, Julia declined to continue therapy. She found that she had achieved enough. While to a certain extent, this discontinuation of therapy again indicated the issue of *submission vs. control*, it may also be considered a developmental gain, since Julia was taking leave of the therapist as a substitute, as it were, for her parents.

13. Structure

The *structure* axis captures the severity of a disorder. It is a sophisticated instrument for planning and organizing treatment. The diagnostic assessment of the various dimensions of the *structure* axis provides evidence as to whether a conflictual pathology or a developmental pathology prevails. If conflict-pathological aspects predominate, a different approach to treatment will be taken than if the child or adolescent is diagnosed with a structural problem or developmental psychopathology.

13.1 Degree of the Disorder

The degree of structural limitations is to be checked according to the structural characteristics listed in **Table 4.** Here it is important to distinguish between occasional limitations in individual dimensions and more general impairments. In children and adolescents, control capabilities may be impaired without a structural pathology being the case (example: simple attention disorder). A more precise classification may then be afforded only with the help of the conflict axis.

The structure axis captures the underlying structural problems in apparently conflict-related psychopathologies. For example, an eating disorder may either exist within a well-integrated structural level during a maturity crisis or serve self-repair in an underlying psychosis. The same applies to obsessive-compulsive disorders, in which there is a deficient boundary between reality and fantasy on all structural levels – the lower the structural level, the more evident the degree of ego-structural limitations will be (Streeck-Fischer, 1988).

A differentiated diagnosis of the structure will yield information for the therapeutic technique, the necessary agreements, and the framework to be arranged. For example, with moderately to well-integrated structural capabilities, conflict-oriented interventions will tend to predominate.

Table 4. Overview of structural abilities

Control	Identity	Interpersonality	Attachment
Affect tolerance	Self-perception	Initiating emotional contact	Access to attachment representations
Self-worth regulation	Self–object differentiation	Fantasies	Secure internal base
Impulse control	Object perception	Affective experience	Capacity to be alone
Controlling instances (conscience formation)	Coherence	Reciprocity	Use of the attachment relationship
	Belonging	Empathy	
		Capacity to separate	

Generally a relationship exists between the central issue of conflict and the existing structural capabilities. It can hardly be expected that the *closeness vs. distance conflict* (formerly: autonomy vs. dependency) will occur with a moderately to well-integrated structural level. On a moderately to well-structured level, conflicts like *taking care of oneself vs. being cared for, submission vs. control,* or an *oedipal conflict* will prevail. In neurotic conflicts on a moderately to well-integrated level, distinct structural (or rather, functional) ego limitations will occur. In contrast, more global structural impairments are usually connected with a structurally and developmentally related psychopathology, ranging from "low to moderate," but also from "low to disintegrated," and possibly combined with a conflict of *closeness vs. distance* (formerly: dependency vs. autonomy), or with an *identity conflict* or *self-worth conflict* or even a *guilt conflict* (formerly: loyalty conflict).

13.2 Treatment Planning and Therapeutic Objectives With Low Level Structural Disorders

In the following, only the therapeutic aspects of disorders with a low-integration level are discussed, as in these cases structural work is especially called for, while conflict pathology is rather secondary in importance. The second step in therapy may focus on the conflict axis if the therapeutic work is no longer challenged by attacks on the framework and relationship.

In structural disorders, abilities such as self-reflection, affect perception and differentiation, reality testing, as well as the ability for self-control exist only to a limited extent. At the fore in therapeutic interventions are not unconscious conflicts, desires, and defence, but developmental limitations on self-regulation and the handling of relationships.

Arrangement of the Setting

The setting must be arranged so as to meet the boundary conditions for the child's or adolescent's development. For example, agreements must be made on keeping appointments, compliance with rules (no destruction of toys, no running away), behavior destructive to self or to others or suicidal in nature, addictive behavior, etc. The therapist may have to arrange the playroom so that the child, given his/her susceptibility to stimuli, is not constantly distracted by the various possibilities of play and can develop his/her own ability to play. Keeping the therapy room more or less bare with locked cabinets may therefore be wise, to help the child concentrate on essentials. The structural limitations of the child or adolescent with his/her deficient self-control should not be viewed as containing some deeper meaning to be uncovered through interpretation (see Diepold, 1995); the aim is rather to establish the boundaries and thus the framework as therapeutic constraints.

Clear agreements with the parents are also required so that the child's or adolescent's development is not hindered by a persistently disorganized family environment (Streeck-Fischer, 2005).

The Therapeutic Attitude

Structurally disturbed children and adolescents require a therapeutic attitude associated with a benevolent, friendly, and open relationship. The different therapeutic concepts require more or less responsive and structure-forming approaches (e.g., Clarkin, Yeomans, & Kernberg, 2001; Foelsch et al., 2013; Rudolf, 2004; Streeck-Fischer & Streeck, 2010) that will lead to a corrective, emotional experience for the child or adolescent. In a supportive relationship experienced as helpful, the therapist can assist the child or the adolescent as a person in the improvement of deficient abilities in impulse control, self-perception, and the perception of others. Important is to keep in mind, for example, that the ability of impulse control must be developed first, before the focus turns to anger affects. Generally the therapist assumes an active therapeutic attitude. Therapeutic abstinence is characterized by the therapist not behaving towards the patient in the same way as the attachment figures (e.g., neglectfully), but rather appearing as an alternative object.

A hierarchy of therapeutic steps is necessary when working on structural limitations. The deeper the structural disorder, the more important it is to work on self-perception and impulse control. Here self-determination and autonomy of the self as well as the development of reality testing are the primary goals (i.e., aspects of self-control and identity). Only later should attention be turned to object perception and interpersonality.

The more severe the structural disorder, the more caution is required with affect-mobilizing techniques. Offers of therapy promoting regression and dependency are not appropriate here. The aim is rather the basal stabilization of the self. Due to the weakness in mentalization, it is important to register nonverbal communications and to respond as the case may be. The work occurs in the "here and now," in coping with everyday problems and conflicts, expectations and demands, and not in the "there and then."

In the process, the following steps should be kept to:

- Along the dimension of self-regulation and self-control the therapist supports the child in establishing an inner distance from his/her own impulses, affects, and addictive behavior.
- Identity concerns a more realistic perception of oneself and others, in view of reality. This occurs through mirroring, differentiation, and confrontation. Peculiarities provide migration-related identity insecurity.
- The interpersonality dimension allows affective contact to be made with the child or adolescent.
- The attachment dimension focusses on observable patterns of handling relationships, with the aim of promoting secure attachments.

Play as the Best Way to Acquire Structural Abilities

Structurally limited children often lack a capacity for play. Two extreme cases illustrate the problem.

1. In the first case, the child avoids fantasizing and fully adheres to concrete representations within which nothing conflictual or even imaginative emerges. Play remains meagre and unrelated. The therapist becomes tired, and no communication like play or psychotherapy gets started.
2. In the second case, fantasy (e.g., also the destructive kind) is excessive, and the patient loses touch with reality. Play gets out of hand and becomes real, forcing the therapist to set boundaries and impose a structure.

In both cases, the therapist must bring missing aspects into the play. What does this mean? In the case of meagre, uninformative play, the therapist would have to check what is preventing fantasies and conflicts from coming to the surface. Does the patient suffer from massive, panicky fears that need to be hidden behind the emptiness and warded off? Does the child possibly have to be activated with imaginative stories presenting nothing threatening (such as Horton the Elephant, etc.)?

In the case of a deficient boundary between reality and fantasy (Example 2) or between play and reality, it will be important to refer to this boundary through making pacts and laying down frameworks. If play exhibits excessive destructiveness, it will be necessary to seek a safer place where protection can be found. A helpful, supportive, and accompanying object should be introduced here that offers an alternative, sets limits, and provides protection.

13.3 The Structure Axis in In-Patient Treatment and in the Overall Multimodal Treatment Plan

Can the OPD-CA-2 Be Usefully Applied in Everyday Clinical Work?

Won't such precise diagnoses require too much expenditure of time?

Since the structure axis in particular can serve as an aid in the therapeutic approach to children and adolescents with very complex disorders, the structure axis can be used fruitfully both in diagnosis and in the evaluation of therapy (Cropp, Salzer, Häusser, & Streeck-Fischer, 2013)). Besides the precise differential diagnostics, use of the structure axis will help avoid discrepancies in the assessment of a child's or adolescent's disorder pattern within the therapeutic team. If the structure axis is employed as recommended by different professional groups for detailed diagnostics, it allows for common strategies in the therapeutic approach to be agreed upon. It may then become clear whether the child or the adolescent in fact behaves differently in different surroundings. This will be the case, for example, if the child or adolescent has no coherent sense of self and exhibits different self-images in different settings. By analysing the structure axis, the different members of a therapeutic team can avoid divisive disputes over which perceptions are the "right" ones. Such a rating, confined to a single axis, can be thoroughly integrated in clinical procedures without great expenditure of time thanks to the depiction of the individual dimensions with their anchor-point descriptions.

The instrument can be used both at the beginning and end of treatment. Any changes in the degree of the structural disorder will then be evident from a structural elevation.

Treatment Planning in the Specialized Therapies

Music, occupational, art, and body therapies have become indispensable in clinical treatment. As they are not focussed on the spoken word or language, they are of great importance when working with children and adolescents.

In this work too, we can distinguish between conflict-centred and structurally related or developmentally oriented approaches. We illustrate this point only with two specialized forms of therapy: occupational therapy and body psychotherapy (Schulze et al., 2009); see the following overview in **Table 5**.

Table 5. Therapeutic approach depending on the structural level

OPD-CA-2-Structure Axis	Occupational Therapy	Body Psychotherapy
Integrated	For example, group work, creating something together, creative representations of internal states, expression-focussed approach	Conflict-focussed work, e.g., group work, integration of body image/self-image
Moderate integration	Support of expression and skills with perception-based aspects, activation of resources	Work on affect perception and affect differentiation on the bodily level, experience of self-effectiveness
Low integration	Support in the search for expression and activity, aid in self-control, frustration tolerance, self-perception in action	Support of work on setting boundaries, perception of self and others, work on self-regulation, relationship between body and space, search for protection
Disintegrated	Structure-providing guidelines in case of freezing up or loss of reality, e.g., craft techniques	Support and promotion of action-oriented approach, self-determination, perception of boundaries

14. Prerequisites for Treatment

As explained in the previous chapters, the *interpersonal relations, conflict,* and *structure* axes are defined and operationalized based on the central psychodynamic constructs of the same names. The diagnoses of the prevailing interpersonal relationship dynamics and the intrapsychic conflict dynamics yield an extensive understanding of disorders and symptoms to form the basis for clinical hypotheses and the resulting substantive focus in treatment planning. If, moreover, the understanding of a mental structure underlying a disorder pattern is integrated in the overall diagnostic picture, we can derive important supplementary clinical working hypotheses both for the phenomenology of the symptomatology and for the therapeutic modalities and preferred intervention techniques to be chosen (primarily structure-related or conflict-coping?), including the treatment setting (to what extent primarily structure-providing?). From the clinical working hypotheses that can be formulated with these three axes, further considerations on the indication for specific methods of treatment and settings as well as considerations for effective treatment planning can be derived. With the *prerequisites of treatment* axis as a basis, these considerations are systematically checked and added to regarding their clinical validity, case-specific suitability, and feasibility. The extensive conceptualization of this axis from the patient's subjective perspective of experience is an important complement to the assessments of relationship dynamics, conflict, and structure formulated from a professional, therapeutic perspective. The application of the *prerequisites of treatment* axis focusses on the indication for treatment and its planning.

As explained in the introductory chapter, the basic need for treatment of a mental disorder in a child or adolescent is determined not with the OPD-CA-2, but on the basis of guideline-governed diagnostics in child and adolescent psychiatry according to the diagnostic criteria of the multiaxial classification scheme (MAS; Rutter et al., 1975) for mental disorders in childhood and adolescence as stated in the ICD-10 (World Health Organisation, 1996) as well as, given the specific disorder, the current guideline recommendations; for instance, the guidelines of the National Institute for Health and Care Excellence (NICE) or the DSM-5 (American Psychiatric Association, 2015). Accordingly, the pathological significance of the problems or symptomatology leading to a presentation must be first determined through confirmation of a corresponding clinical diagnosis. For the differential indication of specific measures of treatment, besides clinical diagnosis (MAS Axis I: Clinically Psychiatric Syndrome), in particular, the severity of the psychosocial impairment caused by the disorder (MAS Axis VI: Global Assessment of the Psychosocial Functional Level) points the way in treatment. The assessment of the psychosocial functional level according to MAS Axis VI does not depend on the assessment of the integration level of the mental structure according to the *structure* axis and is in no way superseded by the latter, although the two types of assessment overlap and a lower level of structural integration usually also determines a lower general psychosocial functional level. While the global level of functioning is operationalized purely descriptively according to social external criteria, the *structure* axis is primarily used to rate intrapsychic abilities and skills. For example, completely independent from the psychodynamic working hypotheses on relationships, conflict, and structure, the question of the retained or no longer existing everyday functioning, which in childhood and adolescence is generally measured in terms of school attendance, already plays a superordinate role in the indication for partial or full in-patient measures of treatment or for an initial primary attempt at out-patient treatment. A special consideration in the differential indication for introductory treatment measures in childhood and adolescence is also that, besides the severity of a symptomatology and the resulting current impairment of the psychosocial level of functioning, it must be checked to what extent that symptomatology hinders or blocks general psychosocial development or possibly supports such development in the service of progression. Conspicuous types of behavior that in themselves have the quality of symptoms may be "frictional noise" accompanying progressive development, whereas a condition with few symptoms may be worrying primarily because of the standstill in coping with pending psychosocial developmental tasks and, therefore, warrant the indication for treatment measures. The criterion for the extent to which a symptomatology is to be rated as inhibiting or blocking development also plays a leading role in the diagnostic assessment of clinical significance of intrapsychic conflict themes (see *conflict* axis). Conflict themes prominently presented are thus not to be considered as clinically significant if they evidently do not hinder development as measured in terms of coping with pending psychosocial developmental tasks. For example, the conflictual or "loud and noisy" problems presented in relationships with symptoms of vehement outbursts of anger inappropriate to the situation may be, all things considered, supportive of pubertal development directed towards separation, whereas in the case of an anxious-depressive development a moderately pronounced lack of contact as well as inhibition in play can lead to a serious standstill in coping with psychosocial developmental tasks.

In summary, *prior* to applying the *prerequisites of treatment* axis we must answer three questions for the differential indication:

1. Is a clinically significant disorder present? What diagnosis can be made according to MAS Axis I (Clinical Psychiatric Syndrome)?
2. What is the impairment of the psychosocial level of functioning, due to the symptomatology of the possibly existing disorder, according to MAS Axis VI?
3. To what extent is coping with pending psychosocial developmental tasks impaired by the existing symptomatology?

The answers to these three questions will usually yield information on the need for therapy, which marks only the first step on the way to differential indication, however. If the need for treatment exists, the motivation for treatment as well as the ability for treatment must be assessed in separate steps. For these steps in the differential indication for treatment measures, utilizing the *prerequisites for treatment* axis is helpful. The superordinated three dimensions of this axis then have the following relevance:

14.1 Subjective Dimensions

Decisive for the assessment of the motivation for treatment is first of all the general *motivation for change*. It results in a more or less pronounced degree from the level of suffering, which, in turn, in a more or less pronounced degree, results from the subjectively felt impairment due to the existing mental or somatic symptomatology. This more or less corresponds to the objectively ascertained severity of a symptomatology as well as to the causally related psychosocial impairment and inhibition of development. The above diagnostic categories thus form a causal functional chain in several steps, with each step possibly containing differently directed discontinuities that may have to be diagnosed in order to derive from such a psychodynamic understanding of a low motivation for treatment suitable interventions for improving that motivation.

In line with the subjective dimensions, the motivation for treatment is assessed in steps (see **Figure 6**). First, the *subjective impairment from the existing psychical and possibly somatic symptomatology*, assessed on the basis of the patient's utterances in the interview, is related to the objectively determined severity of the psychosocial impairment. Should this motivation seem inordinately low, which typically can be the case in anorexia or school phobia, confrontational interventions also involving the parents become necessary in order to clarify the seriousness of the prognosis in the event of inappropriate treatment. The next step checks to what extent an expressed *subjective impairment* is reflected in the corresponding *level of suffering*. If this *level of suffering* is pronounced to an inappropriately low degree, relatively considered, a sufficient motivation for treatment will hardly be possible, usually because of a high *gain from illness* (see below). It will then be necessary to decode the *gain from illness* psychodynamically and through suitable interventions involving the entire family system to try to undo the effect undermining the motivation for treatment as much as possible or at least ameliorate this effect. The next step checks to what extent the existing *level of suffering* is reflected in a corresponding expressed *motivation for change*. A discrepancy in the form of a low *motivation for change* compared with the level of suffering can have various causes. An especially high gain from illness may, in turn, exist (despite the high level of suffering), typically in patients with somatizing disorders, for example. Another possible cause is a highly pronounced fear of change despite a high level of suffering (e.g., fear of losing a relationship by openly addressing conflicts). Still another possible cause may be resistance from the family system for the sake of which the patient, despite his/her high level of suffering, makes sacrifices in a pronounced bond of loyalty by clinging to the role of invalid, in the often unconscious desire to protect the family system from destabilization (for example, by joining in the denial of intrafamilial sexual abuse). Depending on the psychodynamic decoding of a discrepancy in one of the aforementioned steps, suitable interventions can be derived aiming at increasing the level of suffering or motivation for change, in order to effect a sufficient motivation for treatment.

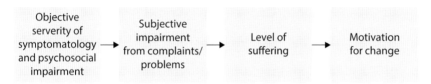

Figure 6. Causal functional relationships between the factors leading to the motivation for change.

14.2 Resources

The diagnostic rating of the resources operationalized along the *prerequisites of treatment* axis is significant primarily for assessing the general ability for treatment as well as for indicating a suitable treatment setting. In addition, treatment planning can be based on a realistic assessment of resources, so that a patient can or will have to be picked up from where he/she stands through suitable interventions in line with his/her perceptible strengths and deficits (including those of his/her social environment). This resource orientation in the assessment of an appropriate ability for therapy in the case of a specific form of treatment (e.g., out-patient analytical psychotherapy) is supplemented by an assessment of the structural abilities according to the *structure* axis as well as by the diagnosis of any well-defined developmental deficits (MAS, Axis II), the level of intelligence (MAS, Axis III), and the associated current abnormal psychosocial circumstances (MAS, Axis V). The assessment of the resources along the lines of the OPD-CA-2 is important in particular for the question of whether out-patient psychotherapy suffices as the sole form of treatment or whether it must be conjoined with socio-educational measures, or whether instead partial or full in-patient treatment is indicated. Out-patient psychotherapy of a child or adolescent as the sole form of treatment typically presupposes sufficiency of intrapsychic and familial resources for supporting or responsibly co-supporting an out-patient treatment setting. In addition, the peer resources should suffice to enable the patient to carry on without anxiety intrapsychic processes, initiated in therapy by corrective emotional experiences and self-reflective processes, as probatory steps towards change in social contexts. If peer resources do not suffice for such a newly experimental social implementation of intrapsychic developmental steps, there is the risk of the therapy becoming a purely intrapsychic "dry run" making no real headway, and one should check the possible indication for at least initial treatment in the more sheltered space of a partial or fully in-patient setting.

14.3 Specific Prerequisites of Treatment

Finally, we employ the items of the *specific prerequisites of treatment* dimension again to assess the motivation for treatment and the ability for treatment with regard to a specific psychodynamically oriented psychotherapy. This should be preceded by an assessment of the level of suffering, the general motivation for change, and the resources. If a motivation for treatment can be assumed to exist on the basis of a sufficient level of suffering and the corresponding motivation for change, and, if psychodynamically oriented psychotherapy (with an initially conflict-coping or structure-giving focus) seems indicated and promising according to the relationship and conflict dynamics captured with the OPD-CA-2, the patient's specific suitability and motivation can be described by means of the items *insight into biopsychosocial interrelations* and *specific motivation for therapy*. The assessment of the *gain from illness* allows a prognosis as to the expected resistance to treatment, i.e., of the patient's inclination to cling to his/her symptom or invalid role. In the case of children and adolescents, the secondary gain from illness in the invalid role must particularly be noted, as this gain can essentially contribute to the maintainance of certain symptomatology, even with a high level of suffering and a high motivation for change. For example, the initial concern that adolescent patients with self-destructive symptoms and a high level of suffering cause their parents may itself initially afford emotional relief to those patients. Therapeutic progress may be forthcoming in the hope of positive changes in the parent–child relationship. In the further course of therapy, the fear that the parents and family could fall back into their old patterns of behavior ("returning to business as usual") if recovery occurs too rapidly can make the patient cling to self-destructive symptoms. The psychodynamic understanding of the *gain from illness* enables the therapist to address this matter at an early stage when planning treatment, in order specifically to counteract this tendency that is to be expected during therapy. The assessment of the ability to form a working alliance and of the use of psychosocial care systems finally completes treatment planning with a specific check of the realistic feasibility of an indicated treatment plan or setting. If, for example, the child's or adolescent's own motivation for treatment and ability for therapy becomes precarious, does not come to pass, or threatens to break down because of the family system's insufficient ability to form a working alliance, the therapist's attention will be drawn at an early stage to the necessity of counteracting this problem through specific interventions (such as more frequent contact with the parents, supplemental sociopsychiatric measures in the case of mentally ill parents, etc.).

In summary, the three main pillars of an indication for therapy and treatment planning, namely the clarification of the need for therapy, the motivation for treatment, and finally the ability for treatment, can be completed and differentiated as steps by means of the *prerequisites of treatment* axis. An absolute prerequisite for the first step is a conventional psychiatric diagnosis with the multiaxial classification scheme according to the guidelines of ICD-10. The rating of the relationship dynamics, conflict dynamics, and structural integration level according to the respective axes of the OPD-CA-2 allows the formulation, from a trained therapeutic perspective, of essential clinical working hypotheses for understanding the disorder, for the differential indication, for the suitable treatment setting, and for the initial focus of treatment (i.e., addressing conflict issues or structural deficits). These clinical working hypotheses are supplemented by assessing the motivation for treatment and the ability for therapy according to the *prerequisites for treatment* axis. A detailed view of individual items and dimensions along this axis will lead to specific considerations about which initial or supplemental interventions may ensure that the differential indication and planning of treatment will rest on all three aforementioned pillars.

15. Training in the OPD-CA-2

The strength of the OPD-CA-2 lies in the possibility of a diagnostic investigation of structure and conflict (structural and conflict-related limitations of behavior and experience) as a supplement to the multiaxial classification system, in the capturing of relationship patterns and in the possibility of assessing the prerequisites of treatment. In addition, the structural and conflictual foci can be formulated for treatment planning and the progress and outcome of treatment can be described (Resch & Koch, 2012).

Given the quality criteria of an operationalization of psychodynamic constructs (reliability, objectivity, validity) and with a view to the possible difficulties with such a complex operationalization of relationship behavior, mental structure, intrapsychic conflicts, and the prerequisites of treatment, seminars are just as necessary for training as they are for the continual exchanges with users for obtaining feedback and for the further development of the instrument.

15.1 Interested Persons and Needs

So far most training seminars have been offered at training institutes for psychodynamic psychotherapy, but also mental healthcare teams have been trained in diagnostics with the OPD-CA axes. Interested individuals and established colleagues have had and continue to have the possibility of continuing their training at conferences and therapy weeks.

Need and demand have been constantly increasing over the last ten years, and so far over 2,000 colleagues have received training.

OPD-CA intervision and supervision groups allow the attainment and preservation of high standards as well as help communication within the training institutes and clinics.

In addition to therapists, physicians, and psychologists engaged in hospital and out-patient care, educational workers in youth welfare are increasingly using the instrument to formulate plans of action for handling and for educationally guiding children and adolescents in a structured way keyed to the OPD-CA axes.

Moreover, the OPD-CA is finding a growing interest among other therapy approaches.

15.2 Previous Experience With the Training Seminars

Over a hundred basic and advance training seminars have been conducted since the publication of the OPD-CA Manual in 2003. Lively exchanges among the participants and their feedback have allowed the continued development of the instrument and its adaptation to the needs of people providing therapy. The Task Force originally assumed that mainly colleagues experienced in clinical work and psychodynamic psychology would use the OPD-CA axes, but experience with the training seminars has shown that beginners can also profit from the courses and apply the acquired knowledge in their work. The feedback from the seminars has continually been incorporated in the improvement and continued development of the instrument, and the basic changes to the OPD-CA-2 are outlined in the theoretical parts and manualizations of the individual chapters on the axes.

15.3 Structure and Content of the Training Seminars

OPD-CA certification requires attendance of a basic course and two advanced courses. The courses build upon one another and each comprises 12 hours attendance time.

Structure of the Basic Course

The basic course provides a theoretical introduction to the development of the operationalization of psychodynamic diagnostics and to the individual axes.

Following a theoretical introduction, we evaluate the subjects of relationship patterns, mental structure, and intrapsychic conflicts in small groups with the aid of video material, and then discuss them in the large group. Assistance with difficulties that may arise in operationalization is also provided. The basic course thus affords an initial insight into the structure and handling of the instrument.

Structure of the First Advanced Course

The first advanced training course begins by refreshing pre-existing knowledge incorporating previous experiences with the tool and expands the assessment possibilities of the interpersonal relations axis by including the examiner's internal resonance. Participants rate and discuss in depth the OPD-CA axes using several videos or case vignettes provided by the participants.

Structure of the Second Advanced Course

The second advanced course serves the further consolidation and planning of treatment focussing on conflicts and structure using the participants' case vignettes. Specific clinical issues in diagnostics and treatment planning can be taken up and discussed as required.

Certification

On successful completion of the second advanced course, participants receive the OPD-CA certificate and are qualified and authorized to independently carry out the assessment of relationships, structures, and conflicts according to the OPD-CA in everyday clinical practice or research. The certificate may be requested from the training coordinator.

Authorized Trainers

Dr. Eginhard Koch (Training Coordinator)
eginhard.koch@med.uni-heidelberg.de

Dr. Oliver Bilke-Hentsch
oliver.bilke-hentsch@somosa.ch

Dr. Heiko Dietrich
hei98die@aol.com

Dr. Rainer Fliedl
Rainer.Fliedl@moedling.lknoe.at

Dr. Florian Juen
florian.juen@uibk.ac.at

Prof. Franz Resch
franz.resch@med.uni-heidelberg.de

Prof. Georg Romer
g.romer@ukmuenster.de

Prof. Inge Seiffge-Krenke
seiffge-krenke@uni-mainz.de

Dr. Susanne Schlüter-Müller
schluetermueller@yahoo.de

Prof. Klaus Schmeck
klaus.schmeck@upkbs.ch

Prof. Annette Streeck-Fischer
annette.streeck@t-online.de

Dr. Matthias Weber
m.weber.bs@sunrise.ch

Dr. Ruth Weissensteiner
rweissensteiner@msn.com

Dr. Klaus Winkelmann
winkelmann@akjp-hd.de

Dr. Sibylle-Maria Winter
Sibylle.Winter@charite.de

16. Applications Across Axes and Outlook

While the four axes of the OPD-CA-2 (*interpersonal relations, structure, conflict,* and *prerequisites of treatment)* are conceptually interrelated, each individual axis can also be used as an independent module in the diagnostic process. This applies to both clinical practice and research, ensuring in particular a need-based efficiency of labor adapted to the respective contexts of these applications. For example, a focussed analysis, based solely on the interpersonal relations axis, of the current relationship dynamics between the patient and therapist can serve as the starting point of case supervision or, if reiterated, capture changes within the therapeutic relationship during the therapeutic process. A pronounced intrapsychic conflict diagnosed exclusively along the conflict axis and plausibly explaining a symptomatology in need of treatment can serve as the key point justifying the indication for analytic therapy in a health insurance request, for example. The differentiated description of a low level of structural integration according to the structure axis can be the key point but also, at the same time, provide a qualified approach in developmental psychopathology in a forensic psychiatric expert report on the criminal responsibility of a youth offender.

The following section offers some suggestions on how the overall instrument can be applied to yield useful diagnostic information from a cross-axis consideration of the findings. Or in other words: How can overall OPD-CA-2 findings be read or interpreted across all axes?

For the psychodynamic understanding of a disorder pattern, an integrated cross-axis diagnostic overview according to the *interpersonal relations, structure,* and *conflict* axes is helpful, whereas the *prerequisites of treatment* axis is to be understood more as a stand-alone module for the differential indication for and planning of treatment in psychotherapeutic approaches (see *Part 3: Clinical Application of the Axes in Diag-*

nosis and Therapy). The following star-shaped diagram (see **Figure 7**) illustrates the intertwined understanding of the relationship dynamics, intrapsychic conflict dynamics, and level of structural integration.

Interpersonal relations

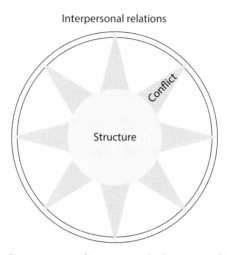

Figure 7. Conceptual intertwining of interpersonal relations, conflict, and structure.

Structure accordingly forms the organizational core of the mental organism. The level of structural integration crucially determines how internalized intrapsychic conflicts organize and define themselves. The more integrated the structure is, the more clearly and inherently coherent can conflicts develop and organize themselves as compromises between the intrapsychic agencies, i.e., their gestalt will be more clearly recognisable. The less integrated the structural level is, the less inherently coherent the organization of mental conflicts will be, with the consequence of their being less clearly defined, which does not mean that they are absent or less effective psychodynamically. If present and significant in a dysfunctional and developmentally inhibitive way, they will be merely more difficult to diagnose according to the operationalizations of the conflict axis, given a low level of structural integration, since the behavioral typologies in question, as described in the anchor-point examples, will be less clearly defined as behavioral strategies representing a compromise between defence and that which is defended against. In order to diagnose clinically significant intrapsychic conflictual themes with a low level of structural integration or disintegrated level of structure, the conflictual theme must be viewed through the lens of the structure in question. For example, virulent conflictual themes regarding *closeness vs. distance* or *submission vs. control* can become evident through dysfunctional affect regulation in dealing with the particular conflictual theme, even if a basically stringent behavioral pattern following the active or passive mode is less evident.

If clinically significant intrapsychic conflicts are present, the interpersonal relationship dynamics in the here and now will form the "outer skin" of the mental organism as a contact surface vis-à-vis the environment, on which these conflicts become visible through re-enactments subject to the repetition compulsion. In the symbolic star-shaped diagram (see Figure 7), vertices of the conflictual triangles thus protrude through this outer layer of the interpersonal relationship dynamics. If we discern these protruding vertices, presented according to subtle patterns of interaction to be carefully differentiated from one another, as they are operationalized along the interpersonal relations axis, we can decode the gestalt of the underlying intrapsychic conflicts, whose definition in turn becomes comprehensible only given the integration level of the structure.

With this understanding across concepts and axes of the effective relationship between interpersonal relations, conflict, and structure according to the star diagram, we can consider, on the basis of an overall view of the three axes, where the most important focus for the beginning of a treatment is to be defined in an individual case, or how different foci are to be arranged in an appropriate hierarchy. Foci in this sense can be defined in terms of relationship dynamics, conflict, or structure. The OPD-2 for adults (Arbeitskreis OPD, 2006) proposes subdivisions and hierarchical rules that, among other things, differentiate between *primarily conflict-related and primarily structure-related disorder patterns*, for which different suitable approaches are respectively recommended. Using the OPD-CA-2, we recommend that the greatest possible indeterminateness in the developmental progression of mental disorders in children and adolescents should be assumed, so that a categorization of disorder patterns according to their appearance in terms of the *interpersonal relations, structure*, and *conflict* axes does not seem advisable. Instead, we recommend viewing the overall picture according to these three axes rather as a psychodynamic "snapshot" of a *psychopathological development pattern*, on the basis of which a clinical decision neverthe-less can be made as to the point where the mental process presents itself most virulently or as to where the initial focus of a therapeutic strategy should lie (according to the principle "first things first").

Focussing on the *relationship dynamics* can be useful, for example, if the dysfunctional handling of relationships in the here and now governs the picture in a particular way and a patient is not receptive or ready to work on the underlying intrapsychic conflict. Of primary importance is the temporary suspension of the repetition compulsion of dysfunc-tional conflict re-enactments in the interpersonal sector by means of an adequate relationship response in the here-and-now therapeutic inter-action. This, for example, occurs in direct response not to the aggres-sive response but rather to the defence against the relationship desire. Focussing on the relationship dynamics may also be indicated if not an intrapsychic conflict but an actual relationship trauma is primarily sup-posed as the cause of the dysfunctional handling of relationships. Work focussing on relationship dynamics in the here and now, with the aim of a corrective emotional relationship experience that will then become available as a new internalizable model, is a path often taken in nonver-bal forms of therapy (e.g., dance and concentrative movement therapy), which can be fruitfully applied in any form of psychotherapy, however.

A *structure-related focus* is useful, for example, if structural deficits primarily govern the current appearance of a disorder so that a con-flict-coping therapy would overwhelm the patient and therefore have a destabilizing effect. In this case, the point is to stabilize the patient's unstable or currently low level of structural integration within the framework of treatment, the setting, and the holding function of the therapeutic relationship, in order to help him/her acquire corrective experiences with *self-control* and *interpersonal relations*, for example, which, in turn, will enable him/her to enter into the therapeutic rela-tionship less anxiously. Generally such a structural focus does not mean settling on a primarily structural disorder in a categorical sense. Follow-ing stabilization, we must rather reassess whether the therapy should continue with a focus on the relationship dynamics or on conflicts.

A *focus on conflicts* seems particularly indicated when we regard intra-psychic conflicts as especially virulent for a disorder pattern and when the patient is suffering in him-/herself and from his/her dysfunctional handling of relationships. If the latter is not (yet) the case, which is often so with contraphobic defence structures characterized by the active processing mode with conflicts, it will be useful first to focus on the relationship dynamics in the here and now of the therapeutic interaction as well as on the everyday relationship experiences. The aim is to give patients emotionally experienced access to their own part in failed relationship experiences through clarifications and confrontations or mirroring interventions, and to afford them the corrective experience that other ways of handling relationships are possible and can succeed. A distinct focus on conflicts along the lines of revelatory ("interpretive") working on conflicts presupposes a minimal ability for introspection and self-reflection (or *insight into biopsychosocial interrelations*). In the absence of this ability, beginning with a focus on the relationship dynamics (actual interaction in the here and now is also useful) again makes sense, which could very well be guided by clinical working hypotheses about prominent intrapsychic conflicts and, through this, implicitly pursue a focus on conflicts.

As illustrated in the previous sections, the described foci can generally merge into one another as well as partly overlap in the course of therapy. This reflects the aforementioned clinical reality of the progression of disorder patterns in children and adolescents, for whom a much greater openness is to be assumed than with adults.

Outlook: Unresolved Questions

In revising the OPD-CA as the OPD-CA-2, we attempted to take up and integrate as many experiences and empirical findings as possible occurring over the last decade, as well as current developments in the discourse on developmental psychopathology and on psychodynamic constructs. However, science is constantly changing. Even at the present time, questions remain open or seem still in need of further clarification. Some issues could only be barely broached by members of the OPD-CA-2 Task Force and had to be set aside for later work. The following topics could be addressed in more detail in the future:

- *Trauma:* In the discourse of developmental psychopathology and psychodynamics, understanding how patients cope with mental traumas as well as understanding the dynamics and phenomenology of their consequences has attracted increasing interest over the last decade. Psychotraumatology has evolved into a separate discipline that explores the specific cause and effect connections in traumatogenic disorders and from these derives specific treatment principles that differ from the approach to conflict-related disorders (Fischer & Riedesser, 1999; Leuzinger-Bohleber, Roth, & Buchheim, 2008; Seidler, Freyberger, & Maercker, 2011; Streeck-Fischer 2006). Traumatically caused psychopathological phenomena can certainly be described using the OPD-CA instrument, in terms of hostile relationship expectations according to the interpersonal relations axis or trauma-related structural deficits according to the structure axis, for example. Such a description of the consequences of mental trauma has so far been strictly phenomenological in the OPD-CA-2 system, however; the OPD-CA-2 (still) lacks a conceptual relation to psychotraumatology or a conceptual anchoring of psychotraumatology. The latter is still far less detailed than the anchoring of the *conflict* axis in psychoanalytic conflict theory. Whether and if so, in what form, psychotraumatological findings can and will be incorporated in a future version of the OPD-CA-2 must remain the subject of our continuing discourse in the future.

- *Identity:* The evolution of the OPD-CA into OPD-CA-2 has expanded the conceptual anchoring of the *identity* construct in line with the central importance of identity development as the core of personality development. In our current discourse, identity development is representable along a separate dimension of the structure axis. In addition, an independent intrapsychic conflict continues to be described as an identity conflict whose presence and, possibly, whose clinical significance should be assessed. This conceptual overlap between the structure axis and the conflict axis in the concept of identity seems to us, for the time being, appropriate to the current state of discussion and to the aforementioned multi-layered significance of identity development and its disorders. In our continuing discourse, we will also have to decide whether to retain this conceptual dichotomy in future versions of the OPD-CA or to supersede it with a more convincing classification.

References

Abelin, E. (1971). The role of the father in the separation-individuation process. In J. B. McDevitt & C. F. Settlage (Eds.), *Separation – individuation* (pp. 229–252). New York, NY: International University Press.

Ainsworth, M. D., Blehar, M. C., Waters, E., & Wall, S. (1978). *Patterns of attachment: A psychological study of the strange situation.* Hillsdale, NJ: Lawrence Erlbaum Associates.

Alamdar-Niemann, M. (1992). *Türkische Jugendliche im Eingliederungsprozess. Eine Untersuchung zur Erziehung türkischer Jugendlicher in Berlin (West) und der Bedeutung ausgewählter individueller und kontextueller Faktoren im Lebenslauf* [Turkish adolescents in the integration process. A study into the upbringing of Turkish adolescents in West Berlin and the importance of specific individual and contextual factors in their life courses]. Hamburg, Germany: Dr. Kovac.

American Psychiatric Association. (2015). *Diagnostic and statistical manual of mental disorders* (5th ed.). Washington, DC: Author.

Arbeitskreis OPD. (Ed.). (1996). *Operationalisierte psychodynamische Diagnostik* [Operationalized psychodynamic diagnosis]. Bern, Switzerland: Huber.

Arbeitskreis OPD. (Ed.). (2006). *Operationalisierte Psychodynamische Diagnostik OPD-2: Das Manual für Diagnostik und Therapieplanung* [Operationalized psychodynamic diagnosis OPD-2: Manual for diagnosis and therapy planning]. Bern, Switzerland: Huber.

Arbeitskreis OPD-KJ. (Ed.). (2003). *Operationalisierte Psychodynamische Diagnostik im Kindes- und Jugendalter* [Operationalized psychodynamic diagnosis in childhood and adolescence]. Bern, Switzerland: Huber.

Arbeitskreis OPD-KJ. (Ed.). (2007). *Operationalisierte Psychodynamische Diagnostik im Kindes- und Jugendalter* [Operationalized psychodynamic diagnosis in childhood and adolescence] (2nd ed.). Bern, Switzerland: Huber.

Arbeitsgruppe OPD-KJ-Institut für Psychotherapie Berlin. (2009). *Interviewsituationen und Formulierungsvorschläge im OPD-KJ-Interview* [Interview situations and formulation suggestions in OPD-KJ Interview]. Unpublished manuscript, IfP – Institut für Psychotherapie e. V. Berlin, Germany.

Bakermans-Kranenburg, M. J., & van IJzendoorn, M. H. (2009). The first 10,000 adult attachment interviews: Distribution of adult attachment representations in clinical and non-clinical groups. *Attachment and Human Development, 11*, 223–263. http://doi.org/10.1080/14616730902814762

Balint, M. (1952). Über Liebe und Hass [About love and hate]. *Psyche, 6*, 19–33.

Ball, J., Lohaus, A., & Miebach, C. (2006). Psychische Anpassung und schulische Leistungen beim Wechsel von der Grundschule zur weiterführenden Schule [Psychological adaptation and educational benefits when changing from primary to secondary school]. *Zeitschrift für Entwicklungspsychologie und Pädagogische Psychologie, 38*, 101–109. http://doi.org/10.1026/0049-8637.38.3.101

Barkmann, C., Romer, G., Watson, M., & Schulte-Markwort, M. (2007). Parental physical illness as a risk for psychosocial maladjustment in children and adolescents: Epidemiological findings from a national survey in Germany. *Psychosomatics, 48*, 476–481. http://doi.org/10.1176/appi.psy.48.6.476

Baumrind, D. (1991). The influence of parenting style on adolescent competence and substance use. *Journal of Early Adolescence, 11*, 56–95. http://doi.org/10.1177/0272431691111004

Benecke, C., Bock, A., Wieser, E., Tschiesner, R., Lochmann, M., Küspert, F., … Steinmayr-Gensluckner, M. (2011). Reliabilität und Validität der OPD-KJ-Achsen Struktur und Konflikt [Reliability and validation of the OPD-CA axes structure and conflict]. *Praxis der Kinderpsychologie und Kinderpsychiatrie, 60*, 60–73.

Bengel, J., Meinders-Lücking, F., & Rottmann, N. (2009). *Schutzfaktoren bei Kindern und Jugendlichen* [Protection factors for children and adolescents]. Cologne, Germany: Bundeszentrale für gesundheitliche Aufklärung.

Benjamin, L. S. (1974). A structural analysis of social behavior (SABS). *Psychological Review, 81*, 392–425. http://doi.org/10.1037/h0037024

Benjamin, L. S. (1982). Use of Structural Analysis of Social Behavior (SASB) to guide intervention in psychotherapy. In J. C. Anchin & D. J. Kiesler (Eds.), *Handbook of interpersonal psychotherapy* (pp. 121–212). New York, NY: Guilford.

Benjamin, L. S. (1987). Use of the SABS dimensional model to develop treatment plans for personality disorders I: Narcissism. *Journal of Personality Disorders, 1*, 43–70. http://doi.org/10.1521/pedi.1987.1.1.43

Benjamin, L. S. (1988). Adding social and intrapsychic descriptors to axis I of DSM-III. In T. Millon & G. Klerman (Eds.), *Contemporary directions in psychopathology* (pp. 599–638). New York, NY: Guilford.

Benjamin, L. S. (1993). *Interpersonal diagnosis and treatment of personality disorders.* New York, NY: Guilford.

Bindernagel, D., Scherrer, A., Winzeler, A. L., & von Wyl, A. (2011). Psychodrama-Gruppentherapie mit Kindern [Psychodrama group therapy with children]. *Zeitschrift für Psychodrama und Soziometrie, 10*, 109–124.

Bion, W. R. (1963). *Container-contained in elements of psychoanalysis.* London, UK: Heinemann.

Blanck, G., & Blanck, R. (1979). *Ego psychology II.* New York, NY: Columbia University Press.

Blos, P. (2001). *Adoleszenz. Eine psychoanalytische Interpretation* [Adolescence. A psychoanalytical interpretation] (7th ed.). Stuttgart, Germany: Klett-Cotta.

Bowlby, J. (1975). *Bindung. Eine Analyse der Mutter-Kind Beziehung* [Attachment. An analysis of the mother-child relationship]. Munich, Germany: Kindler.

Bowlby, J. (1980). *Attachment and loss.* London, UK: Hogarth Press.

Bowlby, J. (1988). Developmental psychiatry comes of age. *The American Journal of Psychiatry, 145*, 1–10. http://doi.org/10.1176/ajp.145.1.1

Bowlby, J. (1998). *A secure base: Clinical applications of attachment theory.* London, UK: Tavistock/Routledge.

Bretherton, I., & Oppenheim, D. (2003). The MacArthur Story Stem-Battery development, administration, reliability, validity, and reflection about meaning. In R. N. Emde, D. P. Wolf, & D. Oppenheim (Eds.), *Revealing the inner world of young children* (pp. 55–80). New York, NY: Oxford University Press.

Bretherton, I., Suess, G. J., Golby, G., & Oppenheim, D. (2011). Attachment Story Completion Task (ASCT): Methode zur Erfassung der Bindungsqualität im Kindergartenalter durch Geschichtenergänzungen im Puppenspiel [Method for capturing attachment at preschool age through supplementing stories with puppet shows]. In G. J. Suess, H. Scheuer-Englisch, & P. Pfeiffer (Eds.), *Bindungstheorie und Familiendynamik: Anwendung der Bindungstheorie in Beratung und Therapie* (pp. 83–124). Gießen, Germany: Psychosozial-Verlag.

Brickman, H. R. (1993). Between the Devil and the deep blue sea: The dyad and the triad in psychoanalytic thought. *International Journal of Psycho-Analysis, 74*, 905–915.

Broderick, P., & Korteland, C. (2002). Coping style and depression in early adolescence: Relationships to gender, gender role, and implicit beliefs. *Sex Roles, 46*, 201–213. http://doi.org/10.1023/A:1019946714220

Burchartz, A. (2012). *Psychodynamische Psychotherapie bei Kindern und Jugendlichen. Das tiefenpsychologisch fundierte Verfahren: Basiswissen und Praxis* [Psychodynamic psychotherapy for children and adolescents. Psychodynamic procedures: Fundamentals and practice]. Stuttgart, Germany: Kohlhammer.

Bühler, K. (1918). *Die geistige Entwicklung des Kindes* [The psychological development of children]. Jena, Germany: Fischer.

Bürgin, D. (1998a). Psychoanalytische Ansätze zum Verständnis der frühen Eltern–Kind Triade [Psychoanalytical approaches to understanding the early parent–child triad]. In K. von Klitzing (Ed.), *Psychotherapie in der frühen Kindheit* (pp. 15–31). Göttingen, Germany: Vandenhoek & Ruprecht.

Bürgin, D. (1998b). Vater als Person und Vater als Prinzip [Father as a person, and father as a concept]. In D. Bürgin (Ed.), *Triangulierung. Der Übergang zur Elternschaft* (pp. 179–214). Stuttgart, Germany: Schattauer.

Caldwell, L. L., & Witt, P. A. (2011). Leisure, recreation, and play from a developmental context. *New Directions for Youth Development, 130*, 13–27. http://doi.org/10.1002/yd.394

Chambers, W. J., Puig-Antich, J., Hirsch, M., Paez, P., Ambrosini, P. J., Tabrizi, M. A., & Davies, M. (1985). The assessment of affective-disorders in children and adolescents by semistructured interview – Test-retest reliability of the Schedule for Affective-Disorders and Schizophrenia for school-age children, present episode version. *Archives of General Psychiatry, 42*, 696–702. http://doi.org/10.1001/archpsyc.1985.01790300 0064008

Cierpka, M. (1992). Zur Entwicklung des Familiengefühls [On the development of the sense of family]. *Forum der Psychoanalyse, 8*, 32–46.

Cierpka, M. (2008). *Handbuch der Familiendiagnostik* [Handbook of family diagnostics]. Heidelberg, Germany: Springer. http://doi.org/10.1007/978-3-540-78475-3

Cierpka, M., Grande, T., Rudolf, G., von der Tann, M., Stasch, M., & OPD Task Force (2007). The operationalized psychodynamic diagnostics system: Clinical relevance, reliability and validity. *Psychopathology, 40*, 209–220. http://doi.org/10.1159/000101363

Clarkin, J. F., Yeomans, F. E., & Kernberg, O. F. (1999). *Psychotherapy for borderline personality*. New York, NY: Wiley & Sons.

Clarkin, J. F., Yeomans, J. F., & Kernberg, O. F. (Eds.) (2001). *Psychotherapie der Border-line-Persönlichkeit* [Psychotherapy of borderline personality disorder]. Stuttgart, Germany: Schattauer.

Connolly, J., & Goldberg, A. (1999). Romantic relationships in adolescence: The role of friends and peers in their emergence and development. In W. Furman, B. B. Brown, & C. Feiring (Eds.), *The development of romantic relationships in adolescence* (pp. 266–290). New York, NY: Cambridge University Press.

Cropp, C., Salzer, S., Häusser, L. F. & Streeck-Fischer, A. (2013). Interrater-Reliabilität und Konstruktvalidität der OPD-KJ-Achse Struktur – Erste Forschungsergebnisse zum Einsatz der OPD-KJ im Rahmen der klinischen Routine [Interrater reliability and construct validity of the OPD-CA axis structure: First study results regarding the integration of OPD-CA into clinical practice]. *Praxis der Kinderpsychologie und Kinderpsychiatrie, 62*, 270–284. http://doi.org/10.13109/prkk.2013.62.4.270

Damasio, A. R. (1999). *The feeling of what happens: Body and emotion in the making of consciousness.* New York, NY: Harcourt.

Diederichs-Paeschke, V., Forkel, C., Held, U., Jaletzke, C., Stafski, B., & Bilke-Hentsch, O. (2011). Psychoanalytisches Erstgespräch und OPD-KJ interview. Kein Spagat! [Psychoanalytical initial consultation and OPD-KJ-Interview. No Balancing act!]. *Praxis der Kinderpsychologie und Kinderpsychiatrie, 60*, 4–26. http://doi.org/10.13109/prkk.2011.60.1.4

Diepold, B. (1995). Borderline-Entwicklungsstörungen bei Kindern [Borderline developmental disorders in children]. *Praxis der Kinderpsychologie und Kinderpsychiatrie, 44*, 270–279.

Dornes, M. (2006). *Die Seele des Kindes: Entstehung und Entwicklung* [The soul of the child: Formation and development]. Frankfurt a. M., Germany: Fischer.

Dührssen, A. (1981). *Die biographische Anamnese unter tiefenpsychologischen Aspekten* [The biographical anamnesis of the aspects of depth psychology]. Göttingen, Germany: Vandenhoeck & Ruprecht.

Egle, U., Joraschky, P., Lampe, S. A., Seiffge-Krenke, I., & Cierpka, M. (Eds.) (2015). *Sexueller Missbrauch, Misshandlung, Vernachlässigung* [Sexual abuse, physical abuse, and neglect]. Stuttgart, Germany: Schattauer.

Eisenberg, N., & Harris, J. D. (1984). Social competence: A developmental perspective. *School Psychology Review, 13*, 267–277.

Erikson, E. H. (1959). *Identity and the life cycle.* New York, NY: International Universities Press.

Erikson, E. H. (1968). *Identity, youth and crisis.* New York, NY: W. W. Norton.

Erikson, E. H. (1982). *The life cycle completed.* New York, NY: W. W. Norton.

Fairbairn, W. R. D. (1952). *Psychoanalytic studies of the personality.* London, UK: Tavistock, Routledge and Keagan.

Faltermaier, T., Kühnlein, I., & Burda-Viering, M. (1998). Subjektive Gesundheitstheorien: Inhalt, Dynamik und ihre Bedeutung für das Gesundheitshandeln im Alltag [Subjective health theories: Content, dynamics and their significance to healthcare in everyday life]. *Zeitschrift für Gesundheitswissenschaften, 6*, 309–326.

Fegert, J. M., & Resch, F. (2012). Risiko, Vulnerabilität, Resilienz und Prävention [Risks, vulnerability, resilience, and prevention]. In J. M. Fegert, C. Eggers, & F. Resch (Eds.), *Psychiatrie und Psychotherapie des Kindes- und Jugendalters* (2nd ed., pp. 131–142). Berlin, Germany: Springer.

Fenichel, O. (1941). *Problems of psychoanalytic technique*. New York, NY: Albany.

Field, T. (1998). Maternal depression effects on infants and early interventions. *Preventive Medicine, 27*, 200–203. http://doi.org/10.1006/pmed.1998.0293

Fischer, G., & Riedesser, P. (1999). *Lehrbuch der Psychotraumatologie* [Textbook of Psychotraumatology]. Munich, Germany: Reinhardt.

Fisher, S., & Greenberg, P. R. (1977). *The scientific credibility of Freud's theories and therapies*. New York, NY: Basic Books.

Fivaz-Depeursinge, E., & Corboz-Warnery, A. (1999). *The primary triangle*. Boulder, CO: Basic Books.

Fivaz-Depeursinge, E., Favez, N., Lavanchy, S., de Noni, S., & Frascarolo, F. (2005). Four-month-olds make triangular bids to father and mother during trilogue play with still-face. *Social Development, 14*, 361–378. http://doi.org/10.1111/j.1467-9507.2005.00306.x

Fivaz-Depeursinge, E., Lavanchy-Scaiola, C., & Favez, N. (2010). The young infant's triangular communication in the family: Access to threesome intersubjectivity? Conceptual considerations and case illustrations. *Psychoanalytic Dialogues, 20*, 125–140. http://doi.org/10.1080/10481881003716214

Foelsch, P., Odom, A. O., Arena, H., Krischer, M., Schmeck, K., & Schlüter-Müller, S. (2010). Differenzierung zwischen Identitätskrise und Identitätsdiffusion und ihre Bedeutung für die Behandlung [Differentiation between identity crisis and identity diffusion and their implications for treatment]. *Praxis der Kinderpsychologie und Kinderpsychiatrie, 59*, 418–434. http://doi.org/10.13109/prkk.2010.59.6.418

Foelsch, P., Schlüter-Müller, S., Odom, A. O., Arena, H., Borzutzky, A., & Schmeck, K. (2013). *Behandlung von Jugendlichen mit Identitätsstörungen (AIT) – Ein integratives Therapiekonzept für Persönlichkeitsstörungen* [Treatment of adolescents with identity disorders (AIT): An integrative therapy concept for personality disorders]. Heidelberg, Germany: Springer.

Fonagy, P., Gergely, G., Jurist, E. L., & Target, M. (2006). *Affect regulation, mentalization and the development of the self*. New York, NY: Other Press.

Fonagy, P., & Target, M. (2003). *Frühe Bindung und psychische Entwicklung* [Early attachment and psychological development]. Gießen, Germany: Psychosozial-Verlag.

Freud, A. (1936). *The ego and the mechanism of defense* (revised edition: 1966). New York, NY: International University Press.

Freud, A. (1965). *Normality and pathology in childhood*. New York, NY: University Press.

Freud, S. (1953). Three essays of the theory of sexuality. In J. Strachey (Trans. & Ed.), *The standard edition of the complete psychological works of Sigmund Freud* (pp. 1457–1552). London, UK: Hogarth Press and the Institute of Psycho-Analysis. (Original work published 1905)

Freud, S. (1959). *Character and anal erotism*. In J. Strachey (Trans. & Ed.), *The standard edition of the complete psychological works of Sigmund Freud* (pp. 1942–1945). London, UK: Hogarth Press and the Institute of Psycho-Analysis. (Original work published 1908)

Freud, S. (1961). Female sexuality. In J. Strachey (Trans. & Ed.), *The standard edition of the complete psychological works of Sigmund Freud* (Vol. 21). London, UK: Hogarth Press and the Institute of Psycho-Analysis. (Original work published 1931)

Freud, S. (2000). Remembering, repeating and working through. In J. Strachey (Trans. & Ed.), *The standard edition of the complete psychological works of Sigmund Freud*

(Vol. 12). London, UK: Hogarth Press and the Institute of Psycho-Analysis. (Original work published 1914)

Frey, C. U., & Röthlisberger, C. (1996). Social support in healthy adolescents. *Journal of Youth and Adolescence, 25,* 17–31. http://doi.org/10.1007/BF01537378

Goth, K., Foelsch, P., Schlüter-Müller, S., Jung, E., Pick, O., Birkhölzer, M., & Schmeck, K. (2012). Assessment of identity development and identity diffusion in adolescence –Theoretical basis and psychometric properties of the self-report questionnaire AIDA. *Child and Adolescent Psychiatry and Mental Health, 6,* http://doi.org/10.1186/1753-2000-6-27

Göttken, T., & von Klitzing, K. (2013). "Da fehlt etwas!" – Die Arbeit mit Vätern in der psychoanalytischen Kurzzeitherapie für Kinder mit Depression und Angststörungen (PaKT) ["Something is missing!" – The work with fathers in psychoanalytical short-term therapy for children with depression and anxiety disorders]. In H. Walter & H. Hierdeis (Eds.), *Väter in der Psychotherapie – Der Dritte im Bunde?* (pp. 131–165). Stuttgart, Germany: Schattauer.

Grieser, J. (2010). Der Körper als Dritter – Psychosomatische Triangulierungsprozesse am Beispiel der Adoleszenz [The body as third element – Psychosomatic triangulation processes using the example of adolescence]. *Praxis der Kinderpsychologie und Kinderpsychiatrie, 59,* 140–158. http://doi.org/10.13109/prkk.2010.59.2.140

Hampel, P., & Petermann, F. (2005). Age and gender effects on coping in children and adolescents. *Journal of Youth and Adolescence, 34,* 73–83. http://doi.org/10.1007/s10964-005-3207-9

Hassenstein, B. (1986). *Verhaltensbiologie des Kindes* [Behaviorial biology of the child]. Munich, Germany: Piper.

Havighurst, R. (1972). *Developmental tasks and education.* New York, NY: McKay.

Heigl-Evers, A., Heigl, F., & Ott, J. (Eds.). (1993). *Lehrbuch der Psychotherapie* [Textbook of psychotherapy]. Stuttgart, Germany: Fischer.

Heimann, P. (1950). On counter-transference. *International Journal of Psychoanalysis, 31,* 81–84.

Herpertz-Dahlmann, B., Resch, F., Schulte-Markwort, M., & Warnke, A. (Eds.). (2008). *Entwicklungspsychiatrie: Biopsychologische Grundlagen und die Entwicklung psychischer Störungen* [Developmental psychiatry: Biopsychological principles and the development of psychological disorders] (2nd ed.). Stuttgart, Germany: Schattauer.

Horowitz, L. M. (1999). *Manual for the Inventory of Interpersonal Problems.* San Antonio, TX: The Psychological Corporation.

Hoza, B., Molina, B. S. G., Bukowski, W. M., & Sippola, L. K. (1995). Peer variables as predictors of later childhood adjustment. *Development and Psychopathology, 7,* 787–802. http://doi.org/10.1017/S0954579400006842

Jacobson, E. (1964). *The self and the object world.* Madison, CT: International University Press.

Jelen-Maboussin, A., Klipsch, O., Pressel, C., Lenz, K., Lehmkuhl, U., & Winter, S. (2013). Operationalisierte Psychodynamische Diagnostik des Kindes- und Jugendalters – Veränderungsmessung mit der Strukturachse bei Kindern und Jugendlichen mit psychiatrischer Störung [Operationalized psychodynamic diagnostics in children and adolescents – Measurement of change in children and adolescents with structural axes]. *Psychotherapeut, 24,* 24–31. http://doi.org/10.1007/s00278-012-0954-4

Kernberg, O. F. (1975). *Borderline conditions and pathological narcissism*. New York, NY: Janson Aronson.

Kernberg, O. F. (1984). *Severe personality disorders. Psychotherapeutic strategies*. New Haven, CT: Yale University Press.

Kernberg, P. F. (1989). Narzißtische Persönlichkeitsstörungen in der Kindheit [Narcissistic personality disorders during childhood]. In O. F. Kernberg (Ed.), *Narzißtische Persönlichkeitsstörungen* (pp. 261–330). Stuttgart, Germany: Schattauer.

Kiesler, D. J. (1983). The interpersonal circle: A taxonomy for complementarity in human transactions. *Psychological Review, 3*, 185–211. http://doi.org/10.1037/0033-295X.90.3.185

Klein, M. (1962). *Das Seelenleben des Kleinkindes* [The mental life of the infant]. Stuttgart: Klett.

Klein, M. (1975). Envy and gratitude. In M. Klein, *The writings of Melanie Klein*, (Vol. III, pp. 176–235). Stuttgart, Germany: Hogarth.

Kogan, I. (2003). On being a dead, beloved child. *Psychoanalytic Quarterly, 72*, 727–767. http://doi.org/10.1002/j.2167-4086.2003.tb00650.x

Kohte-Meyer, I. (2006). Kindheit und Adoleszenz zwischen verschiedenen Kulturen und Sprachen [Childhood and adolescence among different cultures and languages]. In E. Wohlfart & M. Zaumseil (Eds.), *Transkulturelle Psychiatrie – Interkulturelle Psychotherapie* (pp. 81–94). Heidelberg, Germany: Springer.

Kohut, H. (1971). *The Analysis of self: A systematic approach to the psychoanalytic treatment of narcissistic personality disorders*. Madison, CT: International Universities Press.

Köpp, W. (2002). Die Bedeutung des Beziehungserlebens für die differentielle Therapieeindikation [The meaning of relationship perception for different therapy indications]. *Psychotherapie Psychosomatik Medizinische Psychologie, 52*, 173–178. http://doi.org/10.1055/s-2002-24955

Kuhl, J., & Kazén, M. (1997). *Persönlichkeits-Stil- und Störungs-Inventar (PSSI)* [Personality Style and Disorder Inventory]. Göttingen, Germany: Hogrefe.

Laufer, M., & Laufer, M. E. (1984). *Adolescence and developmental breakdown*. New Haven, CT: Yale University Press.

Leary, T. (1957). *Interpersonal diagnosis of personality*. New York, NY: The Ronald Press.

LeDoux, J. (1996). *The emotional brain*. New York, NY: Simon & Schuster.

Leuzinger-Bohleber, M., Roth, G., & Buchheim, A. (Eds.) (2008). *Psychoanalyse – Neurobiologie – Trauma* [Psychoanalysis – Neurobiology – Trauma]. Stuttgart, Germany: Schattauer.

Lichtenberg, J. D. (1983). *Psychoanalysis and infant research*. Hillsdale, NJ: Analytic Press.

Linderkamp, F. (2006). Komorbidität und elterliche Psychopathologie bei externalisierenden Verhaltensstörungen im Kindesalter [Comorbidity and parental psychopathology in external behavioural disorders during childhood]. *Zeitschrift für Entwicklungspsychologie und Pädagogische Psychologie, 38*, 43–52. http://doi.org/10.1026/0049-8637.38.1.43

Loch, W. (1986). *Perspektiven der Psychoanalyse* [Perspectives of psychoanalysis]. Stuttgart, Germany: Hirzel.

Lohaus, A., & Schmitt, G. M. (1989). Kontrollüberzeugungen zu Krankheit und Gesundheit (KKG), Bericht über die Entwicklung eines Testverfahrens [Locus of control for illness and health, report about the development of a testing procedure]. *Diagnostica, 35*, 59–72.

Luborsky, L., & Crits-Christoph, P. (1990). *Understanding transference.* New York, NY: Basic Books.

Mahler, M., & Gosliner, B. (1955). On symbiotic child psychosis: Genetic, dynamic and restitutive aspects. *The Psychoanalytic Study of the Child, 10*, 195–212.

Mahler, M., Pine, F., & Bergman, A. (1973). *The psychological birth of the human infant.* New York, NY: Basic Books.

Mentzos, S. (2005). *Neurotische Konfliktverarbeitung* [Coping with neurotic conflicts]. Frankfurt a. M., Germany: Fischer.

Mertens, W. (1992). *Kompendium psychoanalytischer Grundbegriffe* [Compendium of psychoanalytic fundamentals]. Munich, Germany: Quintessenz.

Mertens, W. (2012). Wie psychoanalytisch ist die OPD (OPD-KJ)? [How psychoanalytic is the OPD (OPD-CA)?]. *Kinderanalyse, 20*, 172–193.

Montada, L. (1987). Themen, Traditionen, Trends [Themes, traditions, trends]. In R. Oerter & L. Montada (Eds.), *Entwicklungspsychologie* (2nd ed., pp. 3–86). Weinheim, Germany: Beltz PVU.

Müller-Knapp, U. (2012). *Operationalisierte Psychodynamische Diagnostik im Kindes- und Jugendalter (OPD-KJ): Eine Untersuchung der Reliabilität, Validität und Änderungssensitivität im stationär kinderpsychiatrischen Alltag* [Operational psychodynamic diagnosis in childhood and adolescence (OPD-CA): An examination of reliability, validity, and responsiveness in in-patient child psychiatric everyday life] (Dissertation). University of Basel, Switzerland.

Nowotny, E. (2006). Psychische Erscheinungsformen von Vernachlässigung und Missbrauch kleiner Kinder [Psychological manifestations due to neglect and abuse of small children]. *Deutsche Arbeitsgemeinschaft für Jugend- und Eheberatung e. V. – Informationsrundschreiben, 212*, 42–50.

Oerter, R. (1995). Kultur, Ökologie und Entwicklung [Culture, ecology, and development]. In R. Oerter & L. Montada (Eds.), *Entwicklungspsychologie: Ein Lehrbuch* (3rd ed., pp. 84–127). Weinheim, Germany: Beltz.

Oerter, R., & Montada, L. (2008). *Entwicklungspsychologie* [Developmental psychology] (6th ed.). Weinheim, Germany: Psychologie Verlags Union.

OPD Task Force. (2001). *Operationalized psychodynamic diagnosis: Foundations and Manual.* Cambridge, MA: Hogrefe & Huber Publishers.

OPD Task Force. (2008). *Operationalized psychodynamic diagnosis OPD-2: Manual of diagnosis and treatment planning.* Cambridge, MA: Hogrefe & Huber Publishers.

Parker, J. G., & Gottman, J. M. (1989). Social and emotional development in a relational context: Friendship interaction from early childhood to adolescence. In T. J. Berndt & G. W. Ladd (Eds.), *Peer relationships in child development* (pp. 95–131). New York, NY: Wiley.

Perrez, M. (2004). Stressoren in der Familie und Familie als Stressor im Vorfeld der Entwicklung von Störungen bei Kindern und Jugendlichen [Stressors in the family and the family as stressor prior to the development of disorders in children and adolescents]. In P. E. Schlottke, G. Lauth, R. K. Silbereisen, & S. Schneider (Eds.), *Enzyklopädie der Psychologie, Band Störungen im Kindes- und Jugendalter* (pp. 193–246). Göttingen, Germany: Hogrefe.

Petermann, F., & Walter, H. J. (2000). Psychologische Interventionen bei chronisch kranken Kindern: Asthma bronchiale [Psychological interventions in chronically ill children: Bronchial asthma]. In F. Petermann (Ed.), *Fallbuch der Klinischen Kinderpsychologie und -psychotherapie* (2nd ed., pp. 299–310). Göttingen, Germany: Hogrefe.

Piaget, J. (1952). *The origins of intelligence in children.* New York, NY: International University Press. http://doi.org/10.1037/11494-000

Plass, A., & Wiegand-Grefe, S. (2012). *Kinder psychisch kranker Eltern* [Children with psychologically ill parents]. Weinheim, Germany: Beltz.

Plutchik, R. (1997). The circumplex as a general model of the structure of emotions and personality. In R. Plutchik & H. R. Conte (Eds.), *Circumplex models of personality and emotions* (pp. 17–45). Washington, DC: American Psychological Association.

Racker, H. (1959). *Übertragung und Gegenübertragung* [Transference and countertransference]. Munich, Germany: Remhardt.

Raithel, J. (2004). Lebensstil und gesundheitsrelevantes Verhalten im Jugendalter [Lifestyle and health relevant behaviour in adolescence]. *Soziale Welt, 55,* 75–94. http://doi.org/10.5771/0038-6073-2004-1-75

Rathgeber, M., Sommer, T., & Seiffge-Krenke, I. (2009). *Halbstrukturiertes Interview zur OPD-KJ* [Semi-structured interview for OPD-CA]. Unpublished manuscript, Johannes Gutenberg University, Mainz, Germany.

Rebok, G., Riley, A., Forrest, C., Starfield, B., Green, B., Robertson, J., & Tambor, E. (2001). Elementary school-aged children's reports of their health: A cognitive interviewing study. *Quality of Life Research, 10,* 59–70. http://doi.org/10.1023/A:1016693417166

Remschmidt, H., & Mattejat, F. (1994). *Kinder psychotischer Eltern* [Children of psychotic parents]. Göttingen, Germany: Hogrefe.

Remschmidt, H., Schmidt, M. H., & Poustka, F. (2008). *Multiaxiales Klassifikationsschema für Psychiatrische Störungen im Kindes- und Jugendalter nach ICD 10 der WHO* [Multiaxial classification schema of child and adolescent psychiatric disorders according to ICD-10 of WHO] (6th ed.). Bern, Switzerland: Verlag Hans Huber.

Resch, F. (1999a). Beitrag der klinischen Entwicklungspsychologie zu einem neuen Verständnis von Normalität und Pathologie [Contribution of clinical developmental psychology to a new understanding of normality and pathology]. In R. Oerter, C. v. Hagen, G. Röper, & G. Noam (Eds.), *Klinische Entwicklungspsychologie: Ein Lehrbuch* (pp. 606–622). Weinheim, Germany: Beltz.

Resch, F. (1999b). *Entwicklungspsychopathologie des Kindes- und Jugendalters* [Developmental psychopathology in children and adolescents] (2nd ed.). Weinheim, Germany: Psychologie Verlags Union.

Resch, F. (2009). Developing mind: Intersubjektivität und die Entwicklung der psychischen Struktur [Developing mind: Intersubjectivity and the development of psychic structure]. In F. Resch & M. Schulte-Markwort (Eds.), *Kindheit im digitalen Zeitalter* (pp. 2–22). Weinheim, Germany: Beltz.

Resch, F. (2012). Die Perspektive der Kindheit und Jugend [The perspective of childhood and adolescence]. In P. Fiedler (Ed.), *Die Zukunft der Psychotherapie* (pp. 93–116). Heidelberg, Germany: Springer.

Resch, F., & Koch, E. (2012). Bedeutung der Strukturachse für Therapieplanung und Behandlung [The importance of the structure axis for therapy planning and treatment]. *Kinderanalyse, 20,* 4–20.

Resch, F., Mattejat, F., & Remschmidt, H. (2006). Entwicklungspsychopathologie [Developmental psychopathology]. In F. Mattejat (Ed.), *Verhaltenstherapie mit Kindern, Jugendlichen und ihren Familien, Lehrbuch der Psychotherapie* (Vol. 4, pp. 73–83). Munich, Germany: CIP-Medien.

Resch, F., & Schulte-Markwort, M. (Eds.). (2008). *Kursbuch für integrative Kinder- und Jugendpsychotherapie. Schwerpunkt: Adoleszenz* [Coursebook for integrative children and adolescent psychotherapy. Focus: Adolescence]. Weinheim, Germany: Beltz Psychologie Verlagsunion.

Resch, F., Schulte-Markwort, M. & Bürgin, D. (1998). Operationalisierte psychodynamische Diagnostik im Kindes- und Jugendalter – Ein Beitrag zur Qualitätssicherung [Operationalized psychodynamic diagnosis in childhood and adolescence – Contribution to quality assurance]. *Praxis der Kinderpsychologie und Kinderpsychiatrie, 6*, 373–386.

Resnick, M. D., Harris, L. J., & Blum, R. W. (1993). The impact of caring and connectedness on adolescent health and well-being. *Journal of Paediatrics and Child Health, 29*, 3–9. http://doi.org/10.1111/j.1440-1754.1993.tb02257.x

Roth, M. (2002). Geschlechtsunterschiede im Körperbild Jugendlicher und deren Bedeutung für das Selbstwertgefühl [Gender differences in the body image of adolescents and their implications on self-esteem]. *Praxis der Kinderpsychologie und Kinderpsychiatrie, 51*, 150–164.

Rotmann, M. (1978). Über die Bedeutung des Vaters in der „Wiederannäherungs-Phase" [About the importance of the father in the "rapproachment phase"]. *Psyche, 32*, 1105–1147.

Rudolf, G. (1995). *Psychotherapeutische Medizin: Ein einführendes Lehrbuch auf psychodynamischer Grundlage* [Psychotherapeutic medicine: An introductory textbook on a psychodynamic basis] (2nd ed.). Stuttgart, Germany: Enke.

Rudolf, G. (2004). *Strukturbezogene Psychotherapie* [Structure-based psychotherapy]. Stuttgart, Germany: Schattauer.

Rudolf, G. (2012). Psychoanalytisch oder psychodynamisch? [Psychoanalytic or psychodynamic?] *Kinderanalyse, 20*, 195–197.

Rutter, M., Shaffer, D. R., & Sturge, C. (1975). *A guide to a multi-axial classification scheme for psychiatric disorders in childhood and adolescence.* London, UK: Institute of Psychiatry.

Sarason, B. R., Sarason, I. G., & Pierce, G. R. (Eds.). (1990). *Social support: An interactional view. Wiley series on personality processes.* Oxford, UK: John Wiley & Sons.

Schauenburg, H., & Cierpka, M. (1994). Methoden zur Fremdbeurteilung interpersoneller Beziehungsmuster [Methods for external assessment of interpersonal relationship patterns]. *Psychotherapeut, 39*, 135–145.

Schepker, R., & Toker, M. (2009). *Transkulturelle Kinder- und Jugendpsychiatrie* [Transcultural children and adolescent psychiatry]. Berlin, Germany: Medizinisch Wissenschaftliche Verlagsgesellschaft.

Schmitz, B., & Wurm, S. (1999). Social relationships, state and trait affect in adolescence. *Zeitschrift für Pädagogische Psychologie, 13*, 223–235. http://doi.org/10.1024//1010-0652.13.4.223

Schreyer-Mehlhop, I., Petermann, F., Siener, C., & Petermann, U. (2011). Ressourcenorientierte Diagnostik des Sozialverhaltens in der Schule. Ein Baustein zur Förderung sozial-emotionaler Kompetenz [Resource-oriented diagnosis of social behaviours at school. A key element for the promotion of social-emotional competence]. *Kindheit und Entwicklung, 20*, 201–208. http://doi.org/10.1026/0942-5403/a000057

Schulte-Markwort, M. (1996). *Krankheitserleben bei psychiatrisch auffälligen Kindern und Jugendlichen* [Illness experiences in children and adolescents who display psychiatric traits]. Munich, Germany: Quintessenz.

Schulze, U., Sukale, T., Pemberger, B., Kepper-Juckenack, I., Pape, P., Reuter, K., … Bünger, S. (2009). Angewandte klinisch relevante Verfahren: Musik-, Ergo-, Kunst- und Körpertherapien [Applied clinically relevant proceedings: Music, ergo, art, and body therapy]. In J. M. Fegert, A. Streeck-Fischer, H. J. Freyberger (Eds.). *Adoleszenzpsychiatrie – Psychiatrie und Psychotherapie der Adoleszenz und des jungen Erwachsenenalters* (pp. 655–672). Stuttgart, Germany: Schattauer.

Seidler, G. H., Freyberger, H. J., & Maercker, A. (Eds.) (2011). *Handbuch der Psychotraumatologie* [Handbook of psychotraumatology]. Stuttgart, Germany: Klett-Cotta.

Seifert, B. (2011). *Eltern-Kind-Beziehung als Prädiktor für die Beurteilung in Obhuts-und Sorgerechtszurteilungen* [Parent–child relationship as a predictor for the judgment of custody allocations]. Unpublished manuscript, University of Innsbruck, Austria.

Seiffge-Krenke, I. (1998). Chronic disease and perceived developmental progression in adolescence. *Developmental Psychology, 34*, 1073–1084. http://doi.org/10.1037/0012-1649.34.5.1073

Seiffge-Krenke, I. (1999). Families with daughters, families with sons: Different challenges for family relationships and marital satisfaction? *Journal of Youth and Adolescence, 3*, 325–342. http://doi.org/10.1023/A:1021684927661

Seiffge-Krenke, I. (2003). Testing theories of romantic development from adolescence to young adulthood: Evidence of a developmental sequence. *International Journal of Behavioral Development, 27*, 519–531. http://doi.org/10.1080/01650250344000145

Seiffge-Krenke, I. (2006). *Nach Pisa. Stress in der Schule und mit den Eltern. Bewältigungskompetenz deutscher Jugendlicher im internationalen Vergleich* [After Pisa. Stress at school and with the parents. Coping skills among German adolescents in a crosscultural comparison]. Göttingen, Germany: Vandenhoeck & Ruprecht.

Seiffge-Krenke, I. (2009). *Psychotherapie und Entwicklungspsychologie* [Psychotherapy and development psychology] (2nd ed.). Berlin, Germany: Springer.

Seiffge-Krenke, I. (2012a). Die Konfliktachse der OPD-KJ. Grundlagen, klinische Anwendung und erste empirische Ergebnisse [The axis of conflict of OPD-CA. Foundations, clinical applications, and first empirical results]. *Kinderanalyse, 20*, 43–59.

Seiffge-Krenke, I. (2012b). *Therapieziel Identität. Veränderte Beziehungen, Krankheitsbilder und Therapie* [Therapeutic target identity: Change in relationships, illness symptoms, and therapy]. Stuttgart, Germany: Klett-Cotta.

Seiffge-Krenke, I., Dietrich, H., Adler-Corman, P., Timmermann, H., Rathgeber, M., Winter, S., & Röpke, C. (2014). *OPD-KJ-2-Konfliktachse: Ein Fallbuch* [OPD-CA-2 Conflict axis: A casebook]. Göttingen, Germany: Vandenhoeck & Ruprecht.

Seiffge-Krenke, I., Fliedl, R., & Katzenschläger, P. (2013a). Diagnosespezifische Strukturdefizite. Konsequenzen für die psychotherapeutische Behandlung von Kindern und Jugendlichen [Diagnosis specific structural deficits. Consequences for the psychotherapeutic treatment of children and adolescents]. *Psychotherapeut, 58*, 15–23. http://doi.org/10.1007/s00278-012-0955-3

Seiffge-Krenke, I., Fliedl, R., & Katzenschläger, P. (2013b). Welche Vorteile bringt eine umfassende Diagnostik mit OPD-KJ bei kinder- und jugendpsychiatrischen Patienten [What advantages does a comprehensive diagnosis with OPD-CA have for psychiatric children and adolescents]. *Zeitschrift für Kinder- und Jugendpsychiatrie und Psychotherapie, 41*, 6–18.

Seiffge-Krenke, I., & Lohaus, A. (2007). *Stress und Stressbewältigung im Kindes- und Jugendalter* [Stress and stress management in childhood and adolescence]. Göttingen, Germany: Hogrefe.

Seiffge-Krenke, I., Mayer, S., Rathgeber, M., & Sommer, T. (2013). Die Konflikt- und Strukturachse der OPD-KJ als Hilfen für die Indikation und Therapieplanung bei stationären und ambulanten Patienten [The conflict and structure axes of the OPD-CA as aids for indication and therapy planning of in-patients and out-patients]. *Psychotherapeut, 58*, 6–14.

Seiffge-Krenke, I., Mayer, S., & Winter, S. (2011). Beurteilerübereinstimmung bei der OPD-KJ: Wovon hängt sie ab und welchen Erfolg bringt das Training? [Inter-rater agreement of the OPD-CA: On what does it depend and what is achieved by training?] *Klinische Diagnostik und Intervention, 4*, 176–193.

Seiffge-Krenke, I., & Pakalniskiene, V. (2011). Who shapes whom in the family: Reciprocal links between autonomy support in the family and parents' and adolescents' coping behaviors. *Journal of Youth and Adolescence, 40*, 983–995. http://doi.org/10.1007/s10964-010-9603-9

Seiffge-Krenke, I., & Seiffge, J. M. (2005). "Boys play sport …?" Die Bedeutung von Freundschaftsbeziehungen für männliche Jugendliche ["Boys play sport …?" The importance of friendships for male adolescents]. In V. King & K. Flaake (Eds.), *Männliche Adoleszenz* (pp. 267–285). Frankfurt a. M., Germany: Campus.

Seitz, P. (1966). The consensus problem in psychoanalytic research. In L. A. Gottschalk & A. H. Auerbach (Eds.), *Methods of research in psychotherapy* (pp. 209–225). New York, NY: Appleton Century Crofts.

Selman, R. L. (1984). *Die Entwicklung des sozialen Verstehens* [The development of social understanding]. Frankfurt a. M., Germany: Suhrkamp.

Siegal, M., & Peterson, C. C. (1999). *Childrens' understanding of biology and health*. Cambridge, UK: University Press. http://doi.org/10.1017/CBO9780511659881

Sollberger, D., Byland, M., & Widmer, G. (2008). Erwachsene Kinder psychisch kranker Eltern – Belastungen, Bewältigung und biographische Identität [Adult children of mentally ill parents – Stress, coping, and biographical identity]. In A. Lenz & J. Jungbauer (Eds.), *Kinder und Partner psychisch kranker Menschen. Belastungen, Hilfebedarf, Interventionskonzepte* (pp. 157–194). Tübingen, Germany: DGVT Deutsche Gesellschaft für Verhaltenstherapie.

Squire, L. R. (1982). The neuropsychology of human memory. *Annual Review of Neuro-science, 5*, 241–273. http://doi.org/10.1146/annurev.ne.05.030182.001325

Stefini, A., Reich, G., Horn, H., Winkelmann, K., & Kronmüller, K.-T. (2013). Interraterreliabilität der OPD-KJ – Die Achsen "Konflikt" und "Struktur" [Inter-rater reliability of the OPD-CA – The axes "conflict" and "structure"]. *Praxis der Kinderpsychologie und Kinderpsychiatrie, 62*, 255–269. http://doi.org/10.13109/prkk.2013.62.4.255

Stern, D. (1985). *The interpersonal world of the infant*. New York, NY: Basic Books.

Stierlin, H. (1970). Familientherapie mit Adoleszenten im Lichte des Trennungsprozesses [Family therapy with adolescents in light of the separation process]. *Psyche, 24*, 50–68.

Streeck-Fischer, A. (1988). Zwang und Persönlichkeitsentwickung im Kindes- und Jugendalter [Compulsion and personality development in childhood and adolescence]. *Praxis der Kinderpsychologie und Kinderpsychiatrie, 38*, 366–376.

Streeck-Fischer, A. (1999). Zur OPD-Diagnostik des kindlichen Spiels [On Operationalized Psychodynamic Diagnostics of child play]. *Praxis der Kinderpsychologie und Kinderpsychiatrie, 8*, 580–588.

Streeck-Fischer, A. (2005). Psychotherapie mit Kindern und Jugendlichen [Psychotherapy with children and adolescents]. In W. Senf & M. Broda (Eds.), *Praxis der Psychotherapie* (pp. 614–624). Stuttgart, Germany: Thieme.

Streeck-Fischer, A. (2006). *Trauma und Entwicklung: Frühe Traumatisierungen und ihre Folgen in der Adoleszenz* [Trauma and development: Early traumatization and their consequences in adolescence]. Stuttgart, Germany: Schattauer.

Streeck-Fischer, A., & Streeck, U. (2010). Die psychoanalytisch interaktionelle Methode in der Behandlung von Jugendlichen [The psychoanalytic interactional method in the treatment of adolescents]. *Praxis der Kinderpsychologie und Kinderpsychiatrie, 6*, 435–452. http://doi.org/10.13109/prkk.2010.59.6.435

Strupp, H. H., & Binder, J. L. (1991). *Kurzpsychotherapie* [Short-term psychotherapy]. Stuttgart, Germany: Klett-Cotta.

Sullivan, H. S. (1953). *The interpersonal theory of psychiatry.* New York, NY: Norton.

Thomä, H., Grünzig, H. J., Böckenförde, H., & Kächele, H. (1976). Das Konsensusproblem in der Psychoanalyse [The consensus problem in psychoanalysis]. *Psyche, 30*, 978–1027.

Thomä, H., & Kächele, H. (1985). *Lehrbuch der psychoanalytischen Therapie. Band 1: Grundlagen* [Textbook of psychoanalytical therapy. Vol. 1: Foundation]. Heidelberg, Germany: Springer. http://doi.org/10.1007/978-3-662-08324-6

Thomä, H., & Kächele, H. (1988). *Lehrbuch der psychoanalytischen Therapie. Band 2: Praxis* [Textbook of psychoanalytical therapy. Vol. 2: Practice]. Heidelberg, Germany: Springer. http://doi.org/10.1007/978-3-662-08322-2

Tress, W. (Ed.). (1993). *Die strukturale Analyse sozialen Verhaltens (SASB)* [The Structural analysis of Social Behaviour]. Heidelberg, Germany: Asanger.

Tronick, E., & Reck, C. (2009). Infants of depressed mothers. *Harvard Review of Psychiatry, 17*, 147–156. http://doi.org/10.1080/10673220902899714

Vernberg, E., & Field, T. (1990). Transitional stress in children and young adolescents moving to new environments. In S. Fisher & C. L. Cooper (Eds.), *On the move: The psychology of change and transition* (pp. 127–152). Chichester, UK: John Wiley & Sons.

von der Stein, B. (2006). Verborgene Traumatisierung und transgenerationelle Traumaweitergabe bei Nachkommen von Migranten [Hidden traumas and transgenerational trauma transfer in the offspring of migrants]. *Psychoanalyse – Texte zur Sozialforschung, 2*, 137–150.

von Klitzing, K. (1998). „Wenn aus zwei drei werden…" Ergebnisse einer prospektiven Studie zur Entstehung der Eltern-Kind-Beziehung ["When two makes three …" Results of a prospective study of the formation of the parent–child relationship]. In D.

Bürgin (Ed.), *Triangulierung – Der Übergang zur Elternschaft* (pp. 104–115). Stuttgart, Germany: Schattauer.

von Klitzing, K., & Bürgin, D. (2005). Parental capacities for triadic relationships during pregnancy: Early predictors of children's behavioral and representational functioning at preschool age. *Infant Mental Health Journal, 26,* 19–39. http://doi.org/10.1002/imhj.20032

von Klitzing, K., Simoni, H., & Bürgin, D. (1999). Child development and early triadic relationships. *International Journal of Psychoanalysis, 80,* 71–89. http://doi.org/10.1516/0020757991598576

von Staabs, G. (1964). *Der Szenotest. Beitrag zur Erfassung unbewußter Problematik und charakterologischer Struktur in Diagnostik und Therapie* [The Sceno-Test: An approach to detect unconscious problems and personality structure in diagnostics and therapy]. Bern, Switzerland: Huber.

Weber, M. (2012). Anwendungsmöglichkeiten der OPD-KJ Achse Beziehung [Applications of the OPD-KJ relationship axis]. *Kinderanalyse, 20,* 21–42.

Weber, M., & Stadelmann, S. (2011). Verwendung von Geschichtenergänzungsaufgaben zur OPD-KJ Strukturdiagnostik [Application of story stems to the diagnosis of the axis "structure" of OPD-CA]. *Praxis der Kinderpsychologie und Kinderpsychiatrie, 60,* 41–59.

Weitkamp, K., Wiegand-Grefe, S., & Romer, G. (2012). Operationalisierte Psychodynamische Diagnostik im Kindes- und Jugendalter (OPD-KJ): Ein systematischer Review zur empirischen Validierung [Operationalized psychodynamic diagnosis in childhood and adolescence (OPD-CA): A systematic review of the empirical validation]. *Kinderanalyse, 20,* 148–170.

Weitkamp, K., Wiegand-Grefe, S., & Romer, G. (2013). Reliabilität und Konstruktvalidität der OPD-KJ-Achsen Struktur und Behandlungsvoraussetzungen [Reliability and construction validity of the OPD-CA axes of structure and prerequisites for treatment]. *Praxis der Kinderpsychologie und Kinderpsychiatrie, 62,* 243–254. http://doi.org/10.13109/prkk.2013.62.4.243

Welter, N., & Seiffge-Krenke, I. (2006). Essstörung oder dissoziative Störung? Diagnostische Probleme und Verschiebung des Konfliktfokus im Verlauf einer Jugendlichentherapie [Eating disorder or dissociative disorder? Diagnostic problems and shift in conflict focus in the course of an adolescent therapy]. *Kinderanalyse, 14,* 307–334.

Werner, E. E. (2013). What can we learn about resilience from large scale longitudinal studies? In S. Goldstein & R. B. Brooks (Eds.), *Handbook of resilience in children* (pp. 87–105). New York, NY: Springer.

Wiehe, K. (2006). Zwischen Schicksalsschlag und Lebensaufgabe – Subjektive Krankheitstheorien als Risiko- oder Schutzfaktoren der Bewältigung chronischer Krankheit im Kindesalter [Stroke of fate or personal challenge – Subjective theories of illness as risk or protective factors in coping with chronic pediatric illness]. *Praxis der Kinderpsychologie und Kinderpsychiatrie, 55,* 3–22.

Wiggins, J. S. (1991). Circumplex models of interpersonal behavior in clinical psychology. In P. C. Kendall & J. N. Butcher (Eds.), *Handbook of research methods in clinical psychology* (pp. 183–221). New York, NY: Wiley & Sons.

Williams, J. M., & Binnie, L. M. (2002). Children's concepts of illness: An intervention to improve knowledge. *British Journal of Health Psychology, 7*, 129–147. http://doi.org/10.1348/135910702169402

Windaus, E. (2012). Die OPD-KJ und die psychoanalytische Therapie [The OPD-CA and psychoanalytical therapy]. *Kinderanalyse, 20*, 203–219.

Winkler Metzke, C., & Steinhausen, H.-C. (2002). Bewältigungsstrategien im Jugendalter [Coping strategies during adolescence]. *Zeitschrift für Entwicklungspsychologie und Pädagogische Psychologie, 34*, 216–226. http://doi.org/10.1026//0049-8637.34.4.216

Winnicott, D. W. (1953). Transitional objects and transitional phenomena. *International Journal of Psychoanalysis, 34*, 89–97.

Winnicott, D. W. (1956). On transference. *International Journal of Psycho-Analysis, 37*, 386–388.

Winnicott, D. W. (1958). *Collected papers. Through paediatrics to psychoanalysis*. London, UK: Tavistock.

Winnicott, D. W. (1965). *The maturational processes and the facilitating environment: Studies in the theory of emotional development*. London, UK: The Hogarth Press and the Institute for Psycho-Analysis.

Winnicott, D. W. (1971a). *Playing and reality*. London, UK: Tavistock.

Winnicott, D. W. (1971b). *Therapeutic consultations in child psychiatry*. London, UK: Hograth.

Winter, S. (2004). *OPD-KJ-Leitfaden* [OPD-CA Guidelines]. Unpublished manuscript, Charité Universitätsmedizin Berlin, Clinic for Psychiatry, Psychosomatics, and Psychotherapy of Children and Adolescents.

Winter, S., Jelen, A., & Lehmkuhl, U. (2007). Ist die Achse „Behandlungsvoraussetzungen" der OPD-KJ ein Prädiktor für den Therapieerfolg? [Is the axis "Treatment prerequistites" of the OPD-CA a predictor for the success of the therapy?] . *Nervenarzt, 78*, 492.

Winter, S., Jelen, A., Pressel, C., Lenz, K., & Lehmkuhl, U. (2011). Klinische und empirische Befunde zur OPD-KJ [Clinical and empirical findings of the OPD-CA]. *Praxis der Kinderpsychologie und Kinderpsychiatrie, 60*, 41–59. http://doi.org/10.13109/prkk.2011.60.1.41

World Health Organisation. (1992). *International Statistical Classification of Diseases and Related Health Problems, 10th Revision (ICD-10)*. Geneva, Switzerland: Author.

World Health Organisation. (1996). *Multiaxial Classification of Child and Adolescent Psychiatric Disorders: The ICD-10 classification of mental and behavioural disorders in children and adolescents*. New York, NY: Cambridge University Press.

Zero to Three. (2005). *Diagnostic Classification of Mental Health and Developmental Disorders of Infancy and Early Chilhood (rev. ed.)*. Washington, DC: Zero to Three.

Zolkoski, S. M., & Bullock, L. M. (2012). Resilience in children and youth: A review. *Children and Youth Services Review, 34*, 2295–2303. http://doi.org/10.1016/j.childyouth.2012.08.009

Appendices

Appendix A:
Interview Guide

General Aspects		
Interview Situation – Objectives	**Suggested Formulations**	**Situational Events/ Dynamics**
Initial contact and opening of the interview: • *Active attempt to establish contact* • *Explanation of the examination situation* • *Discussion of symptomatology and reasons for presentation, with preliminary information handled tactfully*	• You and your parents have said you're all willing to have this talk with me … • Do you know who I am (explanation of function and framework of interview)? • Do you understand the purpose of our meeting here? • Do you know why you're here? • As you know, I've already gotten to know your parents and have spoken with them. They told me about the following problem … • I can understand that it's difficult to talk about this subject …	• Generally children and adolescents don't come to therapy through their own motivation. • Create an atmosphere instilling trust • Explain the situation and your own function • Mention the rules of confidentiality • Addressing the symptoms is a serious initial challenge for a child or adolescent. • Use preliminary information carefully

Joint reflection on making contact: • *Let self-perception take effect in establishing the relationship.* • *Incorporate what is sensed and observed into the dialog. Note the other person's reactions.* • *Avoid interview bias when conducting the interview (due to induced anxieties, for example)*	• I notice that it's a bit difficult for you to be here. This is an unusual situation for you. How are you feeling about this? • I can imagine that you're not feeling especially comfortable. Do you think you can still tell me a few things? • Or: I have the feeling that it's not hard at all for you to be here. So can you tell me what's the matter.	• Reflection on the initial impressions about the way contact was initiated, the relationship dynamics, and the discussion of the subject. • The subject will be what goes on in the relationship itself as the space for inner experiences • In no way should a dialog be forced.
Handling refusals: • *Attempt to address the sensed difficulties and enter into a dialog through a more pro-active approach.*	• You know that you're here so that I can get to know you and get an idea about you and your life. I'll now ask you a few things – maybe this will make it easier for you …. • What sort of things do you like to do? I see that you're interested in that toy. Maybe we can start there. • Take whatever you need for playing. • I'll begin myself since you seem to find it difficult …	• Children and adolescents may develop non-cooperative attitudes from anxiety or a feeling of shame, for example. • In the face of refusal, a more proactive attitude may be helpful. With smaller children you can initiate playing yourself without becoming too intrusive. • Show curiosity about and interest in the problem in order to obtain information and clarification.
Pause for reflection: • *Reduce the pressure to respond*	• Let me now think about what you've said … • I'm just thinking about how I'd like to answer you … • I'm trying now to understand what you've just told me/done … • You want me to … But first I want to understand what you mean/want to show by this …	• Children and adolescents sometimes ask very direct questions or ask the interviewer to join in play or to react in some other way (by setting boundaries, for example). • Eliminate the necessity to respond immediately, as pauses for thought or silence are important for letting the scene and the available materials sink in.

Forming hypotheses about important areas of conflict, reflection on self-perception	• Ah, I've already noticed that you're someone who likes/doesn't like to do this or that … who thinks a lot about this or that … who could quickly become annoyed about this or that … Is that so? • Could you maybe tell me more exactly how that is for you? • I notice that you always react that way in certain situations. • Could this be because …	• Development of initial hypotheses • Focus on subject • Confrontation with these issues • Trial interpretations
Conclusion of the interview	• Thanks a lot for taking part and talking to me (so openly) about yourself …	• Formulate a concluding statement • Express appreciation even in the face of great resistance

Axis-Specific Aspects		
Conflict Axis		
Conflicts	Exploratory Questions	Behavioral Observation/ Internal Resonance
Closeness vs. distance	• Imagine you encounter some children or adolescents you don't yet know and you'd like to play with them. How do you make contact with them? • How do you feel when you're alone? • Do you like being together with other children or adolescents? • Why?	• Does the patient offer closeness and contact in the interview situation or rather keep his/her distance? • Do I feel like accepting this patient into therapy, or would I rather have nothing to do with him/her?
Submission vs. control	• If you think about all the things your parents allow you to do and what they forbid you to do, how satisfied are you with this? • Who actually has the say among your parents and friends? • Is it so that you don't like submitting "playing second fiddle" to others? • Do you insist on being right in differences of opinion?	• Does it become clear in the interview that the patient enjoys contradicting you? • Does the patient let everything be done with him/her in the interview, even if it would be appropriate for him/her to complain? • Do I have the feeling of being dictated to by the patient? • Do I find the patient is willing to submit him-/ herself to me?

Taking care of oneself vs. being cared for	• What do you do when you see that someone needs help? • Do you feel that others often don't listen to you the way they should? • Do you sometimes do things that your parents usually do for you? • Can you give me an example? • Do you sometimes wish you had more comfort and safety, or do you feel that your parents are too concerned about you? Why? • What do you do when you can't manage to do something alone?	• Is the patient demanding or clinging? • Do I experience the desire to especially look after the patient?
Self-worth conflict	• Imagine you find out that another child is saying bad things about you that are not at all true. How would you feel? Would you do something about it? • What do you do when you don't succeed at something? • What could be the reasons for your not succeeding? • Do you sometimes compare yourself to other children? What are these comparisons about? What do you then think about yourself? • Can you remember whether you ever felt very offended by something another person said or did? What exactly happened?	• Is the patient especially bashful? • Does the patient come across as very self-assured on the outside, but very insecure on the inside? • Does the patient seem especially irritated when offended? • Do I feel the impulse especially to support the patient, admire him/her, or make fun of him/her? • Do I feel devalued by the patient?

	• All of us feel insecure at times, when we enter a new situation, for example. If you compare yourself to others – how do you rate your own sense of insecurity? Or do you seldom feel insecure?	
Guilt conflict	• How content are you with your family? Do you think you are better or worse of than other children/adolescents? • Are there things you don't like about your parents? • Is it difficult for you to do something just for you instead of being there for your friends and family? • Do you think it is your fault for what happened to your family (for instance, parental divorce)?	• Does the patient largely blame him-/herself for things or does he/she tend to blame others? • Do I have the feeling of relieving the patient of his/her responsibility or of condemning him/her? • Is the patient able to talk about negative emotions in relation to his/her family/friends or is he/she denying them or is he/she describing friends/family overly negative?
Oedipal conflict	• Sometimes children or adolescents wish a particular girl/boy in their class would pay them more attention. What was this situation like for you? • Did you do anything to make the girl/boy notice you? • Have you ever felt that a girl/boy especially liked you? How did you notice this? • What would you say: How important is your appearance, such as your hairstyle or your clothes? • Who decides what clothes you wear?	• Is the patient rather shy or quite dramatic? • Does the patient dress more "mousey" person or does he or she wear clothing accentuating their attractiveness? • Do I have the feeling of competing with the patient? • Do I have the feeling of being idealized as an expert by the patient and then possibly not ultimately living up to this expectation?

Identity conflict	• Do you already have an idea of what you'd later like to become and what you would like to have as a job? • Do you ever imagine what it would be like to be somebody else? If yes, how often do you imagine this? • What does this other life look like? • *If from an immigration background:* How well are you getting along with your parents' culture and the culture in which you live?	• Do I experience contradictory aspects of the patient? • Is the patient able to move about within two cultures?
Severe stress in life	Are there current or previous stresses of life in the form of acute critical life events or chronic stressors?	

Structure Axis		
Control	**Exploratory Questions**	**Behavioral Observation / Internal resonance**
Impulse control	*Note: The history taken from others is additionally required* • Should things really go bad for you (imagine, for example, you get poor grades or have a fight with a friend), what would you do? Could you control yourself?	• Can the patient adhere to the formal and temporal constraints of the interview? • Am I afraid that the patient might break off the dialog?
Affect tolerance	• I'm sure you've argued with your parents or a friend in the past. How did you react to these fights? If you were very angry, were you able to calm down again?	• How does the patient react when he/she becomes frustrated during the interview? • Am I afraid that the patient won't be able to return to a different emotional state?
Controlling instances	✓ See Clinical Anchor-Point Descriptions	
Self-worth regulation	• Is there anything that others might not find so good about you? • Have you ever gotten a poor grade for school work? How was that for you?	• Is the patient easily offended? • Does the patient radiate self-confidence? • Do I have the feeling that I have to be extra careful when expressing criticism?
Identity	**Exploratory Questions**	**Behavioral Observation/ Internal Response**
Coherence	*Note: This is rather to be determined through self-descriptions in various life situations*	• Can the patient experience different feelings and needs internally as belonging to him-/ herself?

Self-perception	• What sort of boy/girl would you say you are? • What do you find good or not so good about yourself? • What are your hobbies?	• Does the patient seem to be at a loss? • Are the patient's descriptions clichéd or inauthentic? • Or are they vivid or graphic? • Do the descriptions touch me on an emotional level?
Self–object differentiation	• How would you describe your friend as opposed to yourself? Are you both always of the same opinion?	• Am I unsure about whom the patient is speaking – him-/herself or someone else?
Object-perception	• Do you have friends or a best friend? How would you describe him/her or her? • How would you describe your family or brothers and sisters?	• Are the patient's descriptions vivid or graphic? • Do they touch me on an emotional level? • Can the patient describe different objects in a detailed way?
Belonging	• Do you feel comfortable around people your age? • *If from an immigration background:* Do you feel comfortable in your parents' culture and in the culture in which you are growing up?	• Can the patient's peer group provide him/her with support and guidance? • Can the patient easily switch between the culture of his/her parents and the culture of the host society?
Interpersonality	**Exploratory Questions**	**Behavioral Observation/ Internal Resonance**
Fantasies	• Can you talk about your current thoughts and feelings?	• Can fantasies play a regulatory role in replacing actions and contribute to finding creative solutions?
Inititating emotional contact	✓ See Clinical Anchor-Point Descriptions	
Reciprocity	✓ See Clinical Anchor-Point Descriptions	

Affective experience	• Are you aware of your feelings and can you talk about them? Is this true for happy feelings as well as for bad feelings like anger?	• Does the patient's perception of his/her affects correspond to his/her verbalizations? • Do the patient's descriptions make him/her seem alive?
Empathy	• Can you put yourself in other people's shoes? • When you argue with others, do you get an idea of how they might feel?	• Does the patient's perception of his/her affects towards the object correspond to his/her actions? • Do the descriptions touch me on an emotional level?
Capacity to separate	• What happens inside you if someone leaves you?	• Can the patient respond to offers of alternatives in cases of separation?
Attachment	**Exploratory Questions**	**Behavioral Observation/ Internal Resonance**
Access to representations of attachment	• How do you react when someone leaves you?	• Does the patient have self-regulating skills for situations of separation?
Secure internal base	• How do you feel when you're alone?	• Can the patient calm him-/herself down in solitary situations without external regulatory aids?
Capacity to be alone	• What do you do when you're alone? • Do you manage to occupy yourself with something or be creative?	• Are the patient's internal images of significant others detailed and diverse?
Use of attachment relationships	• What do you do when you need help? Can you reach out to others and actively ask for help?	• Can the patient seek and give active assistance?

Prerequisites for Treatment Axis		
Subjective Dimensions	**Exploratory Questions**	**Behavioral Observation/ Internal Resonance**
Subjective impairment through somatic and mental complaints/problems	*Note: As of Age Group 2, use graphic symbols as aids* • Are you sick? Do you have problems? Do you feel sick? • How bad is your problem/your sickness for you? • How serious are your problems in your view? • How would your life be different if you didn't have this problem? What could you do differently if your problems did not exist?	• Are the patient's complaints evident from his/her facial expressions and gestures? • Are the described complaints noticeable during the interview? • Do I perhaps feel pity or rather aversion/ distrust?
Subjective illness theory	• Where do you think your problems or illness comes from? • What do you think could help you feel better again?	• Does the patient have his/her own concept of psychosomatic illness? • Or does he/she insist on a further somatic diagnosis? • Can I develop a clear concept of illness or do I feel helpless?
Level of suffering	*Note: As of Age Group 2, use graphic symbols as aids* • Are you badly off because of your problem/your illness? • Does your illness/your problem weigh down on you? • How badly do you suffer from your problem/ your illness?	• Does the patient give the impression of hardly suffering from even severe symptoms? • Is there a discrepancy between symptoms and level of suffering?

Motivation for change	• Are you unhappy with your current situation? Specifically as of Age Group 2: • Would you like to make a change yourself so that you'll feel better?	• Does the patient show interest in changing the situation? • Do I have the feeling that the patient him-/ herself wants to change things?
Resources	**Exploratory Questions**	**Behavioral Observation/ Internal Resonance**
Relationships with peers	• Do you have friends? • What do you most like doing with your friends? • What is especially important to you in a good friendship? • Do you have a best friend?	• Does the patient enjoy talking about his/her friends or is he/she rather ashamed because he/she has none? • Does the patient create in me vivid pictures of his/her friends?
Family resources	• Who belongs to your family? • Which family member supports you the most?	• Does the patient enjoy talking about his or her family? • Does the patient create in me a vivid picture of his/her family?
Intrapsychic resources	• Can you do something or have you done anything to improve your problem or illness? • How confident are you that you can overcome your problem or illness? Why?	• Does the patient radiate confidence in resolving his/her problems? • Do I have the feeling that I can help this patient?
Extra-familial social support	• Are there people outside the family who support you?	• Does the patient create in me vivid pictures of his/her family's friends, relatives, and acquaintances?

Prerequisites for Treatment	Exploratory Questions	Behavioral Observation/ Internal Resonance
Insight into biopsycho-social interrelations	*Note: Can be assessed only as of age 12* • Do you remember when the problem/illness occurred for the first time? Did anything special happen before the onset of your illness, or was anything different from usual? Did anything particularly pre-occupy you or weigh down on you?	• Is the patient interested in analysing when the symptoms emerged and what feelings could have been associated with them? • Do I have the feeling of being able to explore the relationships together with the patient? Or do I run up against a wall?
Specific motivation for psychotherapy	*Note: Assessment is also made via reactions* • Can you think of specific things about you that you'd like to change? • Can you say what you want from the treatment?	• Is the patient interested in a solution to the problem? • Do I have the feeling of being able to work together with the patient towards resolving his/her problem?
Gain from illness	*Note: Assessment is mainly made through observable behavior* • Has the illness also brought something good into your life?	• Are there any moments in the interview when it becomes clear that it is more advantageous to the patient to remain ill? • Do I develop the feeling that the patient is also making things comfortable for him-/herself?
Ability to form work-ing alliances	*Notes: Can be assessed only as of age 6* *Cannot be assessed from the initial interview; at least two appointments are necessary*	• Initial assessments: Can the patient adhere to the formal framework of the interview?

Utilization of the care system	Note: Assessment is mainly made from discussion with parents • Have you or your parents ever sought help or assistance because of your problem/illness? Where? How often?	• To which degree do you have the impression that the family could benefit from professional services?

Concluding Questions	
	• Are there situations or things you particularly like? • Are there situations or things that you don't like at all or that you're afraid of? • Can you still remember from when you were very little? What is your earliest childhood memory? Can you tell me about your dreams? • Imagine you had three free wishes. What would you wish for? • Do you already know what you'd like to become when you grow up?

Appendix B:
Diagnostic Assessment Sheets

Appendix B.1

Interpersonal Relations Axis – Assessment Sheet A
("Object-Directed Circle" Dyads)

Below you will find 8 circularly arranged items capturing communication directed towards the interlocutor. Described is how influence is exerted on the interaction partner or how a qualifying statement is made about that person.

The assessment is based on the following examination situation:

☐ Observation
☐ History
☐ Symbolized

Assessment scales:

0 Absent
1 Rarely/somewhat present
2 Moderately present
3 Often/strongly present
4 Very often/very strongly present

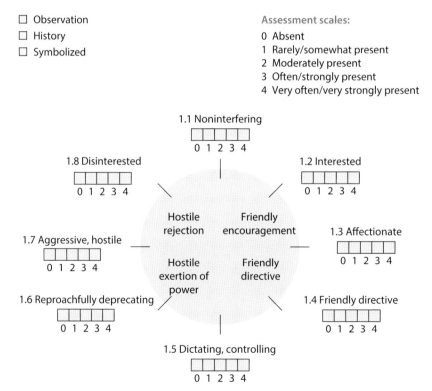

1.1 Noninterfering
0 1 2 3 4

1.8 Disinterested
0 1 2 3 4

1.2 Interested
0 1 2 3 4

Hostile rejection   Friendly encouragement

1.7 Aggressive, hostile
0 1 2 3 4

1.3 Affectionate
0 1 2 3 4

Hostile exertion of power   Friendly directive

1.6 Reproachfully deprecating
0 1 2 3 4

1.4 Friendly directive
0 1 2 3 4

1.5 Dictating, controlling
0 1 2 3 4

From OPD-CA-2 Task Force et al.: *OPD-CA-2 Operationalized Psychodynamic Diagnosis in Childhood and Adolescence: Theoretical Basis and User Manual* © 2017 Hogrefe Publishing

Appendix B.2

Interpersonal Relations Axis – Assessment Sheet A
("Subject-Directed Circle" Dyads)

Below you will find 8 circularly arranged items capturing the person's reactions to the interaction partner or to utterances referring merely to the person's own feelings.

The assessment is based on the following examination situation:

☐ Observation
☐ History
☐ Symbolized

Assessment scales:

0 Absent
1 Rarely/somewhat present
2 Moderately present
3 Often/strongly present
4 Very often/very strongly present

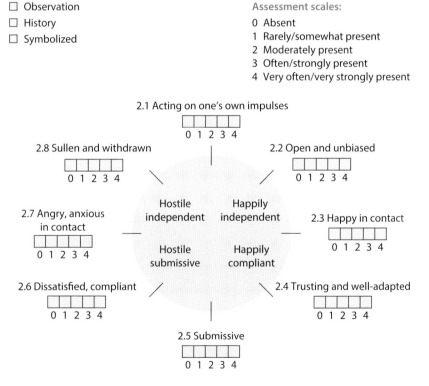

2.1 Acting on one's own impulses
0 1 2 3 4

2.8 Sullen and withdrawn
0 1 2 3 4

2.2 Open and unbiased
0 1 2 3 4

2.7 Angry, anxious in contact
0 1 2 3 4

2.3 Happy in contact
0 1 2 3 4

Hostile independent Happily independent

Hostile submissive Happily compliant

2.6 Dissatisfied, compliant
0 1 2 3 4

2.4 Trusting and well-adapted
0 1 2 3 4

2.5 Submissive
0 1 2 3 4

Appendix B.3

Interpersonal Relations Axis – Assessment Sheet B
Examiner's Internal Resonance (Object-Directed Circle)

Below you will find 8 circularly arranged items for capturing your subjective experience as an examiner in your relation to the patient.

The assessment is based on the following examination situation:

☐ Observation
☐ History
☐ Symbolized

Assessment scales:

0 Absent
1 Rarely/somewhat present
2 Moderately present
3 Often/strongly present
4 Very often/very strongly present

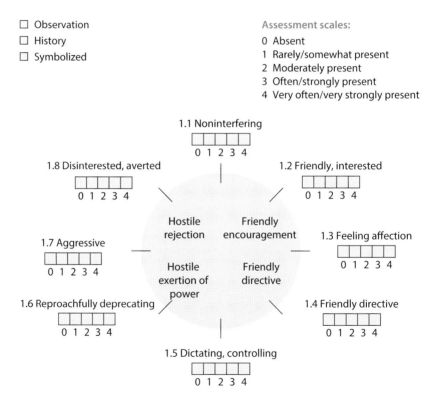

Appendix B.4

Interpersonal Relations Axis – Assessment Sheet B
Examiner's Internal Resonance (Subject-Directed Circle)

Below you will find 8 circularly arranged items for capturing your subjective experience as an examiner in your relation to the patient.

The assessment is based on the following examination situation:

☐ Observation
☐ History
☐ Symbolized

Assessment scales:

0 Absent
1 Rarely/somewhat present
2 Moderately present
3 Often/strongly present
4 Very often/very strongly present

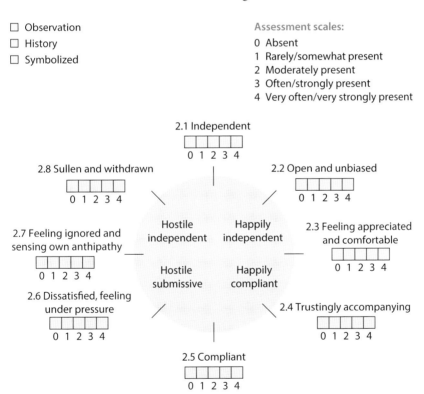

2.1 Independent
0 1 2 3 4

2.8 Sullen and withdrawn
0 1 2 3 4

2.2 Open and unbiased
0 1 2 3 4

Hostile independent   Happily independent

2.7 Feeling ignored and sensing own antipathy
0 1 2 3 4

2.3 Feeling appreciated and comfortable
0 1 2 3 4

Hostile submissive   Happily compliant

2.6 Dissatisfied, feeling under pressure
0 1 2 3 4

2.4 Trustingly accompanying
0 1 2 3 4

2.5 Compliant
0 1 2 3 4

From OPD-CA-2 Task Force et al.: *OPD-CA-2 Operationalized Psychodynamic Diagnosis in Childhood and Adolescence: Theoretical Basis and User Manual* © 2017 Hogrefe Publishing

Appendix B.5

Diagnostic Assessment Sheet for OPD-CA-2

Interpersonal Relations Axis – Assessment Sheet C
(Self-Referential Circle)

Below you will find 8 circularly arranged items **capturing the patient's relationship to him-/herself.**

The assessment is based on the following examination situation:

☐ Observation
☐ History
☐ Symbolized

Assessment scales:

0 Absent
1 Rarely/somewhat present
2 Moderately present
3 Often/strongly present
4 Very often/very strongly present

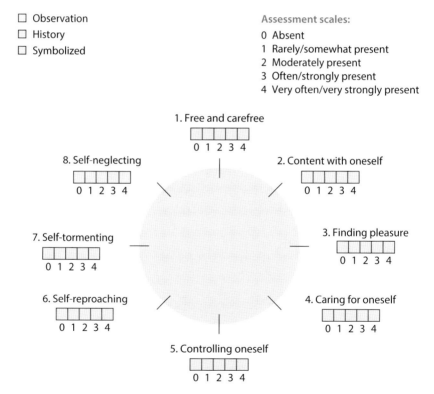

1. Free and carefree
0 1 2 3 4

8. Self-neglecting
0 1 2 3 4

2. Content with oneself
0 1 2 3 4

7. Self-tormenting
0 1 2 3 4

3. Finding pleasure
0 1 2 3 4

6. Self-reproaching
0 1 2 3 4

4. Caring for oneself
0 1 2 3 4

5. Controlling oneself
0 1 2 3 4

From OPD-CA-2 Task Force et al.: *OPD-CA-2 Operationalized Psychodynamic Diagnosis in Childhood and Adolescence: Theoretical Basis and User Manual* © 2017 Hogrefe Publishing

Appendix B.6

Diagnostic Assessment Sheet for OPD-CA-2

Conflict Axis

	Absent	Present but Insignificant	Present and Significant	Present and Very Significant	Processing Mode
1. Closeness vs. distance	0	1	2	3	☐ More active ☐ More passive
2. Submission vs. control	0	1	2	3	☐ More active ☐ More passive
3. Taking care of oneself vs. being cared for	0	1	2	3	☐ More active ☐ More passive
4. Self-worth conflict	0	1	2	3	☐ More active ☐ More passive
5. Guilt conflict	0	1	2	3	☐ More active ☐ More passive
6. Oedipal conflict	0	1	2	3	☐ More active ☐ More passive
7. Identity conflict	0	1	2	3	☐ More active ☐ More passive
8. Current severe stress in life (within the last 6 months)	0	1	2	3	
9. Previous severe stress in life	0	1	2	3	
10. No clear conflict, but a conflict theme called _____ is noticeable.					
11. For formulating the focus: Most important conflict is _____ Possible other important conflict is _____					

From OPD-CA-2 Task Force et al.: *OPD-CA-2 Operationalized Psychodynamic Diagnosis in Childhood and Adolescence: Theoretical Basis and User Manual* © 2017 Hogrefe Publishing

Appendix B.7

Diagnostic Assessment Sheet for OPD-CA-2

Structure Axis

Assessment based on:

☐ Third-party information
☐ Scene
☐ Diagnostic interview

Please choose the integration level for the four different dimensions by marking a cross in the appropriate box. Next to the four levels of intergration: 1 = good integration, 2 = limited integration, 3 = low integration, 4 = disintegration, inbetween values are also possible (1.5, 2.5, 3.5). Please take into consideration the age groups of the Manual.

Name		Age		ICD-10	
Age group		1	2		3

Control Dimension

Ability	Integration level						
Impulse control	1	1.5	2	2.5	3	3.5	4
Affect tolerance	1	1.5	2	2.5	3	3.5	4
Controlling instances	1	1.5	2	2.5	3	3.5	4
Self-worth regulation	1	1.5	2	2.5	3	3.5	4
Overall rating*	1	1.5	2	2.5	3	3.5	4

Identity Dimension

Ability	Integration level						
Coherence	1	1.5	2	2.5	3	3.5	4
Self-perception	1	1.5	2	2.5	3	3.5	4
Self–object differentiation	1	1.5	2	2.5	3	3.5	4
Object-perception	1	1.5	2	2.5	3	3.5	4
Belonging	1	1.5	2	2.5	3	3.5	4
Overall rating*	1	1.5	2	2.5	3	3.5	4

Diagnostic Assessment Sheet for OPD-CA-2

Interpersonal Relations Dimension

Ability	Integration level						
Fantasies	1	1.5	2	2.5	3	3.5	4
Initiating emotional contact	1	1.5	2	2.5	3	3.5	4
Reciprocity	1	1.5	2	2.5	3	3.5	4
Affective experience	1	1.5	2	2.5	3	3.5	4
Empathy	1	1.5	2	2.5	3	3.5	4
Capacity to separate	1	1.5	2	2.5	3	3.5	4
Overall rating*	1	1.5	2	2.5	3	3.5	4

Attachment Dimension

Ability	Integration level						
Access to representations of attachment	1	1.5	2	2.5	3	3.5	4
Secure internal base	1	1.5	2	2.5	3	3.5	4
Capacity to be alone	1	1.5	2	2.5	3	3.5	4
Use of attachment relationships	1	1.5	2	2.5	3	3.5	4
Overall rating*	1	1.5	2	2.5	3	3.5	4

Structure:* Total Score	1	1.5	2	2.5	3	3.5	4

* After the clinical assessment, decide on a Total Score (this can deviate from the arithmetic average).

Appendix B.8

Diagnostic Assessment Sheet for OPD-CA-2

Prerequisites for Treatment Axis

Category	Degree			
	Absent	**Low**	**Moderate**	**High**
Subjective dimensions				
Subjective impairment through somatic complaints/problems	0	1	2	3
Subjective impairment through mental complaints/problems	0	1	2	3
Subjective illness theory (direct quote)				
	Absent	**Low**	**Moderate**	**High**
Level of suffering	0	1	2	3
Motivation for change	0	1	2	3
Resources				
Relationships with peers	0	1	2	3
Family resources	0	1	2	3
Intrapsychic resources	0	1	2	3
Extra-familial social support	0	1	2	3
Prerequisites for treatment				
Insight into biopsychosocial interrelations	0	1	2	3
Specific motivation for psychotherapy	0	1	2	3
Gain from illness	0	1	2	3
Ability to form working alliances	0	1	2	3
Utilization of the care system	0	1	2	3
☹	☹	☺	☺	

Appendix C:
OPD-CA-2 Diagnostic Documentation (General Overview)

Name						
Date of birth:				Sex: m/f		
Examination period				Diagnostican:		
MAS Axis 1:	Axis 2:	Axis 3:	Axis 4:	Axis 5:		Axis 6:

Interpersonal Relations	1–2 items with highest degree	Free text
Object-directed circle		
Subject-directed circle		
Resonance		
Self-referential circle		

	Significance				Processing Mode	
Conflict	0	1	2	3	More active	More passive
Closeness vs. distance						
Submission vs. control						
Taking care of oneself vs. being cared for						
Self-worth conflict						
Guilt conflict						
Oedipal conflict						
Identity conflict						
Severe stress in life						

Integration Level							
Structure	1	1.5	2	2.5	3	3.5	4
Control							
Identity							
Interpersonality							
Attachment							
Total SCORE							

Prerequisites for Treatment	0	1	2	3
Subjective dimensions*				
Resources*				
Prerequisites for treament*				

* Free text for relevant findings in the dimensions

Summary and formulation of focus:

From OPD-CA-2 Task Force et al.: *OPD-CA-2 Operationalized Psychodynamic Diagnosis in Childhood and Adolescence: Theoretical Basis and User Manual* © 2017 Hogrefe Publishing

Advances in Psychotherapy
Evidence-Based Practice

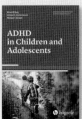

Brian P. Daly /
Aimee K. Hildenbrand /
Ronald T. Brown
**ADHD
in Children and
Adolescents**
Vol. 33, 2016, viii + 90 pp.
US $29.80 / € 24.95
ISBN 978-0-88937-412-6

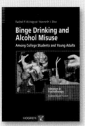

Rachel P. Winograd /
Kenneth J. Sher
**Binge Drinking and
Alcohol Misuse Among
College Students
and Young Adults**
Vol. 32, 2015, vi + 92 pp.
US $29.80 / € 24.95
ISBN 978-0-88937-403-4

Attention-Deficit/Hyperactivity Disorder is a common childhood disorder that can have serious consequences for academic, emotional, social, and occupational functioning. When properly identified and diagnosed, however, there are many interventions for the disorder that have established benefits.

Heavy drinking – and its associated problems – are an integral part of many college students' and other young adults' lives. Though some young drinkers are able to consume alcohol without incident, many face significant negative fallout from their excessive consumption.

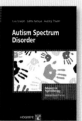

Lisa Joseph /
Latha V. Soorya /
Audrey Thurm
**Autism Spectrum
Disorder**
Vol. 29, 2015, vi + 100 pp.
US $29.80 / € 24.95
ISBN 978-0-88937-404-1

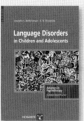

Joseph H. Beitchman /
E. B. Brownlie
**Language Disorders
in Children
and Adolescents**
Vol. 28, 2014, vi + 130 pp.
US $29.80 / € 24.95
ISBN 978-0-88937-338-9

This volume is a straightforward yet authoritative guide to effective diagnosis and empirically supported treatments for autism spectrum disorder. It provides clear guidance on evaluation of autism spectrum disorder and comorbidities, with practical outlines and examples to guide practice.

As many as half of children and adolescents presenting for mental health services have language impairments, often undiagnosed. This book offers a clear and comprehensive description of language impairment emerging in childhood and its implications for clinical practice with children and adolescents.

www.hogrefe.com

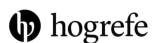

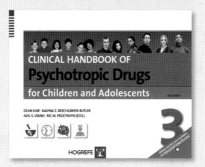
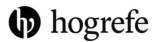